Guide to the
Canadian
Family Medicine
Examination

Guide to the Canadian Family Medicine Examination

Editors

Megan Dash, MD, CCFP

Family Medicine and Enhanced Skills: Sports and Exercise Medicine
University of Saskatchewan, Regina
Regina, Saskatchewan
Canada

Angela Arnold, BASc, MEng, PEng, MD, CCFP(EM)

Family Medicine and Emergency Medicine
University of Saskatchewan, Regina
Regina, Saskatchewan
Canada

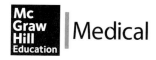 Medical

New York / Chicago / San Francisco / Lisbon / London / Madrid / Mexico City
Milan / New Delhi / San Juan / Seoul / Singapore / Sydney / Toronto

Guide to the Canadian Family Medicine Examination

Copyright © 2013 by McGraw-Hill Education. All rights reserved. Printed in the United States of America. Except as permitted under the United States Copyright Act of 1976, no part of this publication may be reproduced or distributed in any form or by any means, or stored in a data base or retrieval system, without the prior written permission of the publisher.

6 7 8 9 10   DOW   20 19 18 17 16

ISBN 978-0-07-180342-7
MHID 0-07-180342-4

This book was set in Minion by Cenveo Publisher Services.
The editors were Christine Diedrich and Robert Pancotti.
The production supervisor was Sherri Souffrance.
Project management was provided by Vastavikta Sharma, Cenveo Publisher Services.
The cover designer was Thomas De Pierro.
RR Donnelley was printer and binder.

This book is printed on acid-free paper.

Library of Congress Cataloging-in-Publication Data

Guide to the Canadian family medicine examination/editors, Megan Dash, Angela Arnold.
        p. ; cm.
     Includes bibliographical references.
     ISBN 978-0-07-180342-7 (pbk. : alk. paper)—ISBN 0-07-180342-4 (pbk. : alk. paper)
     I. Dash, Megan.   II. Arnold, Angela, 1968-
     [DNLM: 1. Family Practice—Canada—Examination Questions.   2. Family Practice—Canada—Outlines.   WB 18.2]
     610.971—dc23
                                                                                2012040750

McGraw-Hill Education books are available at special quantity discounts to use as premiums and sales promotions, or for use in corporate training programs. To contact a representative, please e-mail us at bulksales@mcgraw-hill.com.

To Saskatchewan family physicians:

You have provided inspiration and have been dynamic and strong role models. Family medicine is the backbone of Canadian healthcare and we owe a debt of gratitude to you and other family physicians for your continual pursuit of excellence in this diverse field of practice.

To our family, friends, and loved ones:

The art of family medicine could not be practiced without the love and support of those in our lives who care for us. We send a special thanks to those who have stuck beside us through the many years of school, long nights of studying, and countless nights of being on-call. This book would never have become a reality without you standing beside us!

Angela Arnold and Megan Dash

Contents

Contributors List

Malyha Alibhai, BMedSci, BMBS, CCFP
Family Medicine Resident
University of Saskatchewan
Regina, Saskatchewan
Chap 5: Pediatrics

Angela J. Arnold, BASc, MEng, PEng, MD, CCFP(EM)
Family Medicine-Emergency Medicine Resident
University of Saskatchewan
Regina, Saskatchewan
Book editor; Chap 15: Preparation for the SOO

Jill A. Blaser, MSc, MD, CCFP
Family Physician
Assistant Professor of Family Medicine
Department of Academic Family Medicine
University of Saskatchewan
Saskatoon, Saskatchewan
Chap 6: Psychiatry

Nicholas Bouchard, MD
Family Medicine Resident
University of Saskatchewan
Regina, Saskatchewan
Chap 1: Emergency Medicine

Kieran Conway, BA, MD
Family Medicine Resident
University of Saskatchewan
Prince Albert, Saskatchewan
Chap 8: Preventative Medicine

James Coruzzi, MB, BCh, BAO, CCFP(EM)
Emergency Physician
Clinical Assistant Professor
Department of Academic Family Medicine
University of Saskatchewan
Regina, Saskatchewan
Chap 2: Internal Medicine

Danielle Cutts, BA, MD, CCFP
Family Physician
Clinical Assistant Professor
Department of Academic Family Medicine
University of Saskatchewan
Regina, Saskatchewan
Chap 5: Pediatrics

Megan Dash, MD, CCFP
Family Medicine and Enhanced Skills: Sports and Exercise Medicine
University of Saskatchewan
Regina, Saskatchewan
Book editor; Chap 6: Psychiatry

Samir Datta, MD, CCFP
Family Medicine Resident
University of Saskatchewan
Regina, Saskatchewan
Chap 6: Psychiatry

Paul S. Dhillon, BA, MBBChBAO, EMDM, DRCOG
Family Medicine Resident
University of Saskatchewan
Regina, Saskatchewan
Chap 13: Travel Medicine

Nicole J. Dressler, MD
Family Medicine Resident
University of Saskatchewan
Regina, Saskatchewan
Chap 7: Chronic Disease

Adam Gruszczynski, MD, CCFP, FCFP
Family Physician
Associate Professor
Department of Academic Family Medicine
University of Saskatchewan
Regina, Saskatchewan
Chap 14: Social Medicine

Jason Hosain, MD, CCFP
Family Physician
Assistant Professor
Department of Academic Family Medicine
University of Saskatchewan
Saskatoon, Saskatchewan
Chap 6: Psychiatry

Jacqueline L. Jenkins, MD, MSc
Family Medicine Resident
University of Saskatchewan
Regina, Saskatchewan
Chap 6: Psychiatry

Rejina Kamrul, MBBS, CCFP
Family Physician
Assistant Professor
Department of Academic Family Medicine
University of Saskatchewan
Regina, Saskatchewan
Chap 7: Chronic Disease

Beverley E. Karras, MD, CCFP
Family Physician
Assistant Professor
Department of Academic Family Medicine
University of Saskatchewan
Saskatoon, Saskatchewan
Chap 12: Care of the Elderly Patient

Lauren E. Kimball, MD, CCFP
Family Medicine Resident
University of Saskatchewan
Regina, Saskatchewan
Chap 9: Sexual Health

Jennifer Kuzmicz, MD
Family Physician
Associate Professor
Department of Academic Family Medicine
University of Saskatchewan
Regina, Saskatchewan
Chap 8: Preventative Medicine

Tara Lee, MD, CCFP
Family Physician
Associate Professor
Department of Academic Family Medicine
University of Saskatchewan
Swift Current, Saskatchewan
Chap 3: Infectious Disease

Mark Lees, MD, CCFP
Family Physician
Associate Professor
Department of Academic Family Medicine
University of Saskatchewan
Saskatoon, Saskatchewan
Chap 3: Infectious Disease

Lise Susan Legault, MD
Family Medicine Resident
University of Saskatchewan
Regina, Saskatchewan
Chap 2: Internal Medicine; Chap 6: Psychiatry

Janice Lising, MBBS
Family Medicine Resident
University of Saskatchewan
Regina, Saskatchewan
Chap 14: Social Medicine

Sarah Patricia Liskowich, BSc, BEd, MD, CCFP
Family Medicine Resident
University of Saskatchewan
Regina, Saskatchewan
Chap 7: Chronic Disease

Amanda D. Loewy, MSc, MD
Family Medicine Resident
University of Saskatchewan
Saskatoon, Saskatchewan
Chap 12: Care of the Elderly Patient

Kish Lyster, BSc, MD, CCFP(EM)
Hospitalist/Emergency Medicine
Clinical Assistant Professor
Department of Academic Family Medicine
University of Saskatchewan
Regina, Saskatchewan
Chap 2: Internal Medicine

Sally C. Mahood, MD, CCFP, FCFP
Family Physician
Associate Professor Family Medicine
University of Saskatchewan & Staff
Women's Health Centre
Regina, Saskatchewan
Chap 10: Women's Health

Milena Markovski, MD, CCFP
Family Physician
Assistant Professor
Department of Family Medicine
University of Saskatchewan
Regina, Saskatchewan
Chap 9: Sexual Health

Raenelle Nesbitt, MD, CCFP
Emergency Physician/Family Physician
Clinical Assistant Professor
Department of Academic Family Medicine
University of Saskatchewan
Regina, Saskatchewan
Chap 1: Emergency Medicine

Michael J. Nicholls, MD, CCFP, FCFP, Dip Sport Med
Family Physician
Associate Clinical Professor
College of Medicine
University of Saskatchewan
Regina, Saskatchewan
Chap 11: Musculoskeletal Medicine

Anna O'Malley II, MBChB
Family Medicine Resident
University of Saskatchewan
Regina, Saskatchewan
Chap 2: Internal Medicine

Jana R. Patenaude, BSc, MSc, MD, CCFP
Family Medicine Resident
University of Saskatchewan
Saskatoon, Saskatchewan
Chap 2: Internal Medicine

Stephen Pomedli, BSc, MSc, MD
Family Medicine Resident
University of Toronto
Toronto, Ontario
Chap 3: Infectious Disease

Randi Ramunno, MD, BSc
Family Medicine Resident
University of Saskatchewan
Regina, Saskatchewan
Chap 1: Emergency Medicine

Jeremy Reed, MD, FRCSC
Orthopedic Surgeon
Associate Clinical Professor of Surgery
University of Saskatchewan
Regina, Saskatchewan
Chap 1: Emergency Medicine; Chap 11: Musculoskeletal Medicine

Clara Rocha Michaels, MD
Family Physician
Assistant Professor
Department of Academic Family Medicine
University of Saskatchewan
Regina, Saskatchewan
Chap 7: Chronic Disease

Dr. Rajeev Sachdeva
Family Medicine Resident
University of Saskatchewan
Regina, Saskatchewan
Chap 11: Musculoskeletal Medicine

Julie Seymour, MBBS
Family Medicine Resident
University of Saskatchewan
Regina, Saskatchewan
Chap 4: Surgery

Sheila Smith, MD, CCFP(EM), FCFP
Emergency Physician
Program Director of Family Medicine -Emergency Medicine
Clinical Assistant Professor
Department of Academic Family Medicine
University of Saskatchewan
Regina, Saskatchewan
Chap 4: Surgery

Beavan Talukdar, BSc, MD, CCFP
Family Medicine Resident
University of Saskatchewan
Regina, Saskatchewan
Chap 11: Musculoskeletal Medicine

Ronald Taylor, MD, CCFP(EM)
Hospitalist/Emergency Medicine
Clinical Assistant Professor
Department of Academic Family Medicine
University of Saskatchewan
Regina, Saskatchewan
Chap 13: Travel Medicine

Damon Tedford, MD, CCFP
Family Medicine Resident
University of Saskatchewan
Regina, Saskatchewan
Chap 10: Women's Health

Kathryn C. Walker, BA, BEd, MD, CCFP
Family Medicine Resident
University of Saskatchewan
Regina, Saskatchewan
Chap 7: Chronic Disease

Cheryl Zagozeski, MD, CCFP, FCFP
Family Physician
Associate Professor
Department of Academic Family Medicine
University of Saskatchewan
Regina, Saskatchewan
Chap 7: Chronic Disease

Preface

Passing the College of Family Physicians of Canada (CFPC) exam is an important milestone for residents and international medical graduates who want to practice family medicine and obtain a full license in Canada. The void in publication material to aid in the preparations for this exam makes the task daunting. With this in mind, we have compiled material from multiple resources to make what we hope is a comprehensive yet relatively concise guide that covers the 99 priority topics suggested by the CFPC. To see the complete list of topics, see the Web site for the College of Family Physicians of Canada:

http://www.cfpc.ca/EvaluationObjectives/. Click on the "Priority topics and key features for assessment in family medicine" link.

The idea for this study guide for the Canadian family medicine exam came from our own study efforts. In our preparations for the exam, Megan and I compiled a collection of notes, lovingly called the "orange book" in reference to the color of the binder that we used to store the notes. These notes became the basis for the book.

This has been a Saskatchewan-driven, and predominantly a Regina-driven, initiative. The editing and revision of the original set of notes has drawn on the experience of many family physicians and residents who have taken the exam, are involved in Canadian family medicine residency programs, or are currently studying for the exam. We feel that the background and experience of the participants have helped to make the material relevant for the exam and for the first few years of clinical practice.

The aim of the study guide is to provide a brief and relatively comprehensive review of the CFPC priority topics, including signs, symptoms, diagnostic measures, and treatment options. In all chapters, the authors as a group have attempted to review recent Canadian clinical practice guidelines and to include relevant information in the diagnostic and treatment aspects. There is wide provincial variability in both the diseases and conditions included in their guidelines and in the clinical practice suggestions: this study guide is in no way meant to replace any of these guidelines.

The CFPC's 99 priority topics are not an exhaustive list of subjects to cover over the course of your study. We have expanded on these topic areas to provide a more exhaustive list of subject material that you may encounter. Additional features of this study guide include:

- Simple formatting style that is consistent in every chapter
- Multiple mnemonics
- Space in the margins for making personal notes and annotations
- Key points highlighted in boxes or margin areas

Mastering family medicine does not result from a single textbook resource: we have tried to blend information from multiple resources into one study guide. However, you may find it necessary to supplement your knowledge in some areas. (Our personal suggestions to supplement your reading: *RxFiles: Drug Comparison Charts* and *Anti-infective Guidelines for Community-Acquired Infections.*) It is also strongly encouraged for readers to begin using this study guide early in their study preparations, to supplement the text with margin notes, and to highlight the items you find most valuable.

We would also be very grateful for any suggestions or recommendations for future editions of the study guide.

Recommended Reading

Anti-infective Review Panel. *Anti-infective Guidelines for Community-Acquired Infections.* Toronto: MUMS Guideline Clearinghouse; 2012.

RxFiles: Drug Comparison Charts. 8th ed. Saskatoon Health Region: RxFiles Academic Detailing Program; 2010.

List of Abbreviations

<	less than		FPG	fasting plasma glucose
A1C	glycated hemoglobin		FT_4	free thyroxine
AAA	abdominal aortic aneurysm		GDM	gestational diabetes mellitus
ABPM	ambulatory blood pressure measurement (24 hour blood pressure monitoring)		GERD	gastroesophageal reflux disease
			GHTN	gestational hypertension
ACE-I	angiotensin converting enzyme inhibitor		HF	heart failure
ARB	angiotensin receptor blocker		HIDA scan	hepatobiliary scintigraphy
ASA	acetylsalicylic acid		HOCM	hypertrophic obstructive cardiomyopathy
BCC	basal cell carcinoma		HR	heart rate
BNP			HTN	hypertension
BP	blood pressure		IUGR	intrauterine growth restriction
BPH	benign prostatic hyperplasia		IV	intravenous
BPM	blood pressure measurement		LOC	loss of consciousness
BSA	body surface area		LT_4	l-thyroxine, levothyroxine
C&M	cross and match		MAOIs	monoamine oxidase inhibitors
CAD	coronary artery disease		MCV	mean corpuscular volume
CDA	Canadian Dermatology Association		MDD	major depressive disorder
CHF	congestive heart failure		MI	myocardial infarction
CI	contraindicated		MMI	methimazole
CN	cranial nerve		MRI	magnetic resonance imaging
CNS	central nervous system		MS	multiple sclerosis
COMT	catechol-*O*-methyltransferase		NSAIDs	non-steroidal anti-inflammatory drugs
COPD	chronic obstructive pulmonary disease		OGTT	oral glucose tolerance test
CRP	C-reactive protein		OH	orthostatic hypotension
CT	computed tomography		PD	Parkinson disease
CVD	cerebrovascular disease		PE	pulmonary embolism
CVS	cardiovascular system		PG	plasma glucose
DM	diabetes mellitus		PHQ-9	preventative health questionnaire 9; a screening questionnaire for depression
DVT	deep venous thrombosis			
DWI	diffusion weighted imaging		PMH	past medical history
ECG	electrocardiogram		PNS	peripheral nervous system
Eg	for example		PO	oral route
EM	erythema multiforme		PPG	post-prandial plasma glucose
ENT	ear, nose, and throat		PPT	postpartum thyroiditis
FH	family history		PTU	propylthiouracil
FNA	fine needle aspiration		PV	per vaginum

R/O	rule out		TEN	toxic epidermal necrolysis
RAI	radioactive iodine		TIA	transient ischemic attach
RAIU	radioactive iodine uptake scan		TOP	termination of pregnancy
RS	respiratory system		TPO	thyroid peroxidase
RUQ	right upper quadrant		TRAP	tremor, rigidity, akinesia, postural instability
Rx	treatment		TRH	thyrotropin releasing hormone
QOL	quality of life		TSH	thyroid stimulating hormone
SCC	squamous cell carcinoma		TSI	thyroid stimulating immunoglobulin
SJS	Stevens-Johnson syndrome		UE	upper extremities
T_3	triiodothyronine		U/S	ultrasound
T_4	thyroxine		VZV	varicella zoster virus
TCA	tricyclic antidepressants		WBC	white blood cells

Top Ten Tips for Writing SAMPS

1. Ensure that you read the questions thoroughly. Sometimes the answer is given within the question.
2. CBC is not an appropriate answer. You must state hemoglobin, white blood cell count, etc. This is the same for all laboratory investigations.
3. Take your time. You will have plenty of time to complete all the questions.
4. Be aware of the environment in which the question places you. Your answer may be different if you are in your office versus the emergency room.
5. Know *classes* of medications and ensure that you know a few options for each condition. For example, classes of medications to treat hypertension include calcium channel blockers, diuretics, beta blockers, and so on.
6. Be specific. Answers usually require only a few words.
7. Go with your gut. The questions are not trying to trick you.
8. Use generic names of medications, not trade names.
9. A table of normal laboratory values is provided on the exam, so do not waste your time memorizing those ranges.
10. Visit the CFPC Web site at http://www.cfpc.ca/EvaluationObjectives to review the objectives for the exam.

1

Emergency Medicine

ACLS

Priority Topic 1

- Please refer to ACLS guidelines for a comprehensive review of ACLS algorithms for ACS, cardiac arrest, and arrhythmias (American Heart Association, 2010).
- Arrhythmias are a frequent problem encountered in the ER. A general approach to arrhythmias is essential (Tables 1-1 and 1-2).

TABLE 1-1	Arrhythmias–Approach and Characteristics		
PATHOLOGY	RHYTHM/CAUSE	CHARACTERISTICS	TREATMENT
Tachycardia (HR >100)	Afib	• Narrow complex • Irregularly irregular • No P waves • With or without rapid ventricular response	• ACLS protocol if hemodynamically unstable Electrical cardioversion (and/or) medical rate conversion with diltiazem or amiodarone (expert consultation)
	SVT	• Narrow complex (< 0.12 s) • Aberrant pacemaker can be atrial, AV node, ectopic • Various P wave anomalies (varied timing, morphology)	• Vagal maneuvers • Adenosine 6 mg IV push; then 12 mg • If does not convert, consider beta blocker or diltiazem (expert consultation)
	V Tach	• Wide (> 0.12 s) complexes • Greater than three ventricular complexes with rate > 100	• If pulseless, defibrillate and then give epinephrine 1 mg q 3-5 min • If wide complex (with pulse), give amiodarone 150 mg IV over 10 min and prepare for synchronized cardioversion (expert consultation)
	V Fib	• No clear QRS complexes • No pulse (too disorganized)	• Defibrillate • Epinephrine 1 mg IV q 3-5 min
Bradycardia (HR <60)	**Various:** Search for causes = 6 Hs and 5 Ts	• Heart rate <60 • May or may not be symptomatic • Rx only if clinically inadequate perfusion	• Transcutaneous pacing • Atropine 0.5 mg IV • Consider epinephrine (2-10 mcg/min) or dopamine (2-10 mcg/min) infusion • Definitive (transvenous) pacing

TABLE 1-1	Arrhythmias–Approach and Characteristics (*Continued*)		
PATHOLOGY	RHYTHM/CAUSE	CHARACTERISTICS	TREATMENT
Asystole/PEA	Various: Search for causes = 6 Hs and 5 Ts (see Table 1-3)	• ECG flat. No rhythm. (Or a rhythm but no pulse is able to be palpated)	• CPR • Do not defibrillate unless shockable rhythm (VF or VT) • Epinephrine 1 mg IV/IO q 3-5 min • May give vasopressin 40 U IV/IO to replace first or second dose epinephrine • May consider atropine 1 mg IV/IO q 3-5 min
Metabolic/drugs	Cocaine toxicity	• Tachycardia +/− ischemic changes	• Do not give beta blocker
	Hyperkalemia	• Peaked T waves	• Decrease potassium with insulin, beta agonist (salbutamol), diuretic
	Digoxin toxicity	• ST depression with inverted T waves (V_5-V_6) • Short QT segment	• Digoxin immune FAB (Digibind)

Abbreviations: A fib, atrial fibrillation; SVT, supraventricular tachycardia; V Tach, ventricular tachycardia; V Fib, ventricular fibrillation; PEA, pulseless electrical activity.

TABLE 1-2	Heart Blocks	
RHYTHM	CHARACTERISTICS	TREATMENT
1st degree AV block	Long PR interval (>200 mS)	No treatment
2nd degree AV block Mobitz 1	Progressive increase in PR interval until a dropped beat, PR then resets	Stop offending drugs
2nd degree AV block Mobitz 2	No change in PR with patterned dropped QRS beats (2:1 or 3:1)	Pacemaker
3rd degree AV block	No relationship between P wave and QRS complex	Pacemaker

TABLE 1-3	6 Hs and 5 Ts (Underlying Causes for Bradycardiac and Tachycardic Arrhythmias)

Hypovolemia **H**ypoxia **H**ydrogen ion (acidosis) **H**ypo/**H**yperkalemia **H**ypoglycemia **H**ypothermia	**T**oxins **T**amponade (cardiac) **T**ension pneumothorax **T**hrombosis (coronary or pulmonary) **T**rauma (hypovolemia, increased ICP)

Bibliography

ASA. American Heart Association guidelines for cardiopulmonary resuscitation and emergency cardiovascular care. *Circulation* 2010:122.

Loss of Consciousness

Priority Topic 59

Definition

The occurrence of a loss of the ability to perceive and respond.

History

Must differentiate between **traumatic** LOC and **non-traumatic** LOC.

- AMPLE history is important
  - **A**—allergies
  - **M**—medication
  - **P**—past medical history
  - **L**—last meal
  - **E**—event, the details of what happened
- History from witnesses is very important
- Seek information on:
  - Trauma
  - Drugs, Rx or illicit
  - Toxins
  - Seizure activity
  - Psychological history

Physical Examination

This is a critical care scenario! Switch into ACLS/ATLS/ICU mode. Do your ABCs. Do a thorough examination and **do not skip** any steps. These people cannot talk to you; it is up to you to glean **all** information available.

- ABCDEs
  - Ensure a patent airway; intubate if necessary
  - Ensure air is moving appropriately
  - Attain accurate vitals, look for signs of shock
  - Check pupils and calculate Glasgow Coma Scoring (GCS)—(see Table 1-4)
    - If less than 8, intubate!
  - Check for, and prevent hypothermia

TABLE 1-4	Glasgow Coma Scoring				
	EYES		VERBAL		MOTOR
4	Open spontaneously	5	Alert and oriented	6	Follows command
3	Open to speech	4	Disoriented	5	Localizes to pain
2	Open to pain	3	Inappropriate words	4	Withdraws from pain
1	No response	2	Moans	3	Decorticate
		1	No response	2	Decerebrate
				1	No response

TABLE 1-5	Neurologic Signs	
	UPPER MOTOR NEURON	LOWER MOTOR NEURON
	Injury above anterior horn cell of spinal cord	Injury below anterior horn cell of spinal cord
	Plantar reflex upgoing	Plantar reflex downgoing
	Tone increased, secondary to unregulated spinal cord reflex arcs	Tone flaccid, secondary to lost muscle innervation
	DTRs increased	DTRs decreased, normal, or absent Atrophy, fasciculations in long term

- Perform a systematic head to toe examination
  - Look for signs of trauma
  - Check for localizing neurologic signs (see Table 1-5)
  - Note smell of alcohol or ketones
  - Look for asterixis, indicating renal or hepatic failure
- Consider various causes of LOC (see Tables 1-6 and 1-7)

TABLE 1-6	Differential Diagnosis–Traumatic			
	SAH	EPIDURAL	SUBDURAL	TRAUMATIC BRAIN INJURY: CONCUSSION–DIFFUSE AXONAL INJURY SPECTRUM
Definition	The presence of blood in the SA space, in the absence of trauma	The presence of blood between the dura and skull	The presence of blood between the dura and arachnoid membrane	Traumatic damage to white matter tracts
Presentation history	"Worst headache ever" "Thunderclap headache" Immediate onset Occasionally confusion Occasionally seizures Occasionally neck stiffness	Altered mental status, changing minutes to hours **May have lucid interval–beware!**	Mental status change over days to weeks May have hemiparesis	Ranging from the mild "fog" of a mild concussion to profound coma secondary to DAI Within minutes of head trauma: "Foggy" Headache Amnesia Transient LOC Coma DAI may declare itself in a delayed fashion on imaging, as majority of damage is biochemical
Physical examination	Decreased GCS Coma May have pupillary dilation if ICP is raised high enough to incite uncal herniation Meningismus	Decreased GCS Coma May have pupillary dilation if ICP is raised high enough to incite uncal herniation	Decreased GCS Coma May have pupillary dilation if ICP is raised high enough to incite uncal herniation	If mild symptoms, sideline concussion assessment and appropriate restriction of activity If comatose, begin critical care style assessment and treatment
Risk factors	Preexisting vascular malformations Trauma	Trauma, especially shearing and rotatory forces	Alcoholism Elderly (falls) Anticoagulation therapy	Trauma Contact sports
Investigation	CBC, renal panel, INR/PTT, serum glucose, ABG, serum EtOH, tox screen, U/A CT head Lumbar puncture if CT is negative	CBC, renal panel, INR/PTT, serum glucose, ABG, serum EtOH, tox screen, U/A CT head	CBC, renal panel, INR/PTT, serum glucose, ABG, serum EtOH, tox screen, U/A CT head	If conscious, perform SCAT 2 assessment If unconscious, perform CT
Treatment	Neurosurgery consultation	Neurosurgery consultation	Neurosurgery consultation	Concussion: activity restriction and graduated return to sport/activity DAI: supportive care in ICU to limit ongoing axonal injury

TABLE 1-7	Differential Diagnosis–Non-Traumatic
Definition	The occurrence of a loss of the ability to perceive and respond, in the absence of a traumatic event
Presentation	Stupor, confusion, unconscious
Physical examination	Recognize a sick patient, record vitals, perform focused, thorough head-to-toe examination as discussed earlier
Etiologies	"The 6 Hs and the 5 Ts" **H**ypovolemia **H**ypoxia **H**ydrogen ion (acidosis) **H**ypo/Hyper K$^+$ **H**ypoglycemia **H**ypothermia **T**oxins **T**amponade **T**ension pneumothorax **T**hrombosis **T**rauma
Investigation	CBC, renal panel, INR/PTT, serum glucose, ABG, serum EtOH, tox screen, U/A, CT head
Treatment	Appropriate recognition of a critically ill patient Supportive critical care management as needed - ABCDE - Warming - Fluid resuscitation Correction of biochemical abnormalities and coagulopathies

Canadian Head CT Rules
- Is a head CT indicated?
- Use mnemonic **BEAN DASH**. CT if any one of following is present:
  - **B**asal skull fracture
  - **E**mesis × 2
  - **A**ge >65
  - **N**euro symptoms (GCS <15)
  - **D**angerous mechanism
  - **A**mnesia (>30 minutes prior)
  - **S**kull fracture (open or depressed)

General Management
1. ABCDEs
   - Manage critical care issues prn
2. Supportive management, prevent ongoing or further damage
   - ICP management
   - Prevent hypoxemia
   - Prevent seizure activity
3. Begin correction of biochemical and coagulation abnormalities
4. Critical care and neurosurgical consultations as needed for definitive management

Bibliography
Stiell IG, Wells GA, Vandemheen K, et al; for the CCC Study Group. The Canadian CT Head Rule for patients with minor head injury. *The Lancet.* 2001 May 5;357(9266):1391-1396.

Yingming A Chen. *Toronto Notes 2011: Comprehensive Medical Reference Review for MCCQE I USMLE II.* 27th ed. Toronto, ON: Toronto Review; 2008.

Trauma
Priority Topic 92

Trauma is one of the leading causes of morbidity and mortality in young age groups.

All primary care providers should consider taking ATLS course. ATLS provides everyone with a systematic way to bring calm to a chaotic scenario, optimize patient outcomes, and at times, save a life. For more information see: http://www.traumacanada.org.

OVERVIEW

- **Be prepared**. Know your facility and your team's capabilities.
- Review what is available, and ensure that necessary equipment is available.
  - Warmed IV fluid
  - Warm blankets
  - Chest tube tray
  - Intubation set
  - Cricothyroidotomy set
  - Appropriate drugs
  - A Broselow tape for peds
  - Fabric pelvic binders
  - Blood, if feasible
  - Appropriate monitoring

MANAGEMENT

- Be as prepared as possible
- Upon arrival:
  - Ensure c-spine immobilization
  - Apply oxygen, monitors, and start **two** IVs—16 g or larger
  - Attain a complete and accurate set of vitals
    - HR
    - Respiratory rate
    - SaO_2
    - Blood pressure
    - Temperature
    - Glucose
  - Attain AMPLE history from patient, family, or EMS
    - A—allergies
    - M—medications
    - P—past medical history
    - L—last meal
    - E—events, what happened?

PRIMARY SURVEY

- Airway—Is it patent? Is intubation required?
- Breathing—Is air moving in both lung fields?
- Circulation—What is the BP? Are they making urine?
- Disability—Assess papillary responses and calculate GCS (*see LOC for GCS*).
- Exposure—Completely uncover the patient. Ensure you are warming them as much as possible—via warmed IV fluid and recovering the patient as soon as possible.

Recheck your ABCDEs constantly. If there is a change in condition, immediately revert back to "A."

ADJUNCTS TO THE PRIMARY SURVEY

- Trauma labs
  - CBC, electrolytes, blood type and crossmatch, toxicology screen, serum EtOH, arterial blood gas
- X-ray
  - AP pelvis
  - CXR
  - In most cases a lateral C-spine view is not required. Leave patient in C-spine precautions if concerned.

SECONDARY SURVEY

- Recheck ABCDEs
- A thorough and systematic examination from head to toe (including log roll and rectal examination) should be performed

ADJUNCTS TO THE SECONDARY SURVEY

- NG or OG tubes—if you are certain there is no sign of basal skull fracture
  - No Battle sign, no otorhinorrhea
- Foley catheter—if you are certain there is no bladder or urethral trauma
  - No blood at meatus, normal rectal examination
- ECG if indicated—that is, if cardiac ischemia or contusion is suspected
- CT scanning if indicated

DEFINITIVE MANAGEMENT

- Stabilize the patient to the best of your, and your facility's, ability.
- Seek help and advice early from a traumatologist.
- Discuss most appropriate mode of transfer—ground versus airplane versus helicopter.
- "Package up" the patient for transfer:
  - Intubation and placement of chest tubes in an ambulance is very unpleasant. It's also unpleasant on the side of a busy highway. It's almost impossible in a plane or helicopter. Anticipate what your patient might need before transferring.
  - If transferring via air, remember that a pneumothorax will progress faster as altitude increases during flight. Also remember that FiO_2 decreases with altitude. If a patient is not maintaining sats at ground level, this will be made worse during flight.

  But......
  - Do not take extra time with procedures or diagnostics (ie, CT scans) unless they contribute appropriately to the patient's stability in preparation for transfer. Do not undertake diagnostics that your facility is not equipped to act upon (ie, if you do not have surgical coverage, don't do a CT scan).
  - Travel with the patient in the ambulance/plane/helicopter if there is ongoing hemodynamic instability.

LIFE-THREATENING EMERGENCY SCENARIOS THAT FAMILY PHYSICIANS SHOULD KNOW

Tension pneumothorax

- **Signs/Symptoms:** hemodynamic instability, respiratory distress, increased HR, asymmetrical chest wall motion, tracheal deviation, hyperresonance to percussion, unilateral absence of breath sounds.

- **Rx**: needle thoracostomy at second intercostal space at mid-clavicular line. Do not delay for X-ray. Follow with chest tube at fifth intercostal space at anterior axillary line.

Cardiac tamponade

- **Signs/Symptoms**: usually with penetrating chest wound. Beck triad (hypotension, distended neck veins, muffled heart sounds), pulsus paradoxus (abnormally large drop in SBP on inspiration), Kussmaul sign (rise in JVP on inspiration).
- **Rx**: confirm with ECHO or bedside U/S if possible; pericardiocentesis (at xiphoid, aim needle at 45 degrees toward nipple).

Bibliography

American College of Surgeons Committee on Trauma. *Advanced Trauma Life Support for Doctors*. 8th ed. Chicago, IL: American College of Surgeons; 2008.

Chen YA, Tran C. *Toronto Notes–Comprehensive Medical Reference & Review for MCCQE I and USMLE II*. Toronto, Canada: Toronto Notes for Medical Students Inc; 2011.

Tintinalli JE, Stapczynski JS, Cline DM, Ma OJ, Cydulka RK, Meckler GD, eds. *Tintinalli's Emergency Medicine: A Comprehensive Study Guide*. 7th ed. New York, NY: The McGraw-Hill Companies; 2011.

Shock

Supplementary Topic

Definition

Inadequate end-organ perfusion resulting in loss of aerobic cellular function

The "end organs" are

- Brain (signs—altered consciousness, loss of consciousness)
- Kidneys (signs—decreased urine output)
- Skin (signs—cool, clammy, dusky, pale)
- Heart (signs—myocardial ischemia, decreased cardiac output, hypotension)

TYPES OF SHOCK

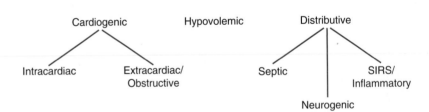

Hypovolemic Shock

Definition

Lack of effective circulating blood volume

- **Beware:**
  - Bleeding might not be external, that is, GI bleed, ruptured ovarian cyst, femur fracture, pelvic fracture.
  - "Blood" isn't just the red stuff. Large serum losses, such as in burn patients, nausea and vomiting, high output ileostomy, and pancreatitis can also lead to hypovolemia.

Signs

Tachycardia; peripheral vasoconstriction leading to cool, clammy skin; acidosis; tachypnea; altered mental status

Decreased urine output is the most sensitive, and simplest, method by which to monitor response to hypovolemic shock resuscitation.

Treatment

- **Stop the bleeding!!!**
- Simultaneously restore blood volume with crystalloid, transfusions
- Vasopressors play **no role** in the initial management of hypovolemic shock. Fill the tank, then optimize the pump and plumbing!!!

Cardiogenic Shock

Definition

- Decreased cardiac output and evidence of tissue hypoxia in the presence of adequate intravascular volume
- Occurs most often due to myocardial ischemia, but can also occur due to valve disease, cardiac trauma, massive pulmonary embolus, or cardiac tamponade

  Intracardiac:
  - Ischemia
  - Valve disease, involves endocarditis, chordae rupture, but is rare
  - Contusion

  Extracardiac:
  - Very rare
  - Cardiac tamponade
  - Massive pulmonary embolism

Cardiogenic Shock—think of this as a pump problem
Distributive shock—think of this as a plumbing problem.

Signs

Distended jugular veins (increased JVP); arrhythmia and/or tachycardia, altered LOC, decreased urine output

Treatment

- Treat ischemia if present.
- If ischemia not present, as evidenced by ECG and troponins, consider another possible diagnosis, valve issue, contusion, tamponade, or massive PE, and **get help!!!!**
- Often there is a role for inotropic medications to temporize until definitive treatment can be reached.
- Consider thrombolysis if massive PE is probable and there are no absolute contraindications.

Distributive Shock

Definition

- Loss of vascular tone, and in turn, poor venous return leading to poor cardiac function and output
- **Distributive shock is of three types:**
  1. **Septic**
  2. **SIRS/Inflammatory**
  3. **Neurogenic**

1. Septic Shock

Definition

Acute circulatory failure characterized by persistent arterial hypotension despite adequate fluid resuscitation or by tissue hypoperfusion (as defined by a lactate concentration >4 mg/dL), and not explained by other causes.

Signs

Fever (not always), hypothermia (if severe sepsis), decreased LOC, decreased urine output

Treatment

Most important step is recognition of a patient as very sick, and that they are in need of the services of a facility that offers critical care services!!

- Attempt to identify a possible focus of infection
- Always draw cultures prior to starting antibiotics
- Start empiric, broad-spectrum antibiotics asap
  - Time of first dose of antibiotics is directly linked to outcome
  - Taper antibiotic choices based on cultures
- Supportive care
  - Think ABCs
  - Oxygen by mask
  - Intubate if necessary
    - To improve oxygenation and/or
    - To reduce the work of breathing
      - Can reduce oxygen needs by up to 30%
  - Fluid resuscitation and monitoring via Foley and urometer
  - Vasopressors have a definite role

2. Inflammatory Shock/SIRS

Definition

A combination of multiple, synergistically destructive, pathophysiologic processes that lead to endothelial dysfunction, fluid losses, and in turn, end organ dysfunction

- Criteria:
  - Two or more of the following factors:
    - Body temperature <36°C or >38°C
    - Heart rate >90 beats/min
    - Tachypnea >20 breaths/min or arterial partial pressure of carbon dioxide <4.3 kPa (32 mm Hg)
    - White count <4000 cells/mm³ (4 × 10⁹ cells/L) or >12,000 cells/mm³ (12 × 10⁹ cells/L) or the presence of >10% bands

Causes

- Anaphylaxis
- Pancreatitis
- Toxins, insect or snake bites
- Bowel ischemia or necrosis
- Burns
- Toxic shock syndrome
- Sepsis

"SIRS" is a bit of an odd classification for the non-intensivist, in that it encompasses some of the rarer causes of shock, but the main causes (hypovolemia, cardiogenic, septic, etc) can cross over into SIRS.

Septic shock is simply SIRS with a known infection.

3. Neurogenic Shock

Definition

Hypotension caused by loss of vascular tone, secondary to loss of sympathetic outflow from the T1 to L2 sympathetic chain.

Common error is to confuse this with "spinal shock." These are completely different.

Spinal shock is a state of transient physiologic (vs anatomic) loss of cord function below the level of injury, with associated loss of all reflex and sensorimotor functions. This lasts somewhere from 1 to 24 hours. It has nothing to do with hemodynamics or end-organ function.

Classic Manifestations of Neurogenic Shock

- Hypotension and bradycardia
  - Versus tachycardia in other types of shock

Treatment

- Recognition of underlying spinal cord injury and transfer to appropriate specialist
  - Vasopressors play a definite role

Beware of concomitant hypovolemia that often occurs along with spinal cord injuries. Car accidents with enough energy to crush a spinal cord often have enough energy to break a pelvis, a femur, or cause a hemothorax. Urine output is your best guide to ensuring proper end organ perfusion.

Bibliography

EMedicine website content. http://www.emedicine.com. Accessed 29 March 2012.

Approach to Poisoning
Priority Topic 74

INITIAL EVALUATION

ABCDEs

- Airway management
  - Give naloxone if considering opioid overdose
    - Respiratory rate <12 breaths/minute is the best predictor of response to naloxone
- Breathing
  - Give 100% oxygen in carbon monoxide poisoning
- Circulation
  - ECG and cardiac monitor
- Drugs
  - Empiric treatment with naloxone, glucose, and thiamine should be considered as they are relatively cheap and safe treatments of three common causes of altered mental status (opioid overdose, hypoglycemia, and Wernicke encephalopathy)
- Decontamination
  - Ipecac syrup for inducing emesis should **not** be used as it has significant potential adverse effects
  - Orogastric lavage should be used in potentially lethal ingestions that present within 1 hour
  - Activated charcoal
    - Indicated if within 1 to 2 hours postingestion
    - Complications include aspiration/vomiting/constipation and diarrhea
    - Dosing: 10:1 (charcoal to drug) or 1 g charcoal/kg body weight, whichever is larger
    - Drugs not bound by charcoal include iron, lithium, lead, hydrocarbons, and toxic alcohols
- Elimination
  - Urinary alkalinization
    - Enhances urinary elimination of certain drugs

INDICATIONS FOR DIALYSIS:

A	Acidosis
E	Electrolytes (increased K)
I	Intoxication (ASA, methanol, ethylene glycol)
O	Overload (fluids)
U	Uremia

DRUGS THAT DO NOT ABSORB ONTO CHARCOAL:

P	Pesticides, Potassium
H	Hydrocarbons
A	Alkali, Acids, Alcohols
I	Iron
L	Lithium, Lead
S	Solvents

FORMULAS TO KNOW FOR POISONED PATIENTS:

Anion gap = Measured −
$[Na^+ − (Cl^- + HCO_3^-)]$
Normal <12

Osmolar gap = Measured −
$[2Na^+ + glucose + BUN + (1.25 × ETOH)]$
Normal <10

ANION GAP−CAUSES:

M	Methanol
U	Uremia
D	DKA
P	Paraldehyde
I	Iron, Ibuprofen, INH
L	Lactate
E	Ethylene glycol
S	Salicylates

- Achieved by IV sodium bicarbonate bolus or infusion (3 amps $NaHCO_3$ in 1 L D5W at 1.5-2× normal maintenance rate)
- Most commonly used in moderate-severe ASA overdose
- Contraindicated in hypokalemia and renal insufficiency
- Hemodialysis
  - Used for removal of potentially life-threatening toxins that have either already been absorbed or do not bind to activated charcoal
  - Common toxins include ASA, lithium, theophylline, toxic alcohols, and carbamazepine

Key Questions to Ask

What was ingested (one drug vs multi drugs)?

When was the ingestion?

How much was ingested?

Was alcohol also consumed?

TABLE 1-8   Common Toxidromes

TOXIDROME	CLINICAL PRESENTATION	TREATMENT
Alcohol (ethanol)	- Disinhibition, slurred speech, ataxia, aggression, hypoglycemia, retrograde amnesia, coma	- Thiamine - Folate - Treat hypoglycemia - Supportive treatments
Opioids	- Triad of miosis, CNS depression, and respiratory depression	- Ventilatory support - Naloxone
Sympathomimetics (cocaine, amphetamines, alcohol withdrawal)	- Agitation/excitation, hypertension, tachycardia, mydriasis, hyperthermia, diaphoresis, sudden death	- Cooling - Benzodiazepines for agitation and hypertension - Treat cocaine-induced MI as per ACS protocol - Avoid beta-blockers in cocaine OD
Anticholinergics	- Hot as a hare−hyperthermia - Dry as a bone−dry skin and mucous membranes - Red as a beet−flushed skin - Blind as a bat−mydriasis - Mad as a hatter−altered mental status - Also dysrhythmias and seizure	- Benzodiazepines - Cooling - Physostigmine in certain situations
Cholinergics (organophosphates, pesticides)	**D**−diarrhea/diaphoresis **U**−urination **M**−miosis **B**−bradycardia/bronchorrhea **E**−emesis **L**−lacrimation **S**−salivation - Also muscle weakness and respiratory failure	- Airway and ventilatory support - Atropine - Pralidoxime
TCA	**3Cs:** **C**ardiotoxicity (wide QRS and prolonged QT) **C**onvulsion/seizure **C**oma/sedation Other: ataxia, dry mouth, urinary retention	- Sodium bicarbonate (for wide QRS) - Circulatory support - Benzodiazepines for seizures
Sedatives (barbiturates, benzodiazepines)	- Decreased level of consciousness, slurred speech, ataxia, respiratory depression	- Supportive
Hallucinogens (phencyclidine hydrochloride [PCP], lysergic acid diethylamide [LSD])	- Psychosis, agitation, hallucination, hyperthermia, mydriasis, nausea	- Supportive - Benzodiazepines

ACETAMINOPHEN OVERDOSE

- The metabolite *N*-acetyl P-benzoquinone imine (NAPQI) causes hepatotoxicity
- **Toxic dose = 150 mg/kg**
- Have high clinical suspicion as it is often found in combination with other drug overdoses
- Appropriate treatment with *N*-acetylcysteine (NAC) has a near 100% success rate if given <8 hours from ingestion

Clinical Features

1. <24 hours	Nausea, vomiting, and diaphoresis
2. 24 to 48 hours	Often asymptomatic or RUQ pain
	Minor increases in transaminases, bilirubin, and prothrombin time may be seen
3. 72 to 96 hours	Peak liver dysfunction, jaundice, pain, encephalopathy, GI symptoms
4. 4 days to 2 weeks	Spectrum ranges from full recovery to death or liver transplant

Treatment

- Initial evaluation and supportive treatment
- Decontamination
  - Consider activate charcoal if within 1 to 2 hours
- Consult poison control
- Serum NAPQI level at 4 hours post ingestion or as soon as possible → plot level on Rumack-Matthew nomogram
- Begin treatment with NAC if:
  - Time of ingestion is known and serum NAPQI level falls above the lower line on the nomogram
  - Serum level not available until >8 hours post ingestion, first dose of NAC should be given
    - NAC may be discontinued if acetaminophen level is subsequently found to be nontoxic
    - Time since ingestion is not known or >24 hours
    - Continue treatment after initial dose if serum acetaminophen >10 mcg/mL or elevated AST/ALT

ASA OVERDOSE

- Mechanism/toxicity caused by direct stimulation of respiratory center and chemoreceptor trigger zone, uncoupling of oxidative phosphorylation, increased fatty acid metabolism, ototoxicity
- Chronic ingestion is associated with higher toxicity for a given salicylate level

Clinical Features

- Nausea, vomiting, tinnitus, hearing loss, tachypnea/hyperventilation, altered mental status
- Mixed acid-base disturbance
  - **Metabolic acidosis**
    - ASA inhibits the Krebs cycle and oxidative phosphorylation leading to increased production of CO_2, heat, and metabolic acids, and enhancing glycolysis and lipolysis
    - Usually will have an elevated anion gap but in the case of co-ingestion it may be normal

- **Respiratory alkalosis**
  - ASA causes direct stimulation of the medullary respiratory center

Diagnosis

- Salicylate levels—repeat Q_2H until level falls and clinical improvement
- Blood gas—follow serially until metabolic acidosis resolves
- Electrolytes, liver function tests, CBC, urinalysis
- ECG
- AXR—concretions may appear on plain abdominal film

Treatment

- ABCs—significant volume depletion is common
- Decontamination—activated charcoal if within 2 hours
- Elimination
  - Urine alkalinization
    - For moderate-severe toxicity
    - Bolus of 1 to 2 mEq/kg $NaHCO_3$ followed by an infusion (three ampules of $NaHCO_3$ added to 1 L of 5% dextrose in water)
    - Follow urine pH Q_1H and titrate infusion to a pH >7.5
    - Monitor for hypokalemia and replace as needed
  - Hemodialysis
    - Indications include serum ASA >100 mg/dL, refractory acidosis, need for respiratory support, renal failure, altered mental status, and severe acid-base disorder

Bibliography

Hall JB, Schmidt GA, Wood LDH, eds. *Principles of Critical Care*. 3rd ed. New York, NY: The McGraw-Hill Companies; 2005.

Longo DL, Fauci AS, Kasper DL, Hauser SL, Jameson JL, Loscalzo J, eds. *Harrison's Principles of Internal Medicine*. 18th ed. New York, NY: The McGraw-Hill Companies; 2012.

Tintinalli JE, Stapczynski JS, Cline DM, Ma OJ, Cydulka RK, Meckler GD, eds. *Tintinalli's Emergency Medicine: A Comprehensive Study Guide*. 7th ed. New York, NY: The McGraw-Hill Companies; 2011.

Chest Pain
Priority Topic 13

Chest pain is one of the most common presenting complaints to the emergency department. It is the responsibility of the clinician to identify those patients at high risk for life-threatening causes of chest pain and manage them accordingly.

Always start with ABCs and address life-threatening issues immediately.
If the patient has any of the following:

- Visceral-type chest pain (difficult to describe, radiates, imprecise location, *heaviness, discomfort, pressure, aching*)
- Abnormal vital signs
- Significant vascular disease risk factors
- Dyspnea

Place patient in treatment room, hook up a cardiac monitor, establish IV access, give O_2, and perform an ECG.

History/Risk Factors

HPI: onset, duration, quality, severity, radiation, associated symptoms

PMHx: DM, previous CV disease, dyslipidemia, HTN

FHx: MI in first-degree relative (female <65, male <55)

SHx: obesity, smoking, EtOH, age

TABLE 1-9	Chest Pain: Causes, Characterstics, and Management			
ETIOLOGY	CLASSIC SIGNS/ SYMPTOMS	CHARACTERISTIC FINDINGS	APPROPRIATE WORKUP	TIMELY MANAGEMENT
Aortic dissection	Sudden, severe pain, described as "tearing," radiates to back	CXR-widened mediastinum, >20 mm Hg difference in BP on right vs left sides	TEE, MRI, or CT	ABCs, straight to OR if dissection otherwise admit to ICU Decrease contractility and arterial BP (BBs, CCBs, nitrates) Surgery if ascending aneurysm or if descending aneurysm > 5 cm
Pulmonary embolism	Pleuritic CP, dyspnea, decreased O_2 saturation, anxiety, tachycardia	ECG (T-wave inversions in V_1-V_4, RBBB, S_1-Q_3-T_3 pattern) CXR-usually normal, 5% show Westermark sign or Hampton hump	D-dimer, ECG, CXR, Doppler U/S (to look for DVT), VQ scan, chest CT Use Wells or PERC score (see Table 1-10)	ABCs Heparin → warfarin
Pneumothorax	Pleuritic CP, dyspnea, tachycardia, tachypnea, hypoxia	Decreased/absent breath sounds on affected side Tension pneumothorax: tracheal deviation away from affected side with mediastinal deviation on CXR CXR: lung markings do not extend to periphery	CXR if patient stable	Tension pneumothorax: needle decompression/chest tube If clinically significant: chest tube/ Heimlich valve May consider watchful waiting if asymptomatic/small pneumothorax
Acute coronary syndromes (UA, NSTEMI, STEMI)	Retrosternal squeezing/ pressure, radiates to arm/ shoulder/jaw/neck, dyspnea, n/v, syncope Remember: DM and women present nonspecifically	Unstable angina: no ST or biomarker elevation NSTEMI: no ST changes, biomarkers elevated STEMI: biomarker and ST elevation	Troponin/CK-MB, ECG, CXR	ABCs Pain control (morphine), oxygen, ASA/ clopidogrel, nitro Call cardio: PCI/angio or thrombolysis
Pericarditis	Anterior, precordial CP, pleuritic, better with leaning forward	ECG: diffuse ST elevation (saddle-shaped), PR interval depression Pericardial friction rub on auscultation	ECG Clinical diagnosis	Supportive treatment, fluids, NSAIDs, steroids
GERD/hiatal hernia/ esophageal perforation	Hx of frequent heartburn, dysphagia, relief with antacid If perforation: fever, dyspnea, subQ emphysema, tachycardia, hematemesis	CXR-pneumomediastinum	Perf: CXR, CT, contrast swallow GERD/HH: Upper GI series, gastroscopy, or barium swallow	GERD/HH: trial of PPI, +/− gastroscopy, lifestyle modification Perf: ABCs, supportive, NPO, Abx, consult surgery
Peptic ulcer disease	Dyspepsia +/− UGI bleed, burning 1-3 hours postprandial, improvement with food	*Helicobacter pylori*, stress Hx of NSAID or EtOH use	*Helicobacter pylori* serology, urea breath testing, gastroscopy	*Helicobacter pylori* eradication (PPI, Amox, Clarithro) Lifestyle modifications. D/C NSAID use, quit smoking, lose weight
Cardiac tamponade	Dyspnea, hypotension, tachycardia, CP	Elevated JVP, narrowed pulse pressure, muffled heart sounds	ECG, ECHO	ABCs, pericardiocentesis, surgery
Varicella zoster (shingles)	Tingling sensation → vesicular rash following a dermatome	Unilateral vesicular rash with dermatomal pattern Risks: immunocompromised (cancer, old, HIV+)	Clinical diagnosis, may do serology if unsure	Acyclovir (within 72 h of pain) Contagious until lesions crusted Post-herpetic neuralgia (NSAIDs, gabapentin, TCAs)
Esophageal spasm	Dysphagia (liquids and solids), CP		Barium swallow, manometry	Anticholinergics, nitrates, CCBs, botulinum toxin injection

TABLE 1-10	Wells Score for PE	
FACTOR		**POINTS**
Suspected DVT		3
Alternative Dx less likely than PE		3
Tachycardia (HR >100 bpm)		1.5
Prior VTE		1.5
Immobilization/surgery within last 4 weeks		1.5
Active malignancy		1
Hemoptysis		1

Score <4 do D-dimer (sensitive, not specific, high NPV).
Score >4 do CT chest or VQ scan. (CT chest less sensitive than VQ scan.)
Score >6 is high probability of PE (78.4%).
Score <2 is low probability of PE (3.4%).

Bibliography

DynaMed. Chest Pain. Ipswich, MA: EBSCO Publishing; January 2012. Retrieved March 7, 2012, from http://search.ebscohost.com/login.aspx?direct=true&db=dme&AN=116633&site=dynamed-live&scope=site.

Green GB, Hill PM. Chest pain: cardiac or not. In: Tintinalli JE, Stapcznski JS, John Ma O, Cline DM, Cydulka RK, Meckler GD, eds. *Emergency Medicine: A Comprehensive Study Guide.* 7th ed. McGraw-Hill Companies, Inc, New York; 2011:361-366.

Hollander JE, Dierks DB. Acute coronary syndromes: acute myocardial infarction and unstable angina. In: Tintinalli JE, Stapcznski JS, John Ma O, Cline DM, Cydulka RK, Meckler GD, eds. *Emergency Medicine: A Comprehensive Study Guide.* 7th ed. McGraw-Hill Companies, Inc, New York; 2011:367-385.

Kline JA. Thromboembolism. In: Tintinalli JE, Stapcznski JS, John Ma O, Cline DM, Cydulka RK, Meckler GD, eds. *Emergency Medicine: A Comprehensive Study Guide.* 7th ed. McGraw-Hill Companies, Inc, New York; 2011:430-441.

Atrial Fibrillation

Priority Topic 8

Definition

- Irregular rhythm (atria quiver, irregular ventricular response)

Symptoms

- May be asymptomatic, especially with chronic Afib
- Palpitations, SOB, lightheadedness/dizziness/presyncope, focal neurological deficit (with stroke)

Risk Factors

HTN	EtOH	Cardiomyopathy (ischemic/HF)
Thyrotoxicosis	Valvular heart disease	MI
PE	Pneumonia	Hypokalemia/hypomagnesemia
Hypoxia	Rheumatic heart disease	ASD
Pericardial disease	Sick sinus syndrome	Post-cardiac surgery
SVT	Familial/genetic	Obstructive sleep apnea
Obesity	COPD	Pulmonary HTN

Classification

Four categories:

1. New onset
2. Paroxysmal (short bursts with spontaneous cardioversion)
3. Persistent (lasts >7 days, requires pharmacological or electrical cardioversion)
4. Permanent (prolonged symptoms [>1 year] or refractory to cardioversion)

CHADS2 Scoring

Used to determine appropriate anticoagulation treatment and to estimate stroke risk (Refer to www.ccpn.ca for more detailed information on stroke prevention in Afib)

C: CHF (1 pt)

H: HTN (1 pt)

A: age >75 (1 pt)

D: diabetes (1 pt)

S: stroke/TIA history (2 pts)

Score:

0: ASA 325 mg po daily

1: ASA, warfarin (INR 2-3) or dabigatran

2+: warfarin (INR 2-3) or dabigatran

Management

- Always start with ABCs and address life-threatening issues first!
- Goal is to alleviate patient symptoms, improve quality of life, and decrease mortality/morbidity and not necessarily the elimination of atrial fibrillation.

Investigations

- CBC, INR/PTT, renal and liver panels, TSH (fasting glucose and lipids should also be done but as an outpatient, not in the ED)
- 12-lead ECG (rate, rhythm, conduction disturbances, signs of previous MI, ventricular hypertrophy, atrial enlargement)
- Echocardiogram (to document ventricular size, wall thickness, EF, left atrial size, presence of valvular pathology, or congenital heart disease)—does not need to be done in ED unless urgent cardioversion required (see electrical cardioversion section)

Rate and Rhythm Control

Goal is resting HR <100 bpm in persistent or permanent Afib

A. Rate control:

- Start with rate control, if symptoms continue then move on to rhythm control
- Initial rate control therapy
  - No history of MI or LV dysfunction—beta-blockers (eg, metoprolol) or nondihydropyridine calcium channel blockers (eg, diltiazem)
  - History of MI or LV dysfunction—beta-blockers

B. Rhythm control (maintenance of sinus rhythm):

a. Nonstructural heart disease:

i. Dronedarone, flecainide, propafenone, or sotalol

b. Abnormal LV function but LVEF >35%:

i. Dronedarone, sotalol, or amiodarone

c. LVEF <35%:

i. Amiodarone

- Digoxin is not recommended as initial rhythm control therapy in an active patient. Reserve use for sedentary or LV systolic dysfunction patients. Digoxin can be used as an adjunct to BBs and CCBs to achieve better rate control, but should not be used on its own.

C. Electric cardioversion
- Initially use 150 to 200 J biphasic waveform
- All patients should be pretreated with antiarrhythmic medications
- Indications
  - For unstable patients
  - If Afib <48 hours or anticoagulation >3 weeks and >4 weeks since previous cardioversion
  - If Afib >48 hour duration and not anticoagulated/subtherapeutic → need TEE to ensure no thrombosis in atria/ventricles prior to cardioversion

Anticoagulation
- Purpose: prevention of thrombus/embolus
- Anticoagulate with ASA or warfarin as appropriate (see above for CHADS2 scoring and anticoagulation determination)

Follow-Up
- Outpatient follow-up with cardiology and family physician

Bibliography

Canadian Cardiovascular Society. 2010 *Atrial Fibrillation Guidelines*. 2011, December. Retrieved March 21, 2012, from http://www.ccsguidelineprograms.ca/images/stories/Artrial_Fibriallation_Program/ExecutiveSummary/2010rec_exec_summary_updated.pdf.

DynaMed. Atrial Fibrillation. Ipswich, MA: EBSCO Publishing; February 2012. Retrieved March 7, 2012, from http://search.ebscohost.com/login.aspx?direct=true&db=dme&AN=115288&site=dynamed-live&scope=site.

Piktel JS. Cardiac rhythm disturbances. In: Tintinalli JE, Stapcznski JS, John Ma O, Cline DM, Cydulka RK, Meckler GD, eds. *Emergency Medicine: A Comprehensive Study Guide.* 7th ed. McGraw-Hill Companies, Inc, New York; 2011:142-143.

Seizures

Priority Topic 81

Definitions
- Seizure
  - An episode of abnormal neurologic function caused by inappropriate electrical discharge of neurons
- Generalized seizure
  - Begin with **loss of consciousness** and are caused by nearly simultaneous activation of the entire cerebral cortex
  - May be generalized tonic-clonic (grand mal), absence (petit mal), or myoclonic
- Partial seizure (focal)
  - Electrical discharges begin in a localized region and may or may not spread to involve other regions or the entire cortex
  - Consciousness not affected = **simple partial seizure**
  - Consciousness affected = **complex partial seizure**

- Status epilepticus
  - Seizure lasting 5 to 15 minutes or multiple seizures without full return of consciousness

History

- History of seizure disorder
- Precipitating factors
- Grand mal seizures will usually begin with the patient becoming very rigid with extremities extended and progress into the clonic phase of rhythmic jerking movements
- Always attempt to determine if the movements were localized or generalized and symmetric
- Duration typically 60 to 90 seconds and often overestimated by witnesses
- Loss of bowel and bladder control, tongue biting
- Apnea and cyanosis
- Gradual return to consciousness and a postictal phase of confusion

Physical Examination

- Vital signs, temperature, serum glucose
- Complete neurologic examination looking for any focal signs
- Examine for injuries that were sustained during the attack

Differential Diagnosis

- Syncope, migraine, narcolepsy, movement disorder, pseudoseizure

Treatment

- Protect airway, oxygen, and prepare for endotracheal intubation if unable to terminate seizure
- IV access if possible
- Bedside glucose
- Terminate seizure
  - First-line agent is a benzodiazepine
    - Lorazepam or diazepam
    - Diazepam may be given by rectal or endotracheal route and midazolam may be given IM if unable to secure IV access
  - Second line
    - Phenytoin (15-20 mg/kg IV, max 50 mg/min)
    - Fosphenytoin—can be given faster (100-150 mg "phenytoin equivalents" per min IV or IM)
    - Consult neurology and consider ICU admission
  - Third line
    - Phenobarbital (30-60 mg boluses to maximum 15 mg/kg)
    - Prepare for intubation with this medication
- Investigations
  - If known seizure disorder:
    - Serum anticonvulsant levels
  - If first ever seizure:
    - CBC, glucose, renal panel, Ca, Mg, β-hCG, toxicology screen, head CT, EEG
- Neurology consult to determine need for long-term treatment

FEBRILE SEIZURE
Criteria:
- Temperature >38°C
- Age <6 years
- No CNS infection/inflammation
- No metabolic abnormality
- No history of afebrile seizure

May be classified as benign (simple) if it lasts <15 minutes, there are no focal signs, and seizure does not recur in 24-hour period.

Febrile seizures do not cause brain damage!

Key Points

■ Patient must be seizure free for 1 year before driving.

■ Warn patient about possible dangers related to swimming, living alone, operating heavy machinery, chewing gum, heights.

■ Anticonvulsants are teratogenic; women should take 4-6 mg/day of folic acid during childbearing years and be on lowest-possible dose of anticonvulsant.

■ Many antibiotics can interfere with anticonvulsant levels.

■ Anticonvulsants can lead to osteoporosis, hematologic complications, liver dysfunction, GI upset, and fatigue.

Bibliography

Chen YA, Tran C *Toronto Notes–Comprehensive Medical Reference & Review for MCCQE I and USMLE II.* Toronto, Canada: Toronto Notes for Medical Students Inc; 2011.

Hall JB, Schmidt GA, Wood LDH, eds. *Principles of Critical Care.* 3rd ed. New York, NY: The McGraw-Hill Companies; 2005.

McPhee SJ, Papadakis MA, eds. *Current Medical Diagnosis & Treatment.* New York, NY: The McGraw-Hill Companies; 2012.

Tintinalli JE, Stapczynski JS, Cline DM, Ma OJ, Cydulka RK, Meckler GD, eds. *Tintinalli's Emergency Medicine: A Comprehensive Study Guide.* 7th ed. New York, NY: The McGraw-Hill Companies; 2011.

Lacerations

Priority Topic 56

History

Ascertain details surrounding the laceration.

■ What is the cause of laceration?

■ How clean are/were the surroundings (ie, dirty cut)?

■ Was a bite involved? If yes, was it human, canine, or feline?

■ How long ago did it occur?

■ Is there any chance that a foreign body may remain deep in the wound?

■ Is there a possibility that there is an underlying compound fracture?

   Must ask about tetanus immunization and booster status.

   Ask about potential allergies to local anaesthetics and antibiotics that may be required.

Physical Examination

■ Use appropriate sterile conditions and good lighting.

■ Use appropriate analgesia (local or otherwise).

■ Note the position of the wound, and what surrounding structures may be injured (nerves, vessels, tendons). Test for the function of the suspected injured structures distal to the injury.

■ Document all findings.

■ Under no circumstances should you blindly probe into a wound with an instrument. Do not snap or clamp bleeding vessels, use direct pressure for hemostasis.

■ X-ray if foreign body or underlying fracture is suspected.

Management

- First classify a laceration as simple or complex, and seek specialist assistance (plastic surgery, orthopedic, general surgery, urology, ophthalmology) if complicating factors are present.
  - A wound is simple if it has following factors:
    - Small (under 10 cm)
    - Time to treatment of <6 hours
    - No neural compromise
    - No vascular compromise
    - No tendon involvement
    - Not involving complex facial anatomy (eyelids, lip margins, globe)
    - No foreign body present
- There are differing opinions on how long a wound can be left open and a safe primary closure can be performed. Factors that weigh in on this decision are:
  - Time from injury
  - Site of injury—face versus periphery—consider blood supply
  - Level of contamination of wound
  - Patient factors—diabetes, immunocompromise, trustworthiness
    - If you are concerned at all, always err on the side of safety. Irrigate and dress the wound open, start IV antibiotics, and perform a delayed primary closure in 48 hours. A gas-producing, necrotizing, anaerobic infection almost always results in a loss of limb, and sometimes a loss of life.
- If decision is made to close wound:

1. Ensure that appropriate tetanus prophylaxis and antibiotics are given if required.
2. Ensure that appropriate analgesia is provided:
   - Lidocaine (Xylocaine)
     - Without Epinephrine
       - Duration 30 to 60 minutes
       - **Maximum dose 5 mg/kg,** not to exceed 300 mg
     - With Epinephrine
       - Duration 2 to 6 hours
       - **Maximum dose 7 mg/kg**
   - Bupivicaine (Marcaine)
     - Without Epinephrine
       - Duration 30 to 60 minutes
       - Maximum dose 2 mg/kg, not to exceed 175 mg
     - With Epinephrine
       - Duration 3 to 7 hours
       - Maximum dose 3 mg/kg, not to exceed 225 mg
3. Ensure that the wound has been irrigated and debrided appropriately. Use copious amounts of irrigation (ie, >1 L of NS for a 5 cm wound).
4. Close the wound accurately using a suture technique and material appropriate for the area to be closed.
   - Close in layers with absorbable suture (ie, Vicryl) if warranted.
   - Choice of skin closure based on cosmetic requirements (ie, small, nonabsorbable suture around the eyelid, eg, Prolene) or need for rapid closure (ie, stapler in an intoxicated or hemodynamically unstable patient), etc.

Always withdraw the plunger on your syringe before injecting to ensure you do not inject local anaesthetic intravascularly. This can be deadly.

5. Dress wound appropriately and arrange for necessary follow-up.
   - Immobilize the area with a splint if needed to keep tension off the wound. Remember to use the position of safety if splinting a hand.
   - Consider more frequent follow-up for wounds at higher risk of infection. Use the criteria above to make this decision.

TETANUS IMMUNIZATION

- Td (tetanus toxoid) and TIG (tetanus immunoglobulin) are safe in pregnancy.
- Provide booster if last tetanus update was >5 years ago.
- Only give TIG if unsure of immunization status (unknown if had childhood series) and high-risk wound. TIG is never required in non–tetanus-prone wounds (see Table 1-11).

TABLE 1-11	Guidelines for Treatment of Tetanus-Prone Wounds		
HISTORY		TOXOID REQUIRED	TIG REQUIRED
Dirty wound +	Unknown baseline immunization status	Yes	Yes
Dirty wound +	Booster >10 years	Yes	No
Dirty wound +	Booster >5 years	Yes	No
Dirty wound +	Booster <5 years	No	No

SPECIAL CONSIDERATIONS

1. Small puncture wounds over flexor tendon area and injection injuries (paint guns, sandblasters) often result in gross deep contamination with minimal superficial evidence of this. Be very aware.
2. Bite wounds:
   a. Canine, feline, mammalian, or human in origin
   b. Often infected with organisms that live in the mouth (*Pasteurella multiocida, Staphylococcus aureus, Bacteroides, Streptococcus viridans*)
   c. Often do not close and consider starting on prophylactic amoxicillin/clavulanate 500 mg TID
   d. Consider possibility of HIV or Hepatitis B/C transmission from human bites
   e. Update tetanus
3. Animal wounds can be at risk of transmitting rabies
   a. Send animal to appropriate laboratory if available
   b. Consider rabies vaccine and RIG treatment

Generally *do not* close cat or human bites. May close facial wounds (due to scar risk) with close follow-up.

80% of cat bites and 5% of dog bites become infected. Consider this when deciding if antibiotic is needed.

Bibliography

Anti-infective Review Panel. *Anti-infective Guidelines for Community-Acquired Infections.* Toronto: MUMS Guideline Clearinghouse; 2010:53.

Anti-infectives for common infections—overview. *Drug Comparison Charts.* 8th ed. Saskatoon, Canada: Rx Files; 2010:54.

Pepid website content. http://www.pepid.com. Accessed 26 March 2012.

UpToDate website content. http://www.uptodate.com. Accessed 26 March 2012.

Yingming A, Tran C, eds. Wound closure. *Toronto Notes.* 27th ed. Toronto, ON: Toronto Notes for Medical Students Inc; 2011: PL5-PL10.

Epistaxis

Priority Topic 36

Symptoms

- Bleeding from nose
- With or without associated symptoms such as hematemesis, pain, headache, rhinorrhea, itchy/watery eyes, lightheadedness/dizziness, nausea

Risk Factors

Risk factors include the following:

- Nose picking
- Trauma
- Foreign bodies
- Dry environment
- Blood dyscrasias URTI/infection/inflammatory neoplasm
- Polyp
- Deviated septum
- AV malformation
- Chemical irritants
- Chronic nasal cannula O_2 use
- Recent surgery
- Hereditary hemorrhagic telangiectasia
- Alcohol or cocaine abuse
- von Willebrand disease
- Hemophilia
- NSAIDs/ASA/warfarin/heparin
- HTN (esp. for posterior bleeds)

Management

1. **History**
    - History of present illness (HPI): onset, duration, timeline, pattern, amount of bleeding, associated symptoms, event/trauma, prior/recurrent nosebleeds
    - Personal or family history of bleeding/bruising/coagulopathy
    - Medications: specifically NSAID, warfarin, heparin, and ASA use; chemotherapy
    - Alcohol or cocaine abuse
    - History of HTN

2. **Physical Examination**
    - ABCs/vitals
    - In "sniffing" position use a speculum to visualize bleeding source. Area of bleeding: most commonly involved are anterior nasal septum/Little area/Kiesselbach plexus
    - Check whether there is any fracture or instability

Note: In the ER, the diagnosis of a posterior bleeding source is probable when there has been failure to control an anterior bleeding source. Other features that suggest a posterior source include elderly patients with a coagulopathy, significant hemorrhage seen in posterior nasopharynx, bilateral hemorrhage, hematemesis/hemoptysis.

3. **Laboratories/Investigations**
   - Only necessary if hemodynamically unstable, suspicion of bleeding diathesis, or use of anticoagulation
   - CBC, coagulation, crossmatch
   - X-ray if suspect fracture/trauma history

4. **Treatment**
   - Address airway compromise if present
   - Obtain IV access and cross-match if hemodynamic instability
   - Reassure patient and address their fear or anxiety
     1. Apply direct nasal pressure by pinching nares for 10 to 15 minutes
     2. Topical cocaine, lidocaine, and epinephrine can be used for vasoconstriction
     3. Chemical cauterization with silver nitrate (may anesthetise nasal mucosa first). Electrocautery should be left to ENT due to risk of septal perforation.
     4. Thrombogenic foams/gels (if available)
     5. Anterior nasal packing with layering of ribbon gauze, an anterior epistaxis balloon, or a nasal tampon/sponge
     6. Posterior packing—use longer lengths of anterior packing materials or a 14F to 16F Foley catheter with a 30 cc balloon and call ENT

5. **Follow-up**
   - In case of anterior epistaxis with hemodynamic stability and hemorrhage control for >1 hour, discharge home with clear instructions on what to do if nosebleed recurs, use of humidifier, and avoidance of nose blowing
   - Patients with therapeutic warfarin levels may continue their medication
   - D/C NSAIDs for 3 to 4 days
   - If anterior packing is placed in both nostrils, give Rx for staphylococcus coverage (first dose in ER)
   - Remove nonabsorbable packing in 2 to 3 days

Bibliography

DynaMed.. Nosebleed. Ipswich, MA: EBSCO Publishing; November 2009. Retrieved March 7, 2012, from http://search.ebscohost.com/login.aspx?direct=true&db=dme&AN=115407&site=dynamed-live&scope=site.

Summers SM, Bey T, Epistaxis, nasal fractures, and rhinosinusitis. In: Tintinalli JE, Stapcznski JS, John Ma O, Cline DM, Cydulka RK, Meckler GD, eds. *Emergency Medicine: A Comprehensive Study Guide*. 7th ed. McGraw-Hill Companies, Inc., New York; 2011: 1564-1567.

Red Eye
Priority Topic 79

CONJUNCTIVITIS

■ Most common cause of red eye (see Table 1-12)

Topical steroids should be avoided as treatment of red eye by family physicians.

TABLE 1-12	Red Eye: Causes and Management				
	BACTERIAL	**GONOCOC-CAL AND CHLAMYDIAL**	**VIRAL**	**HERPES**	**ATOPIC/ALLERGIC**
Clinical presentation	- Rapid onset - One or both eyes involved - Discharge is mucopurulent. "Eye glued shut in morning" - Can progress to peri-orbital cellulitis - Photophobia signals involvement of cornea	- Consider in neonates and sexually active persons - Rapid progression - Copious purulent discharge - Unilateral - Tender pre-auricular lymph nodes - May lead to corneal perforation	- Rapid onset - Usually becomes bilateral at 24-48 h - Often associated with a viral respiratory tract infection - Watery discharge - Itchy, foreign body sensation	- Red, irritated eye - Watery discharge - Vesicles on face and eyelid - May have corneal involvement	- Very itchy eyes - Tearing - Redness - Associated with other atopy symptoms - Bilateral - No exudate
Etiology	*Staphylococcus* aureus, *Streptococcus pneumoniae*, *Haemophilus. influenzae*, *Mycoplasma catarrhalis*	*Neisseria gonorrhoeae*, *Chlamydia trachomatis*	- Usually adenovirus - Coxsackie virus	Herpes simplex type 1 or 2	
Treatment	- Most often self-limited (day 2-5) - Topical antibiotics controversial - Contagious for 48-72 h *Use antibiotics if corneal involvement or contact lens user.	- Emergent referral - GO: Ceftriaxone 1 g IM ×1 - CH: Azithromycin 1 g PO ×1 - May add topical antibiotics *Treat for both GO and CH when initiating management.	- Resolves spontaneously without specific treatment - Cold compress for comfort - Very contagious so proper hand hygiene and avoidance of direct contact is important	- Refer to ophthalmology - Topical or systemic antivirals	- Warm or cold compress - Antihistamines

GLAUCOMA

Definition

■ Progressive optic neuropathy involving characteristic structural changes to optic nerve with associated visual field changes

• Usually have increased intraocular pressure (IOP), but this is not required for diagnosis

• Loss of peripheral vision precedes central vision loss

Causes, Presentation, and Management (See Table 1-13)

TABLE 1-13	Glaucoma: Causes, Presentation, and Management	
	PRIMARY OPEN ANGLE GLAUCOMA	PRIMARY ANGLE-CLOSURE GLAUCOMA
Risk factors	- Increasing age - African descent - Diabetes - Family history - Increased IOP	- Increasing age - Asian and Inuit descent - Female - Shallow anterior chamber of eye
Clinical features	- Gradual onset - Initially asymptomatic - *Painless* increase in IOP - Bilateral loss of peripheral vision - Optic disc cupping - No acute attacks	- Rapid onset - Fixed, mid-dilated pupil - *Painful*, red eye - Unilateral - Decreased vision, "halos around lights" - Nausea and vomiting - Usually IOP >50 mm Hg
Diagnosis	- Consistent and reproducible abnormalities in two of the following: - Optic disc, IOP, and visual field	- Clinical presentation and measurement of IOP
Treatment	- Topical prostaglandins, beta-blockers, cholinergics, osmotic diuretics - Prevention is important by screening high-risk patients	- Emergent ophthalmology consult - Medical and surgical treatments aimed at lowering IOP - Beta-blockers, cholinergics, osmotic diuretics

ANTERIOR UVEITIS (IRITIS)

Definition
■ Inflammation of the iris

Etiology
■ Immunologic
  • Ankylosing spondylitis, Reiter syndrome, psoriasis, Crohn's disease, ulcerative colitis, reactive arthritis
■ Infectious
  • Syphilis, Lyme disease, tuberculosis, herpes simplex, herpes zoster, toxoplasmosis
■ Other
  • Sarcoidosis, trauma

Clinical Features
■ Photophobia, decreased visual acuity
■ Pain
■ Miosis
■ Inflammatory cells seen within the anterior chamber
■ Hypopyon (layer of white cells)

Treatment
■ Urgent referral to Ophthalmology
■ Topical corticosteroids
■ Mydriatics

TEMPORAL ARTERITIS (GIANT CELL ARTERITIS)

Definition
■ A systemic inflammation of medium and large arteries which typically involves the temporal artery

Risk Factors

- Female
- Age >60

Clinical Features

- Abrupt unilateral vision loss
- Pain over temporal artery
- Jaw claudication
- Scalp tenderness

Diagnosis

- Elevated ESR
- Temporal artery biopsy

Treatment

- Immediate initiation of high-dose systemic steroids is required in all suspected cases
  - Do not wait for biopsy to be performed before starting treatment
- Give prednisone 40 to 60 mg daily and begin tapering after 2 to 4 weeks

AGE-RELATED MACULAR DEGENERATION

- Degenerative disease of the central retina resulting in loss of central vision
- Many risk factors including age, smoking, family history, and cardiovascular disease
- Patients have vision loss but are otherwise asymptomatic
- Red eye is not a feature
- Should be suspected and investigated for in patients who present with gradual blurring of vision in one or both eyes
- Diagnosis is made clinically on slit lamp examination

CATARACTS

- An opacity of the lens which is the leading cause of blindness in the world
- Risk factors include age, smoking, alcohol use, sun exposure, DM, and poor lifestyle habits
- Presentation is highly variable, but usually begins with an increase in nearsightedness followed by problems with night driving and reading fine print
- Vision loss is painless and red eye is not a feature
- No preventative strategies have been proven effective
- The only treatment includes surgical removal of the opacified lens
- Delay of surgical intervention does not lead to worse outcomes

Bibliography

Anti-infective Review Panel. *Anti-infective Guidelines for Community-Acquired Infections*. Toronto: MUMS Guideline Clearninghouse; 2012.

Longo DL, Fauci AS, Kasper DL, Hauser SL, Jameson JL, Loscalzo J, eds. *Harrison's Principles of Internal Medicine*. 18th ed. New York, NY: The McGraw-Hill Companies; 2012.

McPhee SJ, Papadakis MA, eds. *Current Medical Diagnosis & Treatment*. New York, NY: The McGraw-Hill Companies; 2012.

Tintinalli JE, Stapczynski JS, Cline DM, Ma OJ, Cydulka RK, Meckler GD, eds. *Tintinalli's Emergency Medicine: A Comprehensive Study Guide*. 7th ed. New York, NY: The McGraw-Hill Companies; 2011.

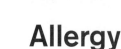

Allergy

Priority Topic 3

Definitions

Allergy: an exaggerated immune response mediated by histamine, leukotriene, C4, and prostaglandins (IgE).

Anaphylaxis: severe life-threatening allergic syndrome involving multiple organs, in a previously sensitized patient. Usually presents as respiratory insufficiency and hypotension.

History

- Differentiate allergy from anaphylaxis
- Patient may be able to share with you a history of severe allergy
- Look for MedicAlert bracelet or necklace

Physical Examination

- Dyspnea, stridor, wheeze, hoarseness
- Erythema
- Generalized urticaria
- Edema
- Pruritus, itchy eyes
- Conjunctival injection
- Tachycardia
- Hypotension
- Syncope
- Nausea, vomiting, diarrhea
- Consider allergy in the differential diagnosis when patients present with recurrent respiratory symptoms otherwise unexplained

Preventative Management and Education

- Always document allergies in chart, and update regularly.
- Clarify true allergy (angioedema, stridor, anaphylaxis, hives) versus intolerance (rash, GI upset, nausea).
- Educate all involved.
- Have patient acquire a MedicAlert bracelet.
- Advise patient to keep on hand epinephrine (EpiPen), antihistamine (H1 blocker +/− H2 blocker), and prednisone (for delayed reaction).
- Refer to allergist if reaction is significant and/or allergen unclear.

Acute Management of Anaphylaxis

- Remove causative agent if possible
- ABCs—secure airway; intubate if necessary but do not delay epinephrine to do so
- **Epinephrine**
  - **Adult dose 0.3 to 0.5 mL 1:1000 IM (0.3-0.5 mg)**
  - **Pediatric dose: 0.01 mL/kg 1:1000 IM (0.01 mg/kg)**
- Diphenhydramine (Benadryl) 50 mg IM or IV

- Ranitidine 50 mg IV or cimetidine 200 mg IV (these offer an added benefit to H1 blocker alone)
- Corticosteroid (methylprednisolone 50-100 mg IV if severe allergy), or concern over possible delayed or recurrent reaction
- Salbutamol nebulizer 2.5 mg if airway concerns present
- Observe for 2 to 3 hours post-epinephrine to ensure no delayed or recurrent reaction

Bibliography
Pepid website content. http://www.pepid.com. Accessed 26 March 2012.

UpToDate website content. http://www.uptodate.com. Accessed 26 March 2012.

Yingming A, Tran C, eds. *Toronto Notes*. 27th ed. Toronto, ON: Toronto Notes for Medical Students Inc; 2011: ER30-ER32.

Deep Vein Thrombosis
Priority Topic 21

Definition
- A blood clot causing blood flow obstruction, usually in a deep vein of the leg
- Distal: thrombi are confined to deep calf veins
- Proximal: thrombi involve popliteal, femoral, or iliac veins, and are more likely to cause pulmonary embolus
- Pathogenesis: Virchow triad, which consists of:
  - Endothelial damage
  - Stasis
  - Hypercoagulability

Risk Factors
- Surgery, fractures, cancer, estrogen therapy, obesity, inflammatory bowel disease, oral corticosteroids
- Likely risk factors: family history of DVT, pregnancy, trauma, sepsis, hematological disorders

Presentation
- Swelling, pain, and erythema of the involved limb
- Consider massive DVT with buttock or groin pain, thigh swelling, or collateral superficial veins

Physical Examination
- See Wells criteria (Table 1-14), as well as:
  - Homan sign: pain during dorsiflexion of foot
  - Superficial venous distension with prominent superficial veins

TABLE 1-14	Wells Criteria for DVT (Used to Assess Pre-test Probability)

CRITERIA	SCORE
Localized tenderness along the deep venous distribution	1
Entire leg swollen	1
Calf swelling ≥ 3 cm larger than on asymptomatic side (measure 10 cm below tibial tuberosity)	1
Pitting edema confined to symptomatic leg	1
Collateral non-varicose superficial veins	1
Paralysis, paresis, or recent plaster immobilization of the lower extremities	1
Recently bedridden for ≥ 3 days, or major surgery within the previous 12 weeks requiring general or regional anesthetic	1
Previously documented DVT	1
Malignancy—on treatment, treated in past 6 months or palliative	1
Alternate diagnosis is at least as likely as DVT	−2

Low risk <1, moderate risk 1-2, high risk > 3. If both legs are symptomatic, score the more severe leg.

Diagnosis

Also see the diagnostic algorithm that follows.

Assess for pre-test probability using the Wells criteria for DVT, and follow the steps in order below:

■ In **low-risk** patients with Wells DVT score <1 and low clinical suspicion
  • D-dimer should be ordered
    ○ If negative—DVT excluded
    ○ If positive—order duplex ultrasound with compression
      □ If the ultrasound is positive—DVT is confirmed and treatment should begin as given under the head level "Treatment (for DVT and PE)"
      □ If the ultrasound is negative—DVT can be excluded
■ In **moderate/high-risk** patients with Wells DVT score of 1 or more
  • In the absence of contraindications, it is appropriate to start treatment immediately
  • Duplex ultrasound should be ordered
    ○ If positive—DVT is confirmed, and treatment should continue as given under heading "Treatment (for DVT and PE)"
    ○ If negative—order D-dimer
      □ If negative—DVT is excluded
      □ If positive—unable to rule out DVT; repeat duplex ultrasound in 3 to 7 days, *or* assess with venography
■ Consider underlying coagulopathy in all patients, especially with unprovoked DVT

Treatment

■ See "Treatment" under "Pulmonary Embolus" for further information

Pulmonary Embolus

Definition

- A mechanical obstruction of the pulmonary vasculature
- Usually due to thromboembolism from DVT
- Massive PE is an acute PE in the presence of:
  - Sustained hypotension with systolic BP < 90, and not due to any other cause
  - Persistent profound bradycardia, HR < 40
  - Pulselessness

WELLS CRITERIA FOR PE (USED TO ASSESS PRE-TEST PROBABILITY)	
Criteria	Score
Clinical signs of DVT	3
Alternate diagnosis is less likely than PE	3
Heart rate >100	1.5
Previous DVT/PE	1.5
Immobilization ≥3 days or surgery in past 4 weeks	1.5
Malignancy—on treatment, treated in past 6 months or palliative	1
Hemoptysis	1
PE unlikely: score ≤ 4; PE likely: score > 4.	

PE RULE OUT CRITERIA (PERC SCORE)
• Age < 50 years
• Heart rate < 100
• Oxygen saturation ≥ 95%
• No unilateral leg swelling
• No hemoptysis
• No recent surgery or trauma requiring hospitalization in the past 4 weeks
• No previous DVT/PE
• No estrogen use
• **All** PERC criteria must be met
Carpenter, CR, et al. Differentiating Low-Risk and No-Risk PE Patients: The PERC Score. *J Emerg Mgmt* 2009; 36(3):317-322. Reprinted with permission of Elsevier.

Diagnosis

Also see the diagnostic algorithm that follows.

- Assess for pre-test probability using the Wells criteria for PE, and follow the steps in order below
- In **low-risk** patients with **Wells PE score ≤ 4 and low clinical suspicion**
  - Assess using PERC
    - If all PERC criteria are met, then PE can be excluded and no further testing is required
    - If any PERC criteria are positive, order a D-dimer
      - If D-dimer negative, PE can be excluded
      - If D-dimer positive, order a V/Q or CTPA scan
        - If scan negative, can exclude PE
        - If scan positive, then PE is confirmed and treatment should begin as given under the heading "Treatment (for DVT and PE)"
- In **high-risk** patients with **Wells PE score >4** and/or **high clinical suspicion**
  - Consider starting treatment immediately (recommended if Wells score ≥ 6)
  - Order CTPA or V/Q scan (see "Notes")
    - If scans are diagnostic, PE is confirmed and treatment should begin as given under the heading "Treatment (for DVT and PE)"

- If scans are not diagnostic of PE, then duplex ultrasound with compression of bilateral legs should be performed
  - If ultrasound negative, follow-up with repeat ultrasound in 3 to 5 days
  - If ultrasound positive for DVT, treat for PE
- Other tests:
  - Arterial blood gas: not useful to diagnose or exclude PE
    - Typically show hypoxemia, hypocapnia, and respiratory alkalosis
  - ECG: typically see non-specific ST changes
    - Historically taught changes of S1Q3T3 pattern with right ventricular strain and new incomplete RBBB are rarely seen in acute PE, but may be seen with massive PE and cor pulmonale
    - Poor prognosis in patients with atrial arrhythmias, RBBB, inferior Q waves, precordial T and ST changes
  - CXR: commonly see abnormalities (atelectasis, pleural effusion), but nothing diagnostic of PE
- Notes on imaging and D-dimer
  - CTPA (CT pulmonary angiography)
    - Contraindicated with renal failure or contrast allergy; high specificity, but reader expertise is required
  - V/Q scan (ventilation/perfusion scan)
    - Consider for patients with contrast allergy or renal failure
    - Reported as: normal, low probability, intermediate probability, or high probability
    - Rules out PE in the following situations:
      - Normal scan with any level of clinical probability
      - Low probability scan **and** low clinical probability
    - Diagnoses PE if high probability scan **and** high clinical probability
    - For any other scan result/clinical probability combination, further testing with angiogram, CTPA, or duplex ultrasound should be done
  - Pulmonary angiogram
    - Gold standard, involves contrast injection into pulmonary artery branch after percutaneous catheterization
  - Bilateral duplex ultrasound with compression
    - Presence of a proximal DVT in a patient with suspected DVT is sufficient to start treatment
    - Negative test insufficient to rule out PE
  - D-dimer (a degradation product of cross-linked fibrin)
    - Elevated post-surgery, and with severe infection, malignancy, DIC
    - Good negative predictive value; can rule out PE with normal D-dimer and low clinical suspicion
    - Normal D-dimer levels are seen in only 40% to 68% of patients without PE; poor specificity

Treatment (for DVT and PE)

- Certain patients will require inpatient management
  - Massive DVT, PE, bleeding risk, comorbidities
- Anticoagulation
  - Start treatment immediately (ie, prior to investigation results) if there is a high index of suspicion of DVT or PE
    - Intermediate index of suspicion and results are likely to take >4 hours, treatment is recommended

- Low index of suspicion, it is reasonable not to start treatment if results are expected within 24 hours
- Bridge anticoagulation for at least 5 days and until INR ≥ 2 for 24 hours
  - Low molecular weight heparin (LMWH)
  - Unfractionated heparin (UFH); IV is preferred to subcutaneous
  - In the absence of renal failure, LMWH is preferred
- Long-term anticoagulation
  - Long-term treatment is recommended for at least 3 months in patients with a transient risk factor (eg, surgery)
  - For patients with an unprovoked DVT or PE, evaluate risk/benefit of continuing therapy as these patients may benefit from a longer course of anticoagulation
  - Warfarin (see "Notes")
    - Start dosing at the same time as initiating bridging of anticoagulation or diagnosis of DVT
    - Target INR is 2 to 3
      - Dabigatran: has been shown to be as effective as warfarin, not yet recommended in Canada for DVT or PE treatment
      - LMWH: in patients with malignancy, long-term anticoagulation with LMWH is preferred to reduce recurrence risk, and duration is typically longer than 3 months
- Thrombolytics should be considered in patients with PE and hypotension where there is no increased bleeding risk
- Early ambulation is not harmful
- Elastic compression stockings may reduce risk of post-thrombotic syndrome
- Inferior vena caval filters are only recommended for patients in whom anticoagulation is contraindicated

Clinical Signs and Symptoms of Lower Extremity DVT

Assess clinical pretest probability using Wells model	
Criteria	**Score**
Active cancer (on treatment for last 6 months or palliative)	1
Paralysis, paresis, or recent plaster immobilization of the lower extremities	1
Recently bedridden for 3 days or more, or major surgery within the previous 12 weeks requiring general or regional anaesthetic	1
Previously documented deep vein thrombosis	1
Localized tenderness along the distribution of the deep venous system	1
Entire leg swollen	1
Calf swelling at least 3 cm larger than that on the asymptomatic side (measured 10 cm below tibial tuberosity)	1
Pitting edema confined to the symptomatic leg	1
Collateral superficial veins (non-varicose)	1
Alternative diagnosis *at least as likely as* deep vein thrombosis	−2

SCORING: Low risk: <1; moderate risk: 1-2; high risk: >3
If both legs symptomatic, score the more severe leg.
Wells, PS, et al. Value of assessment of pretest probability of deep-vein thrombosis in clinical management. *Lancet* 1997; 350(9094):1795-1798. Reprinted with permission of Elsevier.

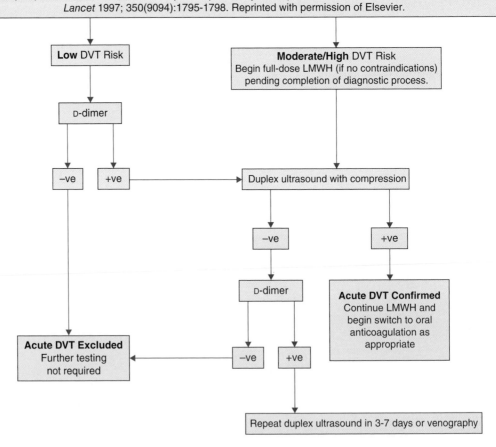

Low DVT Risk

D-dimer

−ve   +ve

Moderate/High DVT Risk
Begin full-dose LMWH (if no contraindications) pending completion of diagnostic process.

Duplex ultrasound with compression

−ve   +ve

D-dimer

−ve   +ve

Acute DVT Excluded
Further testing
not required

Acute DVT Confirmed
Continue LMWH and
begin switch to oral
anticoagulation as
appropriate

Repeat duplex ultrasound in 3-7 days or venography

© The Foundation for Medical Practice Education, www.fmpe.org, August 2010.

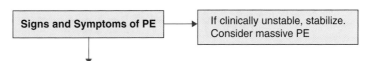

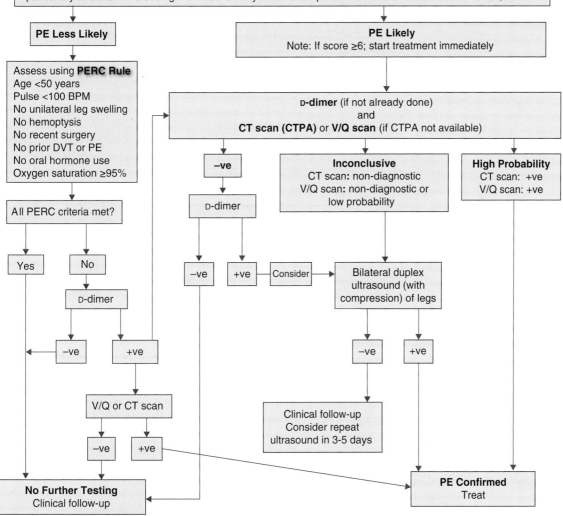

Signs and Symptoms of PE → If clinically unstable, stabilize. Consider massive PE

Assess clinical pretest probability using modified Wells model

Criteria	Score
Clinical signs and symptoms of DVT (minimum of leg swelling and pain with palpation of the deep veins)	3
Heart rate >100	1.5
Hemoptysis	1
Previous DVT/PE	1.5
Immobilization or surgery in previous 4 weeks	1.5
Malignancy (on treatment, treated in last 6 months or palliative)	1.5
An alternative diagnosis is **less** likely than PE	1

SCORING: PE less likely: ≤4; PE likely: >4

Wells PS, Anderson DR, Rodger M, et al. Derivation of a simple clinical model to categorize patients' probability of pulmonary embolism: Increasing the model's utility with the SimpliRED D-dimer. *Thromb Haemost* 2000;83:418.

PE Less Likely

PE Likely
Note: If score ≥6; start treatment immediately

Assess using **PERC Rule**
Age <50 years
Pulse <100 BPM
No unilateral leg swelling
No hemoptysis
No recent surgery
No prior DVT or PE
No oral hormone use
Oxygen saturation ≥95%

D-dimer (if not already done)
and
CT scan (CTPA) or **V/Q scan** (if CTPA not available)

All PERC criteria met?

−ve

Inconclusive
CT scan: non-diagnostic
V/Q scan: non-diagnostic or low probability

High Probability
CT scan: +ve
V/Q scan: +ve

Yes   No

D-dimer

D-dimer

−ve   +ve

−ve   +ve → Consider → Bilateral duplex ultrasound (with compression) of legs

V/Q or CT scan

−ve   +ve

−ve   +ve

Clinical follow-up
Consider repeat ultrasound in 3-5 days

No Further Testing
Clinical follow-up

PE Confirmed
Treat

†Exclusion criteria for algorithm: pregnancy; oral anticoagulant Rx for >24 hours; age <18 years; suspected upper extremity DVT as source of PE

© The Foundation for Medical Practice Education, www.fmpe.org, August 2010.

Warfarin Notes

- Target INR is 2 to 3 for most conditions, including DVT and PE (goal of 2.5)
- Target INR of 2.5 to 3.5 (goal of 3)
  - Indicated for: recurrent VTE (venous thromboembolism) despite anticoagulation; mechanical aortic or mitral valve in the presence of Afib, some STEMIs, left atrial enlargement, low ejection fraction, hypercoagulable state, certain mechanical mitral valves, or older caged ball or caged disc valves
- Risk factors for bleeding are as follows:
  - Elderly
  - Malnourished
  - Congestive heart failure
  - Liver disease
  - Recent surgery
  - Alcohol use
  - Previous gastrointestinal bleed
- Start warfarin
  - Typical starting dose is 5 mg
  - Take an average of the doses over the previous 3 to 5 days in a patient with fluctuating doses to get a picture of the average daily dose that has produced an INR
  - It is preferable to have same dosing every day to avoid confusion
- Medication interactions—increase INR monitoring with the following:
  - Increased warfarin response is caused by factors such as acetaminophen, NSAIDs, alcohol, amiodarone, allopurinol, fibrates, omeprazole, some statins, many antibiotics, thyroid hormone, some herbal preparations, for example, chamomile
  - Decreased warfarin response is caused by factors such as antithyroid medication, barbiturates, carbamazepine, rifampin, phenytoin, St John wort, increased vitamin K intake (brussel sprouts, spinach, avocado, green tea, spinach, mayonnaise)
- Perioperative warfarin management
  - Consider bridging anticoagulation (eg, LMWH)
    - High-risk patients should receive bridging
    - For moderate risk patients consider bridging
  - Discontinue warfarin 5 days prior to surgery
  - Check INR 1 to 2 days prior to surgery
    - Give 1 to 2 mg of oral vitamin K if INR >1.5
    - Resume warfarin 12 to 24 hours after surgery if there is adequate post-surgical hemostasis
- Low-risk procedures not requiring discontinuation of warfarin are diagnostic endoscopy, ERCP, cataract surgery, minor dermatological procedures, joint or soft tissue injections
- For dental procedures obtain INR prior to procedure, and there is no need to discontinue warfarin
- Delay procedure if INR is supratherapeutic

Bibliography

DynaMed. Deep vein thrombosis (DVT). Ipswich, MA: EBSCO Publishing; 2012. Retrieved from http://search.ebscohost.com.cyber.usask.ca/login.aspx?direct=true&site=DynaMed&id=113862.

DynaMed. Periprocedural management of patients on long-term anticoagulation. Ipswich, MA: EBSCO Publishing; 2012. Retrieved from http://search.ebscohost.com.cyber.usask.ca/login.aspx?direct=true&site=DynaMed&id=113862.

DynaMed. Pulmonary embolism (PE). Ipswich, MA: EBSCO Publishing; 2012. Retrieved from http://search.ebscohost.com.cyber.usask.ca/login.aspx?direct=true&site=DynaMed&id=113862.

Jensen B, Downey L, Regier L. Oral antiplatelet and antithrombotic agents. *RxFiles Drug Comparison Charts*. 8th ed. Saskatoon, SK: Saskatoon Health Region; 2010: 10-11.

Landaw SA, Bauer KA. Approach to the diagnosis and therapy of lower extremity deep vein thrombosis. In: Basow DS, ed. *UpToDate*. Waltham, MA: 2012. Retrieved from http://www.uptodate.com/.

Righini M, Le Gal G, Perrier A, Bounameaux H. The challenge of diagnosing pulmonary embolism in elderly patients: influence of age on commonly used diagnostic tests and strategies. *J Am Geriatr Soc*. 2005;53(6):1039-1045.

Thompson BT, Hales CA. Diagnosis of acute pulmonary embolism. In: Basow DS, ed. *UpToDate*. Waltham, MA: 2012. Retrieved from http://www.uptodate.com/.

2

Internal Medicine

Headache
Priority Topic 44

RED FLAGS FOR NEW HEADACHES

- Fever or rash
- Neck stiffness
- Change in consciousness/mentation
- Sudden onset
- Papilledema
- Head trauma
- Headache started after age 50
- Change in headache pattern
- Risk factors for HIV or cancer
- Focal neurological signs (other than typical aura)
- Worse in AM

DIFFERENTIAL DIAGNOSIS AND WORK UP (SEE TABLE 2-1)

TABLE 2-1	Headache: Type and Workup
DIFFERENTIAL DIAGNOSIS	**WORK UP**
Temporal arteritis,[a] mass lesion	ESR, imaging, biopsy
SAH,[b] vascular malformation, hemorrhage, stroke	Imaging, lumbar puncture
Meningitis[c]	Imaging, lumbar puncture, serology
Collagen vascular disease	Antiphospholipid antibody
Trauma (epidural, subdural)	Imaging–brain, skull +/− c-spine

[a]In temporal arteritis give steroids before diagnosis is confirmed.
[b]In suspected SAH if imaging is negative do lumbar puncture.
[c]In meningitis give antibiotics before diagnosis is confirmed.

Also, consider chronic causes of headache (Table 2-2)

SIGNS, SYMPTOMS AND TREATMENT

DIAGNOSIS OF MIGRAINE

1. ≥5 attacks
2. 2-72 hours duration
3. ≥2 of:
   Unilateral
   Pulsatile
   Worse with activity
   Moderate to severe intensity
4. ≥1 of:
   Nausea/vomiting
   Phono/photophobia

TABLE 2-2	Headache–Signs/Symptoms and Treatments	
	SIGNS/SYMPTOMS	ACUTE TREATMENT
Migraine (+/– aura)	2-72 h duration Unilateral Pulsatile Worse with activity Nausea/vomiting Phono/photophobia	See Table 2-3 NSAIDs Triptans Ergots Metoclopramide
Tension	Bilateral (frontal and occipital pain) Bandlike Exacerbated by stress, fatigue, noise Can be related to neck muscle pain	NSAIDs
Cluster	Unilateral and excruciating Peri-orbital 15 min to 3 h duration Conjunctival injection and lacrimation	High-flow O_2 Triptans Ergots
Medication overuse	Bilateral and bandlike Muscle contraction, tenderness Photosensitivity Occurs nearly everyday	Discontinue analgesics Use Triptan and ergots–during withdrawal

TABLE 2-3	Step-Wise Approach to the Treatment of Migraines	
Acute	Mild to moderate Moderate to severe	NSAIDs or acetaminophen Triptans Ergots Tylenol #3 Metoclopramide (dopaminergic)–evidence to support support use alone and as adjunct
Prophylaxis	If >3 per month or decreased quality of life	β-blocker (propranolol) TCA (amitriptyline, nortriptyline) Anticonvulsant (divalproex, topiramate) Riboflavin Calcium channel blocker (verapamil)

Bibliography

Chen YA, Tran C. *Toronto Notes—Comprehensive Medical Reference & Review for MCCQE I and USMLE II*. Toronto, Canada: Toronto Notes for Medical Students Inc; 2008.

Rx Files. Migraine: agents for acute treatment. *Drug Comparison Charts*. 8th ed. 2010:80.

Rx Files. Migraine: agents for prophylaxis. *Drug Comparison Charts*. 8th ed. 2010:81.

Anemia
Priority Topic 4
Definition
- Low hemoglobin (normal range: men 130-180 g/L; women 120-160 g/L)
- Categorized into microcytic, normocytic, and macrocytic based on MCV

TABLE 2-4	Causes of Anemia		
	MICROCYTIC	**NORMOCYTIC**	**MACROCYTIC**
MCV (fL):	<80	80-100	>100
Causes	**S**ideroblastic	**H**emolytic	B_{12} deficiency
	Iron deficiency	**A**plastic	Folate deficiency
	Thalassemia	**A**nemia of chronic disease	Alcohol
	Anemia of chronic disease	**R**enal failure	Hypothyroidism
		Pregnancy	Myelodysplasia
Key Test	Ferritin	Reticulocyte count	Blood smear

ANEMIA MNEMONICS
Microcytic - SITA
Normocytic - HAARP

MEGALOBLASTIC ANEMIAS
B12 deficiency
Folate deficiency*

*After diagnosis, routine testing of folate levels not required

Symptoms
- Fatigue
- Pallor
- Tachycardia
- Dyspnea
- Postural lightheadedness
- Worsening angina or CHF

Treatment
- Transfusion if symptomatic and Hgb <70 g/L; at risk of decomposition (eg, hypovolemic, CHF, angina)
- If unstable vitals, consider fluids before blood transfusion

IRON DEFICIENCY ANEMIA

Symptoms
- Angular cheilitis
- Pica
- Atrophic glossitis
- Koilonychia
- Plummer–Vinson syndrome (esophageal web, atrophic glossitis, dysphagia)

Diagnosis

TABLE 2-5	Diagnosis–Fe Deficiency vs. Anemia of Chronic Disease						
LABS	**MCV**	**RDW**	**FE**	**TIBC**[a]	**FERRITIN**[b]	**FE/TIBC**	**TRANSFERRIN**
Fe deficiency	↓	↑	↓	↑	↓	<18%	↑
Anemia of chronic disease	↓or N	N	↓	↓	↑	>18%	N

[a]TIBC–only measure if ferritin is normal and clinically suspicious for iron deficiency or in kidney failure.
[b]Ferritin–best diagnostic test; iron deficient if <15 mcg/L.

Etiologies
- Chronic blood loss
- Decreased absorption (Celiac disease; Crohn's disease)
- Pregnancy
- Malignancy (Note: low Hgb +/– iron deficiency may be first sign of malignancy)

Treatment
- Elemental Fe 180 mg PO OD
  - A rise in Hgb of 10 to 20 g/L in 2 to 4 weeks supports diagnosis
- Anemia should be corrected in 2 to 4 months of treatment. However, treat for a total of 4 to 6 months to replenish iron stores

VITAMIN B_{12} DEFICIENCY ANEMIA

Symptoms
- Symmetric peripheral neuropathy
- Paresthesias
- Ataxia
- Glossitis
- CNS: memory loss, personality changes, and dementia
- Late stage: severe weakness, spasticity, clonus

Diagnosis
- Serum B_{12} level and clinical picture
- Pernicious anemia tests: anti-intrinsic factor antibody or Schilling test

Etiologies
- Malnutrition
- Fish tapeworm
- Drugs (eg, metformin, PPI, H_2 blocker)
- Bacteria overgrowth at terminal ileum
- GI tract abnormality
- Pernicious anemia—most common cause of vitamin B_{12} deficiency

Treatment
- Vitamin B_{12} (IM for pernicious anemia)

INFANT PRESENTATION OF ANEMIA

Symptoms
- Pallor
- Poor weight gain

Risk Factors
- Poverty
- Non–iron-fortified formula
- Ethnicity
- Whole cow's milk diet
- Exclusive breastfeeding after 6 months of age
- Born to a poorly controlled diabetic mother

Bibliography
Chen YA, Tran C. Toronto Notes—Comprehensive Medical Reference & Review for MCCQE I and USMLE II. Toronto, Canada: Toronto Notes for Medical Students Inc; 2011.

Stroke

Priority Topic 88

Definitions

Transient ischemic attack (TIA): Brief episode of neurological dysfunction without evidence of acute infarction. Returns to baseline in <24 hours.

- Signs/symptoms: typically lasts <1 hour but by definition resolves in <24 hours; motor, sensory, speech/language, vision, or cerebellar dysfunction
- TIA is an important warning sign→ 10% of TIA go on to stroke, half of these occur within 2 days

Stroke: Sudden onset focal neurological dysfunction from infarction or hemorrhage in the brain lasting >24 hours.

- Signs/symptoms: same as TIA but symptoms persist >24 hours

Signs/Symptoms

- Acute or abrupt onset
- Motor weakness
- Sensory deficits
- Decreased reflexes
- Mental status changes
- Hemiparesis
- Neglect
- Amaurosis fugax
- Slurred speech
- Inattention
- Impulsivity

Risk Factors

- Smoking
- Sedentary lifestyle
- High fat diet
- Increased alcohol intake
- Hypertension
- Diabetes
- Cardiovascular disease
- Hyperlipidemia
- Prior TIA
- Prior stroke
- Atrial fibrillation
- Coagulopathy
- Obesity
- Age (risk doubles with every 10 years after age 55)
- Aboriginal or black

Diagnosis

- **History and physical examination:** look for the signs/symptoms listed earlier—may also help to identify a hemorrhagic stroke
  - Increased likelihood of hemorrhage if blown pupil, history of trauma

ABCD2 SCORE—PREDICTION OF EARLY STROKE RISK AFTER TIA (AT DAY 2, 7, AND AFTER 90 DAYS)

	Score
A–Age >60	1
B–BP >140/90	1
C–Clinical features	
Focal weakness	2
Speech impaired only	1
D–duration 10-59 min	1
>60 min	2
D–DM	1

Score: ≤3 = low risk; 4-5 = moderate; 6-7 = high

Score >3 needs admission to hospital.

RISK OF STROKE AFTER TIA

3%—in first 2 days

5%—in first 7 days

12%—in first 90 days

BELL'S PALSY
- Peripheral (lower motor neuron) CNVII palsy
- Abrupt onset: unilateral facial paralysis
- Includes the forehead (central causes will spare the forehead)
- Treatment: steroids and antiviral therapy

See http://www.acls.net/acls-suspected-stroke-algorithm.htm for ACLS stroke algorithm.

CI TO FIBRINOLYTICS

A–AVM/aneurysm

B–Bleeding: active internal or diathesis (INR >1.7; platelets <100000/mm³)

C–cancer (intracranial)

D–dissection of aorta suspected

H–hemorrhagic stroke/HTN uncontrolled

I–ischemic stroke in last 3 months or large stroke on CT

S–seizure at stroke onset/SAH suspected

T–trauma (head) or stroke in last 3 months

■ **Imaging**
  - Non-contrast CT—useful to rule out hemorrhage; infarcts often do not show until 24 to 48 hours
  - MRI—ischemic changes appear within hours
  - Cerebral angiography—gold standard
■ **Laboratory investigations**
  - CBC, INR, PTT, glucose, ECG, Na^+, K^+

Differential Diagnosis

■ Seizure

■ Migraine

■ Subdural hematoma

■ Mass/tumor

■ Hypoglycemia (most common stroke mimic)

■ CNS infection

■ Bell palsy

■ Subarachnoid hemorrhage

Treatment

■ ABCs

■ **Establish time of onset**

■ Rule out hemorrhage with CT scan
  - In case of hemorrhage—consult neurosurgery
  - No hemorrhage—likely ischemic; **consider fibrinolytics if <3 hours from onset of symptoms**

■ Contraindications to fibrinolytics
  - Cranial hemorrhage on CT
  - Clinical presentation of SAH
  - Large infarction
  - Uncontrolled hypertension (>185/110)
  - Known AV malformation
  - Arterial line at a noncompressible site in the last 7 days
  - History of intracranial hemorrhage
  - Witnessed seizure at stroke onset
  - Active internal bleeding or acute trauma
  - Bleeding diathesis
    ○ Platelet <100,000
    ○ Heparin or warfarin—INR >1.7
  - Previous stroke or head trauma in the last 3 months

■ If candidate for fibrinolytics—give tPA, no anticoagulation for 24 hours

■ If not a candidate for fibrinolytics—give ASA and clopidogrel

Prevention

Primary Prevention

Please refer to www.ccpn.ca for more information on stroke prevention in Afib.

■ Determining the need for anticoagulation in Afib based on stroke risk: **$CHADS_2$ score**

■ Risk factor reduction

Secondary Prevention

- ASA +/ − clopidogrel
- Antihypertensive
- Anticoagulation (warfarin, etc)—if Afib or increased risk of cardiac source
- Statin—not in first 48 hours, but long term
- Patient education: smoking, lifestyle, weight loss
- Carotid Doppler and endarterectomy if >70% stenosis of ICA and >5 years life expectancy
  - Carotid ultrasound: if carotid territory presentation of TIA/stroke assess for carotid blockage/source (Canadian 2006 Best Practice Standards state that TIAs need carotid imaging within 24 hour of a carotid distribution TIA)
  - Echocardiogram/transesophageal echocardiogram (TEE)—assess for cardioembolic source
- Early mobilization (<24 hours post stroke) and positioning leads to better outcomes

Medical Complications of Stroke

- Cardiac—common in the first 3 months post stroke
- Depression—occurs in approximately one-third of stroke patients
- Dysphagia—malnutrition/increased risk of aspiration
- Ulcers
- Venous thromboembolus (~ 25% of early death post-stroke is from pulmonary embolism)—consider heparin or leg compression stockings
- Pain—often associated with hemiplegia

Bibliography

Canadian Cardiovascular Pharmacist Network. www.ccpn.ca.

Tintinalli JE, Stapczynski JS, Cline DM, Ma OJ, Cydulka RK, Meckler GD. *Tintinalli's Emergency Medicine: A Comprehensive Study Guide* (Eds.). 7th ed. New York, NY: The McGraw-Hill Companies; 2011.

CHADS2 SCORE: ANTICOAGULATION IN AFIB	
• CHADS$_2$ Score	
• CHF	1
• Hypertension	1
• Age >75	1
• Diabetes	1
• Stroke/TIA (prior)	2
• Total score	
• 0 to 1	ASA
• 2 to 3	Warfarin or ASA
• >4	Warfarin

Insomnia

Priority Topic 53

Definition

Sleep disorder resulting in difficulty falling asleep, difficulty staying asleep, or early morning awakening despite adequate opportunity for sleep. This lack of sleep causes impairment in daily functioning.

History

- Ask people about their **sleep habits**:
  - Bedtime, time to fall asleep, quality of sleep, number of awakenings
  - Distractions in the room: TV or computer in the bedroom
  - Activities before bed including exercise, caffeine, alcohol, medications
- Ask about recent stressors including travel, shift work
- Assess impact on quality of life: fatigue, sleepiness, driving, concentration at work
- Ask patients to complete a **sleep diary** including bedtime, sleep latency, total sleep time, awakenings, and quality of sleep

- Get a collateral history from the **sleep partner**.

- Depression and anxiety are the most common comorbidities in insomnia.

MEDICATIONS THAT AFFECT SLEEP

Caffeine

Nicotine

Alcohol

Diuretics

Antihypertensives

Antidepressants

Bronchodilators

Decongestants

Steroids

INSOMNIA—FIRST-LINE MEDICATIONS

Zopiclone

Temazepam

Trazodone

Differential Diagnosis

The history will give clues to underlying sleep-related disorders that require further investigation and treatment:

- Psychiatric: depression, anxiety, grief, PTSD
- Sleep apnea
- Restless leg syndrome
- CHF
- Pain
- Parasomnias: sleep walking/talking
- Other: central sleep apnea, hyperthyroidism, GERD, COPD, BPH

Advice for Good Sleep Hygiene

- Use an alarm clock to get up at the same time each day
- **No** daytime naps
- Use the bedroom for sleep and sex only
- If not asleep in 20 minutes, get up and do something relaxing; return to bed only when tired
- Relax before bed
- Exercise during the day
- Stop/limit caffeine and alcohol 6 hours before bed
- No smoking for 1 to 2 hours before bed

Treatment

Behaviour and cognitive strategies = foundation of treatment

1. Treat and manage any suspected medical or psychiatric cause
2. Nonpharmacologic (see Sleep Hygiene discussed above)
3. Sleep restriction: time in bed should match total hours slept
4. Medication
   - Best if specific stressor identified: eg, traveling, divorce, returning military
   - Use only if affecting daytime functioning
   - Use for short term only; after stopping expect two to three nights of poor sleep
   - Avoid benzodiazepines and amitriptyline in elderly as the risk outweighs the benefit
5. If no improvement after 3 months:
   - Reassess for secondary causes
   - Consider sleep study/polysomnography
   - Consider referral for cognitive behavioural therapy
6. Polysomnography suggested if:
   - High suspicion of sleep apnea or movement disorder
   - Initial diagnosis uncertain
   - Treatment failure
   - Violent or dangerous behaviour during sleep

Bibliography

Chen AY, Tran C. *Toronto Notes*. Toronto, ON: Type & Graphics Inc; 2011.

Insomnia. *DynaMed*. Ipswich, MA: EBSCO Publishing; 1995. Updated 2012 Mar 29; cited 2012 Mar 29. http://dynamed.ebscohost.com/user/login.

Jensen B, Regier L, RxFiles drug comparison charts. *Sedatives: A Concise Overview*. 8th ed. Saskatoon, SK: Saskatoon Health Regina; 2010: 110-111. Available at www.RxFiles.ca.

Thyroid

Priority Topic 91

Screening for Thyroid Disease

- TSH considered the most sensitive screening test
- Free T_4 should be done if TSH is abnormal
- Free T_3 may be helpful if thyrotoxicosis is suspected
- Screen all symptomatic patients
- Recommended for patients with nonspecific sign and symptoms of thyroid disease and risk factors

Risk Factors for Thyroid Disease

- Woman >50 (female to male ratio is 5:1)
- Elderly
- Strong family history
- Autoimmune disease
- Goiter
- Postpartum (6weeks–6 months)
- Lithium and amiodarone use
- Past history of neck radiation
- Down's and Turner's syndrome
- Infertility
- Hyperlipidemia, HTN, DM

HYPOTHYROIDISM

Definition

- Clinical syndrome caused by cellular responses to insufficient thyroid hormone production

Symptoms and Characteristics: "HIS FIRM CAP"

TABLE 2-6	Symptoms of Hypothyroidism
H	Hypoventilation
I	Intolerance to cold
S	Slow HR
F	Fatigue
I	Impotence
R	Renal impairment
M	Menorrhagia/amenorrhea
C	Constipation
A	Anemia
P	Paraesthesia

MYXEDEMA COMA
- Decompensated hypothyroidism (rare)
- Decreased mental status
- Hypothermia
- ↓ BP and HR plus hypoventilation
- Rx: hydrocortisone IV and LT_4 until stable–then LT_4 PO daily

COMMON ETIOLOGIES
- Hashimoto/s (most common)
- Iatrogenic
- Hypothyroid phase of thyroiditis

SICK EUTHYROID SYNDROME
- Acute, reversible abnormalities in TSH/T_4/T_3 due to non-thyroid illness.
- Occurs commonly after surgery, MI or with fasting, malnutrition, febrile illnesses, renal and cardiac failure, hepatic diseases, uncontrolled DM, CVD and malignancy
- Does not require treatment, consider retesting!

POTENTIAL BENEFITS OF TREATMENT
- Improves patient well-being
- Avoids patient from becoming symptomatic
- Protects fetus in pregnant woman
- Improves lipid profile

Diagnosis: See Table 2-7

TABLE 2-7	Thyroid Diagnosis: Clinical and Biochemical Findings		
	TSH	FREE T_4	ANTIBODIES
Primary hypothyroid	↑	↓	TPO (Hashimoto's)
Subclinical hypothyroid	↑	Normal	
Secondary hypothyroid (insufficiency of pituitary TSH)	↓ or not appropriately elevated	↓	

T3 not used to determine hypothyroidism
Tertiary hypothyroidism: hypothalamic hypothyroidism / decreased TRH from hypothalamus (rare)

Subclinical Hypothyroidism
■ Prevalence 4–8% and every year 2–5% progress to overt hypothyroidism

Therefore treatment is recommended:
1. TSH >10mU/L
2. TSH is above the upper reference interval limit but <10mU/L and any of the following present
3. Elevated TPO
4. Goiter
5. Strong family history of autoimmune disorder

Treatment
Start low and go slow!
■ L-thyroxine (dose range 0.05–0.2 mg PO OD)
■ Elderly patients and those with CAD: start at 0.025mg daily and increase gradually

Monitoring TSH
■ 6–8 weeks after initiating treatment and adjust dose until TSH returns to normal reference range. (TSH may remain abnormal for months. Free T_4 may be more reliable initially.)
■ After a change of weight ≥10 lbs or clinical status
■ 4–6 weeks following a change in medication dose
■ Every 6–12 months once maintenance dose achieved
■ Thyroxine doses may increase by 25–50% during pregnancy, particularly in the first trimester, measure TSH in each trimester

Key Points
■ Remember your high-risk populations and who warrants screening
■ Screen with TSH. Check free T_4 if TSH abnormal.
■ For treatment–start low and go slow!
■ Perform judicious follow-up testing of TSH

99 TOPICS
■ Limit testing for thyroid disease to appropriate patients, namely those with a significant pre-test probability of abnormal results, such as:
  • Those with classic signs or symptoms of thyroid disease
  • Those whose symptoms or signs are not classic, but who are at a higher risk for disease (eg, the elderly, postpartum women, those with a history of atrial fibrillation, those with other endocrine disorders)

- In patients with established thyroid disease, do not check TSH levels too often, but rather test at the appropriate times, such as:
  - After changing medical doses
  - When following patients with mild disease before initiating treatment
  - Periodically in stable patients receiving treatment
- When examining the thyroid gland, use proper technique (ie, from behind the patient, ask the patient to swallow), especially to find nodules (which may require further investigation).

Note: The investigation of thyroid nodules is not covered here.

Bibliography

Chen AY, Tran C. *Toronto Notes.* Toronto, ON: Type & Graphics Inc; 2011.

Guidelines & Protocols Advisory Committee. *Thyroid Function Tests: Diagnosis and Monitoring of Thyroid Function Disorders in Adults.* (2010). Retrieved from http://www.bcguidelines.ca/pdf/thyroid.pdf.

McDonald T, Milosevic V, Singer W. Guideline for the Use of Laboratory Tests to Detect Thyroid Dysfunction.(2007). *Ontario Association of Medical Laboratories.* Retrieved from http://www.oaml.com/res_pract.html.

RxFiles. Drug Comparison Charts, 8th ed. 2010. Retrieved from www.RxFiles.ca.

HYPERTHYROIDISM

Definition

- Hyperthyroid: excess production of thyroid hormone
- Thyrotoxicosis—denotes the clinical, physiologic and biochemical findings in response to elevated thyroid hormone

Symptoms/Characteristics: "Thyroidism"

TABLE 2-8	Symptoms/Characteristics of Hyperthyroidism
T	Tremor
H	Heart rate up
Y	Yawning (fatigue)
R	Restlessness
O	Oligo/Amenorrhea
I	Intolerance to heat
D	Diarrhea/decrease weight
I	Insomnia
S	Sweating
M	Muscle wasting/mood change

May have hematological disturbances: leukopenia, lymphocytosis, splenomegaly, lymphadenopathy (occasionally in Graves' disease)

THYROID STORM
- Life threatening!
- Decompensated thyrotoxicosis
- Fever, tachycardia, dehydration, delirium, coma, N/V diarrhea
- Causes: trauma, surgery, RAI
- Rx: B-Blockers, PTU, iodine, high-dose IV Hydrocortisone

ELDERLY PRESENT ATYPICALLY
- Symptoms maybe less obvious: confusion, dementia, apathy, or depression
- May only have cardiovascular symptoms—commonly new onset Afib, CHF

GRAVES
- Goiter: +/− thyroid bruit
- Opthalmopathy: proptosis/exopthalmous, lid lag/retraction, diplopia
- Acropachy: clubbing and thickening of phalanges
- Dermopathy: pretibial myxedema— non-pitting edema

Physical Examination

Inspection:
- Scars, swellings (goiter, lump, nodule) or any other abnormalities
- Ask patient to swallow—goiter will move
- Ask patient to stick out tongue—thyroglossal cyst will move

Palpation (from behind)
- Feel for isthmus (anterior to cricoid cartilage—retract SCM and feel each lobe
- Feel for nodules, tenderness, consistency and surface
- Ask patient to swallow again—goiter will move

Auscultate with bell for bruits!

Diagnosis: See Table 2-9

COMMON ETIOLOGIES
- Grave's
- Thyroiditis
- Toxic nodular goiter
- Toxic nodule

TABLE 2-9	Determining The Cause of Hyperthyroidism				
PRIMARY CAUSES	**TSH**	**FT3/4**	**THYROID ANTIBODIES**	**RAIU**	**OTHER**
Graves	↓	↑	TSI	↑	
Toxic nodular goiter	↓	↑		↑	
Toxic nodule	↓	↑		↑	
Thyroiditis	↓	↑	Approx. 50% of cases	↓	Elevated ESR in painful thyroiditis
SECONDARY CAUSES					
Extrathyroidal sources of thyroid hormone Endogenous (struma ovariae, ovarian teratoma, metastatic follicular carcinoma) Exogenous (drugs)	↓	↑		↓	
Excessive Thyroid Stimulation Pituitary Thyrotrophoma/ Pititary hormone receptor resistance	↑	↑			A pituitary MRI should be done to look for a pituitary mass (TSH-secreting adenoma)
Increased hCG (ie, pregnancy)	↓	↑			

TSH may be suppressed as a normal finding in the first trimester, check Free T4 for hyperthyroidism

Imaging Goitres
- RAIU: confirms Graves' and exclude other causes (ie, painless thyroiditis)
- Thyroid U/S: assess size
- Other investigations: thyroid Scan (Technicium 99)

GOITRE ETIOLOGY
Diffuse
- Graves
- Hasimoto's
- Subacute thyroiditis (painful)

Nodular
- Multi-nodular goiter
- Adenoma
- Carcinoma

Investigating Nodules
All patients require serum TSH and U/S
- TSH to asses thyroid status and USS to determine size, solid/cystic
- Thyroid scan if TSH is low to determine if the nodule is hot (significant 131 I uptake into the nodule) which signifies very low malignant potential or cold
- FNA for all nodules >1 to 1.5cm/ 5mm +/− suspicious features on U/S

THYROID NODULES
- Benign tumors (ie, follicular adenoma)
- Malignancy (ie, thyroid carcinoma)
- Hyperplastic area in multi-nodular goiter
- Cyst

Treatment

- Graves
  - Thionamides: PTU or MMI
  - Beta-blockers for symptomatic treatment
  - Radioactive ^{131}Iodine if PTU or MMI does not produce disease remission
  - Opthalmopathy: high dose prednisolone in severe cases, orbital radiation, surgical decompression
- Thyroiditis—painful
  - High-dose anti-inflammatories (NSAIDs), prednisolone may be required for severe pain, fever, or malaise
  - Beta blockers for symptomatic treatment
- Postpartum thyroiditis—painless
  - Often self-limiting but monitor TSH every 6–8 weeks as at risk of hypothyroidism
- Toxic adenoma/toxic multi-nodular goiter
  - RAI done over weeks
  - Thionamides may be used initially to attain euthyroid state and avoid radiation thyroiditis
  - Surgery may be used as first-line treatment
  - Propranolol for symptomatic treatment prior to definitive therapy

Monitoring TSH

- Check 4–6 weeks after initiating or changing treatment. TSH can be abnormal for months, free T_4 maybe more reliable.
- Check every 2–6 months once maintenance dose achieved

Key Points

- Screen with TSH. Check free T_4 if abnormal and free T_3 if thyrotoxicosis is suspected
- Have high index of suspicion in elderly who often present atypically
- Examine the thyroid gland thoroughly for a goiter or nodules
- Limit checking TSH testing to 4–6 weeks postinitiation or change in treatment and 2–6 monthly in stable, treated patient

Bibliography

Chen AY Tran C. *Toronto Notes*. Toronto, ON: Type & Graphics Inc; 2011.

Guidelines & Protocols Advisory Committee. *Thyroid Function Tests: Diagnosis and Monitoring of Thyroid Function Disorders in Adults*. 2010. Retrieved from http://www.bcguidelines.ca/pdf/thyroid.pdf.

McDonald T, Milosevic V, Singer W. *Guideline for the Use of Laboratory Tests to Detect Thyroid Dysfunction*. Ontario Association of Medical Laboratories. 2007. Retrieved from http://www.oaml.com/res_pract.html.

Ross. D. Diagnosis of hyperthyroidism. 2012. Retrieved from http://www.uptodate.com.

Ross. D. Overview of clinical manifestations of hyperthyroidism in adults. 2012. Retrieved from http://www.uptodate.com.

RxFiles. *Drug Comparison Charts*. 8th ed. 2010. Retrieved from www.RxFiles.ca.

Dizziness

Priority Topic 29

The term *dizziness* is a nonspecific term used to describe different sensations.

It is important to distinguish (**A**) **true vertigo** from (**B**) **non-vertiginous** *"dizziness,"* (pre-syncope, syncope, and disequilibrium).

Definitions

1. **Vertigo**—illusion of motion: rotational, linear, or tilting movement of self or environment
2. **Disequilibrium**—sense of imbalance, occurs primarily when walking, "unsteady on feet" (eg, peripheral neuropathy, cerebellum or posterior column disease, Parkinson disease)
3. **Pre-syncope**—prodromal symptoms of fainting, "nearly fainted/blacked out"
4. **Syncope**—LOC and postural tone due to decrease in cerebral perfusion with spontaneous recovery

TRUE VERTIGO

There are two types:

1. Peripheral—inner ear/vestibular nerve dysfunction (80%)
2. Central—brain stem–cerebellum dysfunction

Vertigo with any CNS symptoms—assume a central cause!!

Other Key Questions:
- Is there difficulty walking?
- Is the speech slurred?
- Are there visual disturbances (diplopia, poor vision, etc.)?

TABLE 2-10	True Vertigo–Signs and Symptoms	
SYMPTOMS/SIGNS	PERIPHERAL VERTIGO	CENTRAL VERTIGO
Onset	Sudden	Sudden or progressive
Duration	Paroxysmal, intermittent	Constant
Severity	Intense	Less intense
Aggravated by movement	Yes	Variable
Position dependent (typically head)	Yes	No
Associated nausea/vomiting	Frequent	Variable
Associated fatigue	Yes	No
Hearing loss/tinnitus	May occur	No/rare
Nystagmus: Direction Fatigable (with visual fixation)	Unidirectional, horizontal +/− torsional Yes	Bidirectional, vertical No
CNS signs (ie, diplopia, dysphagia, dysarthria, ataxia)	Absent	Usually present
Gait: postural instability/imbalance	Mild to moderate	Severe, falls when walking

TABLE 2-11 Peripheral Vertigo–Causes, Symptoms, Diagnosis, and Treatment

CAUSES	VERTIGO	HEARING LOSS/ CHANGE	TINNITIS	ASSOCIATED SYMPTOMS	DIAGNOSIS	TREATMENT
BPPV Otolithic debris in semicircular canals	Sudden onset with change in head position <30 seconds Intermittent: may last for weeks-months	No	No	Nausea and rarely vomiting	Dix–Hallpike test (negative test does not rule out condition)	Epley maneuver (canalith reposition-ing) Anticholinergics, ie, SERC/Gravol
Vestibular Neuronitis/ Labryithitis Post-viral inflammatory disorder affecting the eighth CN	Sudden onset: worse with head movement Severe: lasting hours to days Often resolves after 1 to 2 days	Possibly unilateral	No	Imbalance Nausea and vomiting	• Associated with viral infection • Rombergs test: patient falls toward affected side	Steroids may hasten recovery Hydration Antihistamines, eg, Benadryl
Meniere Disease Excess endolymphatic fluid pressure causes inner ear dysfunction	Severe Multiple episodes lasting hours to days Exacerbations may last months with frequent weekly episodes	Yes, can be bilat-eral	Brief, intense	Nausea and vomiting Imbalance Aural fullness	CT only to rule out other conditions	Anticholinergics, diuretics Avoid salt/sugar, caffeine, tobacco, alcohol Remission spontane-ously or with treat-ment but can recur
Acoustic Neuroma	Mild and continuous	Gradual, unilateral sensorineural loss	Mild and continuous	Imbalance or vague feeling of swaying or tilting	CT scan	Surgery

Other causes: perilymphatic fistula, herpes zoster octicus (Ramsay Hunt syndrome), aminoglycoside toxicity
Dix–Hallpike: move the patient quickly from a sitting position to a supine position with the head turned to one side and extended over the end of the bed. Look for nystag-mus and ask about vertigo. Repeat with head turned to the other side.

TABLE 2-12 Central Vertigo–Causes, Symptoms, Diagnosis, and Treatment

CAUSES	VERTIGO	HEARING ASSOCIATED SYMPTOMS	PERTINENT HISTORY	DIAGNOSIS
Vertebral Artery Dissection	May be present as part of lateral medullary syndrome[a]	Severe occipital headache or neck pain Lateral medullary syndrome[a]	Hx of recent head or neck trauma (may be minor)	CT, MRI/MRA, or cerebral angiography
Vertebrobasilar Insufficiency/TIA	Single to recurrent episode–lasting several minute to hours	Usually other brain stem symptoms Dysmetria/dysarthria/facial palsy/ severe ataxia	Older patient, vascular RF, and cervical trauma	MRI may demonstrate vascular lesion
Cerebellar Infarction or Hemorrhage	Sudden onset, persis-tent symptoms over days to weeks	Severe gait impairment Headache, limb dysmetria, dyspha-gia may occur	As above	Urgent MRI, CT will demon-strate lesion

Other causes: MS, migraine, intoxications, tumors.
[a]**Lateral medullary syndrome/Wallenberg syndrome:** vertigo, disequilibrium, nystagmus, Horner syndrome, ipsilateral ataxia, ipsilateral facial dysthesia (pain and numbness), contralateral loss of pain, and temperature.

Key Points

- Divide vertigo into peripheral and central causes
- Have a high index of suspicion for central causes in the elderly
- Consult neurologist or neurosurgeon with central causes of vertigo or peripheral vertigo lasting >2 weeks

NON-VERTIGINOUS "DIZZINESS"—SYNCOPE/PRE-SYNCOPE

TABLE 2-13	Syncope/Pre-syncope: Causes, Signs/Symptoms, Diagnostic Investigations		
CAUSE/ORIGIN	**SIGNS/SYMPTOMS/ FEATURES**	**PMHX**	**DIAGNOSTIC INVESTIGATIONS**
Cardiac	• Sudden onset, no prodrome • Palpitations/chest pain • Syncope with exertion (aortic stenosis, HOCM) • Family hx: sudden cardiac death or cardiomyopathy	Heart disease	ECG Echocardiography 24 h Holter monitor
Neurologic	Rare cause of syncope— distinguish from seizure activity, confusion	Epilepsy Narcolepsy	
Reflex 1. Vasovagal	• Young, healthy • Prolonged standing, heat exertion, emotional stress • Prodrome: sweaty, lightheaded, tinnitus, pallor, slow onset, nausea, blurry vision		Tilt-table testing Predominantly clinical diagnosis
2. Situational	Syncope immediately follows cough, sneeze, defecation, micturition		
3. Carotid sinus hypersensitivity	• Elderly (more common) • Often associated with head turning, tight shirt collars, taking of carotid pulse		Carotid massage (avoid if previous TIA/stroke/carotid bruits)

Orthostatic Hypotension	• Postural change = prodrome
	• Contributing factors:
	  ○ Volume depletion (diarrhea, vomit, anemia, bleeding)
	  ○ Drug induced (vasodilators/ antihypertensives, diuretics, anti-depressants, alcohol)
	  ○ Autonomic failure
		Parkinson, DM, spinal cord injury	Postural BP (drop in systolic BP >20 mm Hg or diastolic >10 mm Hg with a postural change from supine/sitting to erect)

CAUSES OF SYNCOPE

H	Hypoxia/Hypoglycemia
E	Epilepsy
A	Anxiety/anemia
D	Drugs/dysfunctional brain stem
H	Heart attack
E	Embolism (PE)
A	Aortic dissection
R	Rhythm disturbance
T	Tachycardia/tamponade
V	Vasovagal (most common)
E	ENT
S	Situational
S	Subclavian steal
e	
L	Low systemic vascular resistance
S	Sensitive carotid sinus

Risk Factors

- Age >70
- CVD or previous TIA/CVA
- Low BMI
- DM
- Alcohol

Differential Diagnosis

- Vertigo, AAA, stroke/CVA, DVT/PE, MI

Treatment

- Treat underlying cause
- Educate avoiding triggers for orthostatic or situational syncope
- Patients with recurrent syncope should avoid high-risk activities (driving)

Key Points

- All syncopal episodes warrant an ECG
- Syncope is most often benign and self-limiting
- Vasovagal response to a trigger is the most common cause
- Have high index of suspicion for a cardiac cause
- Syncope is unlikely to have neurologic sequelae

Bibliography

Chen AY, Tran C. *Toronto Notes*. Toronto, ON: Type & Graphics Inc; 2011.

Furman JM, Barton J. Approach to patients with vertigo. Retrieved from UpToDate website: http://www.uptodate.com.

Furman JM. Pathophysiology, etiology and differential diagnosis of vertigo. Retrieved from UpToDate website: http://www.uptodate.com.

Olshansky B. Evaluation of syncope in adults. Retrieved from UpToDate website: http://www.uptodate.com.

Olshansky B. Pathogenesis and etiology of syncope. Retrieved from UpToDate website: http://www.uptodate.co.

Skin Disorders

Priority Topic 84

Key Points

- Evaluating a skin lesion:
  - Inspect **all areas of the skin** including scalp, nails, palms of the hands, soles of the feet, oral cavity, perineum
  - Always consider a **life-threatening condition** such as, melanoma, necrotizing fasciitis, Stevens-Johnson syndrome
  - Use **biopsy or excision** to rule out serious pathology
  - Use history, physical examination, and investigations to rule out a **systemic disorder**
    - Autoimmune: such as lupus, ulcerative colitis
    - Endocrine: such as diabetes, thyroid disorders
    - Infectious: such as HIV, viral illness
    - Malignancy: such as Paget disease of the breast
    - Other: liver or renal disease
  - Take a **medication** history and consider a drug reaction
  - Determine the **impact on the patient's life**, including **sleep** in pruritic disorders
  - In **high-risk** patients such as diabetics, bed- or chair-bound patients, peripheral vascular disease **assess for skin lesions at every visit** and treat minor lesions aggressively
- Treating a skin lesion:
  - When the lesion is not responding to treatment:
    - **Modify your treatment,** that is, for acne
    - **Reconsider your diagnosis,** that is, dandruff may be psoriasis
  - In chronic diseases focus on optimizing control
  - Provide education and psychological support
    - Scars can be both physical and emotional
    - Depression, anxiety, social isolation, and lack of self-confidence are not uncommon
  - Provide information about support groups; for example, Psoriasis Society of Canada

COMMON SKIN DISORDERS

Acne Vulgaris

Definition

A common inflammatory pilosebaceous disease categorized with respect to severity.

Clinical Categories

- Type I: comedonal, sparse, no scarring
- Type II: comedonal, papular, moderate +/− little scarring
- Type III: comedonal, papular, and pustular with scarring
- Type IV: nodulocystic acne, risk of severe scarring
- Predilection sites: face, neck, upper chest, and back

Treatment

- Mild (Type I and II)—topical treatment
  - Topical antibiotics (clindamycin, erythromycin) and/or benzyl peroxide
  - Retinoid (tretinoin)
- Moderate (Type III) or after topical treatments have failed
  - Systemic antibiotics: tetracycline, doxycycline, or erythromycin for at least 2 to 3 months
  - Hormonal therapy: Alesse, Diane 35/CyEstra 35, or Yasmin for at least 3 to 6 months
- Severe (Type IV) or after above treatments have failed
  - Isotretinoin (Accutane) for 4 to 6 months

Eczema Dermatitis—The Itch That Rashes

Definition

An inflammatory, chronically relapsing, noncontagious, pruritic skin disorder

Characteristics

- Xerosis and pruritis—"the itchy rash"

Physical Examination

- Skin Findings:
  - Inflammation, erythema
  - Excoriation secondary to pruritus
  - Lichenification
  - Weeping, crusting—secondary bacterial infection
- Distribution varies according to age
  - Infants (2-6 months): face, scalp, extensor surfaces
  - Childhood (>18 months): flexural surfaces
  - Adult: hands, feet, flexures, wrists, face, forehead, eyelids, neck

Treatment

I. Moisturize: emollients restore the skin's protective barrier and maintain hydration (Vaseline>creams>gels). "The oilier the better!"

II. Avoid triggers! Consider antihistamines to break the itch-scratch cycle.

III. Steroids for flares: topical corticosteroids (least potent dose that is effective). Advise about finger-tip unit, avoiding face and to use sparingly for 2 weeks at a time to avoid skin atrophy.

IV. Antibiotics for secondary bacterial infection: topical fusidic acid (Fucidin), mupirocin, oral cephalexin, cloxacillin. Antivirals for superseding viral infections.

MYTH BUSTER: ACNE
- Diet is not associated with acne
- Not a disease of poor hygiene
- Black tip of a comedone is oxidized sebum not dirt.

ECZEMA: TRIGGERS
- Irritants: detergents, soaps, clothing—wool, loose cotton
- Contact and environmental allergens: dust mites, pets
- Long hot showers
- Sweating
- Stress

Eczema of the nipple: suspect Paget disease of the breast!

ECZEMA CLASSIFICATIONS:
Atopic: often associated with family history of atopy (asthma, allergic rhinitis)
Contact dermatitis: precipitated by a particular irritant or allergen
Nummular: often in elderly, annular, coin-shaped lesions

Psoriasis

Definition

A chronic, recurring inflammatory dermatosis of which a number of different presentations occur.

Plaque psoriasis (most common)

- Characterized by well-circumscribed erythematous papules/plaques with sliver-white scales
- May be mildly pruritic or painful
- Distribution: scalp, extensor surfaces, trunk, intergluteal folds, pressure areas

Other causes include guttate, pustular, and erythrodermic

Treatment

Plaque psoriasis treatment is based on disease severity (CDA Guidance)

- Mild: 5% of BSA
    - First line: topical corticosteroids
    - Other first-line options: topical vitamin D analogues (calcipotriol) that can be used in combination with corticosteroids
    - Second line: topical retinoids (tazarotene), salicylic acid (removes scales), anthralin, and coal tar

(Emollients can be used in combination with the above agents to help restore the barrier function of the skin.)

- Moderate–severe: BSA >10% or significant affect on QOL, distribution of disease (face, hands, feet, or genitals), or uncontrolled pain +/− pruritus
    - Phototherapy
    - Systemic therapies (oral retinoids, cyclosporin, methotrexate) or biologics (costly)

OTHER SKIN DISORDERS KEY POINTS

Lichen Planus

Characteristics

- Six Ps: purple, pruritic, polygonal, peripheral, papules, penis
- Wickham striae: greyish lines over surface
- Commonly presents on flexural surfaces, mucosa, and genitalia
- Associated with stress and Hepatitis C virus infection

Treatment

- Spontaneously resolves over weeks or may persist for years
- Topical corticosteroids +/− intralesional steroid injections
- Chemo phototherapy for resistant cases

SKIN INFECTIONS

Dermatophytosis

- Fungal infection of the skin
- Defined by infected location
- Microscopic diagnosis: Skin scrapings prepared with KOH will demonstrate hyphae
- Treat with topical antifungals. Use systemic antifungals for resistant cases or nail involvement

PSORIASIS: TRIGGERS

Trauma (Koebner phenomenon)

Infection

Alcohol

Stress

Drugs: beta blockers, NSAIDs, lithium

PSORIASIS: WHEN TO REFER?

- Severe disease or significant impact on QOL
- Involving face, scalp, hands/feet, or intertriginous area
- Pustular, guttate, erythrodermic psoriasis
- Psoriatic arthritis (+ rheumatology referral)
- Inadequate response to Rx according to physician and/or patient
- Patient request

When treatment fails; consider an alternative diagnosis (eg, eczema could be a fungal infection).

DERMATOPHYTOSIS–DEFINED BY LOCATION OF INFECTION

Head: *Tinea capitis*

Body: *T. corporis*

Groin: *T. cruris*

Feet: *T. pedis*

Cellulitis

- Skin infection involving dermis and subcutaneous tissues
- Causative organism:
  - Common **beta-hemolytic Streptococcus** (group A more than group B, C, or G) or **Staphylococcus aureus**
  - Cat or dog bite: *Pasteurella multocida*
  - Saltwater exposure: *Vibrio vulnificus*
- Treatment
  - First-line treatment includes: cephalexin PO or cefazolin IV
  - Demarcate areas of redness with pen to monitor progression

Erysipelas

Type of superficial cellulitis presents as erythema with defined and elevated borders due to lymphatic involvement

Impetigo

Infection of epidermis only. Often in children, **honey-coloured** crusted lesions around mouth. May treat with topical antibiotics.

Necrotizing Fasciitis

Severe, aggressive, and life-threatening form of skin infection. Most often polymicrobial. High fevers and severe systemic toxicity are seen. Treatment requires urgent **surgical debridement** +/− amputation and early broad-spectrum antibiotics! (Use bacteriostatic regimens.)

Herpes Simplex Virus (HSV)

- Affects more than one-third of the world's population
- Presents with multiple painful orolabial or genital vesicles and ulcerations
- Patients are the most sick with their first episode; many patients have fever, headache, malaise, and myalgias
- Lifelong latent infection in sensory ganglia is standard
- Subsequent recurrences are less severe. Prodrome of itching and burning often precedes the rash.
- Maternal-fetal transmission is associated with significant morbidity
- Treatment:
  - Antivirals are needed early to be effective, for example, acyclovir, famciclovir, valacyclovir
  - Chronic suppressive therapy is reserved for those with more than 4 to 6 outbreaks per year

Varicella Zoster Virus (VZV)

- Manifests as Varicella (chicken pox) and Herpes zoster (shingles)
- Rash: pruritic, papular changing to vesicular to pustular and finally to crusting
- Vaccination is available (12 months and 4-6 year old) including vaccination for zoster for those over 60
- Chicken pox:
  - Disease of childhood, highly contagious
  - Incubation period of 14 to 21 days
  - Fever and malaise just before or with skin eruption
- Herpes zoster:
  - More common in elderly and immunocompromised

TREATMENT
Abscesses require incision and drainage.

Consider abuse in preadolescents presenting with genital herpes.

Dewdrops on a rose petal: classic rash of VZV.

COMMON COMPLICATIONS
Second bacterial infection
Post-herpetic neuralgia

- After primary infection, latent virus develops in spinal dorsal root ganglia
- Reactivation causes a rash along the dermatomal distribution
- Pain precedes rash and can be severe
■ Treatment:
  - Antivirals (Acyclovir for 7 days)
  - Treat within 24 to 72 hours of rash appearing
  - Prophylaxis: treat household contacts
■ Herpes zoster ophthalmicus:
  - VZV infection of ophthalmic division of trigeminal nerve
  - Presents with lesions of nose, corner of eye
  - Risk of loss of vision, chronic ocular inflammation, and eye pain
  - Antivirals within 72 hours of rash help to prevent ocular complications
  - Urgent referral of ophthalmologist if ocular involvement suspected
    ○ For example, conjunctivitis, keratitis, uveitis, ocular-motor nerve palsies

SKIN DISORDERS: SERIOUS DIAGNOSES NOT TO MISS!

Hypersensitivity Syndromes

■ Erythema multiforme (EM)
  - Rapid onset of red macules to target-like papules with erythematous border and central sparring
  - Unlike urticaria, the lesions remain fixed 7 to 14 days
  - Rx: Stop causative drug, oral antihistamines
■ Stevens-Johnson syndrome (SJS)/Toxic epidermal necrolysis (TEN)
  - A severe expression of EM, though not as severe as TEN
  - Severe cutaneous reaction often caused by drugs
  - Believed to be same disorder as EM but more severe
  - Presents as sick patient with fever >39°C, blisters on dusky macules, and **involvement of mucous membranes** (**mouth, eyes, genital lesions**)
  - Diagnosis is made based on the percentage of skin involved
    ○ SJS <10%   TEN >30%
  - Mortality is due to fluid loss
  - Treat aggressively! Hospitalize, stop causative drug, IV fluids++, consider IVIG

Skin Cancer

■ Pay attention to sun-exposed areas: face, lips, ears, scalp, and extremities
■ Always consider a life-threatening condition such as malignancy
■ Treatment generally involves excision +/− lymph node dissection for invasive disease

Basal Cell Carcinoma (BCC)

■ Eighty percent of skin cancers are BCC
■ Spread locally and rarely metastasize
■ Nodular BCC (most common) presents as raised pearly white nodule with telangiectasia >6 mm
■ Superficial BCC presents as red scaling plaques with thready border

Squamous Cell Carcinoma (SCC)

■ Five percent develop metastasis
■ Tumor of keratinocytes

RASHES ON THE PALMS
- EM
- Rocky mountain spotted fever
- Drug eruption
- Secondary syphilis
- Scabies
- Hand, Foot & Mouth disease

HSV—Herpes simplex virus is associated with EM in at least 60% of cases.

Use **biopsy or excision** to rule out serious pathology.

SKIN CANCER RISK
Factors
Sun exposure
Age >50
Fair skin
Male gender
Family history
Multiple nevi (melanoma)

- Presents as persistent areas of ulceration, crusting, hyperkeratosis, or erythema
- Common in fair-skinned and organ transplant patients
- Actinic keratosis: premalignant form
  - Presents as rough, scaly spots on sun-exposed skin
  - Often treated with cryotherapy; topical therapy includes: 5-fluorouracil, diclofenac, imiquimod

Malignant Melanoma

- Malignant neoplasm of pigment-forming cells
- ABCDE: to distinguish benign nevi versus malignant lesions (see sidebar)

Leukoplakia

- White lesion seen on oral mucosa which cannot be rubbed off
- Thought to be a premalignant lesion
- Associated with tobacco and alcohol use
- Requires biopsy and close follow-up +/− excision or cryotherapy

Cutaneous T-Cell Lymphoma (Mycosis Fungoides)

- Rare disease, more common in African Americans
- Malignant lymphoma of T cells that usually remains confined to skin and lymph nodes
- Diagnosis: biopsy shows distinctive pathology
- Ninety-five percent are mycosis fungoides (limited superficial type)
  - Presents as erythematous, scaling patches or plaques that are often pruritic
  - Hypo- and hyperpigmented lesions are common
  - Lymphadenopathy is common
- Five percent of cases are Sézary syndrome (widespread systemic type)
- Treatment includes:
  - Topical: high-potency steroids, retinoids, or chemotherapy
  - Phototherapy: UVA/UVB

Pemphigus

- Rare but serious **autoimmune** disease—**refer to dermatologist!**
- **Bullous lesions** of skin and mucosa that quickly erode to **vesicles and ulcerations**
- Most common form is pemphigus vulgaris
- **Nikolsky sign:** superficial detachment of the skin with pressure
- Treatment: goal of treatment is initial remission
  - Systemic steroids, that is, prednisone 40 mg to 80 mg/day
  - Adjuvants/steroid sparring: azathioprine, cyclophosphamide, mycophenolate, gold, methotrexate

MELANOMA VS MOLE

A: asymmetry
B: border, irregular
C: colour, varied
D: diameter, >6 mm
E: evolving, elevation

Think of pemphigus vulgaris when an oral ulceration lasts >1 month.

Bibliography

Chen AY, Tran C. *Toronto Notes*. Toronto, ON: Type & Graphics Inc; 2011.

Canadian Dermatology Association. *Canadian Guidelines for the Management of Plaque Psoriasis*. 1st ed. 2009. http://www.dermatology.ca/guidelines/cdnpsoriasisguidelines.pdf.

Feldman SR. *Epidemiology, Pathophysiology, Clinical Manifestations, and Diagnosis of Psoriasis*. 2012. http://www.uptodate.com.

Feldman SR. *Treatment of Psoriasis*. 2011. http://www.uptodate.com.

McPhee SJ, Papadakis MA, eds. *Current Medical Diagnosis and Treatment*. 49 ed. New York, NY: McGraw Hill Medical; 2010.

Shaikh S, Ta CN. Evaluation and management of herpes zoster ophthalmicus. *Am Fam Phy*. Nov 1 2002;66(9):1723-1730.

Simon C, Everitt H, van Dorp F. *Oxford Handbook of General Practice*. Oxford, UK: Oxford University Press; 2010.

Usatine RP, Smith MA, Chumley H, Mayeaux EJ, Jr, Tysinger J, eds. *The Color Atlas of Family Medicine*. New York, NY: McGraw Hill Medical; 2009.

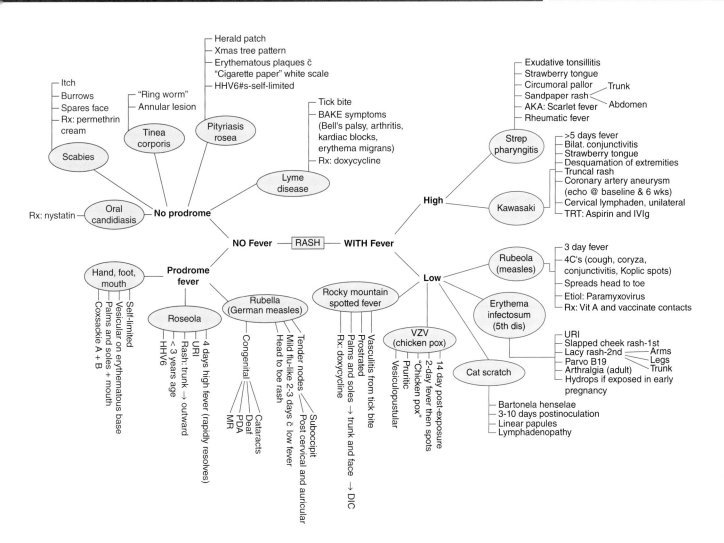

Cancer

Priority Topic 12

Use each visit as an opportunity to provide counseling regarding cancer prevention (eg, quit smoking, practice safe sex).

Use the most up-to-date Canadian Cancer Screening Guidelines to screen all patients in your practice.

In patients who have been given a diagnosis of cancer:

- Provide emotional support and inquire about personal and social consequences of the illness
- Provide close follow-up
- Remain involved in the circle of care. Continue to stay involved in the specialist-driven treatment plan.
- Use each visit to ask about side effects of cancer treatments (eg, diarrhea, swelling, hair loss, paresthesias)
- Be realistic and honest when discussing prognosis with the patient

In patients with a distant history of cancer, have a high index of suspicion for return/new cancer when presenting with new symptoms (eg, new shortness of breath [SOB], back pain) and investigate appropriately

Bibliography

Canadian Cancer Society. *Cervical Cancer*. 2012. http://www.cancer.ca/Canada-wide/Prevention/Getting%20checked/Cervical%20cancer%20NEW.aspx?sc_lang=en.

Canadian Task Force on Preventative Health Care. *Screening for Breast Cancer*. 2012. http://www.canadiantaskforce.ca/recommendations/2011_01_eng.html,

Izawa JI, Klotz L, Siemens DR, et al. *Prostate Cancer Screening: Canadian Guidelines 2011*. Dorval, Quebec: The Canadian Urological Association; 2011. http://www.cua.org/userfiles/files/CUA%20PCa%20Screening%20Guidelines%20v3(4).pdf.

Levin B, Lieberman DA, McFarland B, et al. Screening and surveillance for the early detection of colorectal cancer and adenomatous polyps, 2008: a joint guideline from the American Cancer Society, the US Multi-Society Task Force on Colorectal Cancer, and the American College of Radiology. *Cancer J Clin*. 2008;58:130-160. doi: 10.3322/CA.2007.0018.

Loss of Weight
Priority Topic 60

- Unexplained, unintentional weight loss should be investigated through a thorough history, physical examination, and appropriate investigations as indicated
- Patients' weights should be recorded on a regular basis (eg, annual basis for all patients but more frequently if weight loss is suspected). Persistent weight loss may indicate the need to work the patient up again for a possible cause

Bibliography

The College of Family Physicians of Canada. http://www.cfpc.ca/uploadedFiles/Education/Priority%20Topics%20and%20Key%20Features.pdf.

Parkinsonism
Priority Topic 71

TABLE 2-14	Tremor Definitions		
	RESTING	**POSTURAL**	**INTENTION**
Body part	Distal UE	UE/head/voice	Anywhere
Characteristics	3-7 Hz pill rolling	6-12 Hz fine tremor	<5 Hz coarse tremor
Worse with	Inactivity	Sustained posture/ outstretched arms	Activity (eg, finger to nose)
Associated symptoms	TRAP	+/− autosomal dominant family history	Cerebellar findings
DDx	IPD, Parkinsonism, Wilson disease	Physiologic, benign essential tremor, drugs, hyperthyroid, hyperglycemia	Cerebellar disorders, Wilson disease, alcohol, MS

Adapted with permission from TO notes Table 29 (N34).

KEY PARKINSONIAN FEATURES: "TRAP"

Tremor
Rigidity
Akinesia/bradykinesia
Postural instability

Symptoms/Characteristics

- Older age >60 years—number one risk factor
- Resting tremor—often unilateral
- Muscle rigidity/cogwheeling
  - Increase in resistance to passive movement
- Bradykinesia/akinesia
  - Slow movements
  - Difficulty initiating movements

- Gait
  - Small shuffling steps, decreased arm swinging, unsteady turning, and difficulty stopping
  - Flexed posture
- Postural instability—late feature
- Mask-like face, infrequent blinking
- Seborrhea of face/scalp (dandruff)

Also look for:

- Changes in speech: hypophonia, monotonous speech, dysarthria, decreased spontaneous speech
- Micrographia: small handwriting
- Sleep disturbances, personality changes, anxiety
- Falls

PEARL
Consider Parkinson in an elderly patient with functional status deterioration.

Etiology

- Diopathic decrease in dopaminergic neurons in the pars compacta of the substantia nigra.

Diagnosis

- Classic 80%: bradykinesia + unilateral asymmetric signs, pill rolling resting tremor, and good treatment response to L-dopa.

DRUGS THAT CAUSE PARKINSONISM
Antipsychotics
Metoclopramide
Prochlorperazine
Amphotericin B
Calcium channel blockers
Chemotherapy
Cholinergics
Lithium, manganese

Differential Diagnosis

When atypical features (below) are present → suspect secondary Parkinson or other syndromes

- Young age <60 years or Wilson disease
- Abrupt onset of symptoms
- Rapid progression
- Absent resting tremor
- Poor response to levodopa
- Ocular movement disorder: r/o supranuclear palsy
- Early autonomic dysfunction (eg, urinary incontinence, syncope): r/o multisystem atrophy parkinsonism
- Early dementia

WHEN TO REFER?
All patients should be referred to a neurologist.

Treatment

- General
  - Aim: improve quality of life and functional status
  - Physical/occupational/speech therapy
    - For example, rails, large-handled cutlery, devices to amplify the voice
    - Physiotherapy is helpful to prevent falls due to postural instability
  - Early referral to neurology
  - Ongoing care
    - Assess functional status frequently
    - Anticipate and monitor for medication side effects
    - Recognize associated problems
      - Depression, dementia, falls, and constipation
      - Urinary retention, sexual dysfunction, dysphagia, sleep changes

Dyskinesia is the #1 side effect of levodopa.

- Medical
  - First-line: levo/carbidopa—dopamine replacement
    - Carbidopa decreases the peripheral breakdown of dopamine
  - Amantadine
  - MAOIs: adjunct to dopamine, inhibits degeneration of levodopa
  - Dopamine agonists: best effect in early disease (eg, pramipexole)
  - COMT inhibitor: inhibits breakdown of dopamine (eg, tolcapone)
- Medication side effects:
  - Dopaminergic:
    - Dyskinesias
    - Brief duration of action—needs multi-dose regimen
    - Orthostatic hypotension/dizziness
    - Gastric upset
    - Depression/psychosis/hallucinations/disinhibition
  - MAOIs:
    - Arrhythmia
    - Hypertensive crisis with tyramine (cheese, wine)
- Surgical Treatment Options:
  - Thalamotomy, pallidotomy, deep brain stimulation
  - Reserved for unresponsive patients and late disease

Key Points

- Parkinson disease is the most common cause of bradykinesia
- Distinguish idiopathic from atypical Parkinson disease (young age, drug related)
- Use a team approach, by involving other health care professionals including early referral to neurology
- In an elderly patient with functional status deterioration, consider parkinsonism

Bibliography

Chen AY, Tran C. *Toronto Notes*. Toronto, ON: Type & Graphics Inc; 2011.

Jensen B. Parkinson's disease: drug comparison chart. *RxFiles Drug Comparison Charts*. 8th ed. Saskatoon, SK: Saskatoon Health Region; 2010. 82-83. www.RxFiles.ca.

Lees AJ, Hardy J, Revesz T. Parkinson's disease. *Lancet*. 2009 Jun 13;373(9680):2055-2066. Correction can be found in *Lancet*. 2009 Aug 29;374(9691):684.

McPhee SJ, Papadakis MA, eds. *Current Medical Diagnosis and Treatment*. 49th ed. New York: McGraw Hill Medical; 2010.

Restless Legs Syndrome

Supplementary Topic

Diagnostic Criteria

Must have all four criteria

1. Urge to move the legs usually with dysesthesia
2. Onset or exacerbation with rest
3. Relief with movement
4. Circadian pattern

   Supportive clinical features: family history, response to dopaminergic therapy, periodic leg movements

   No routine testing recommended, consider checking blood work (eg, for anemia) and for underlying medical conditions based on clinical judgment

Causes

Idiopathic (primary) vs underlying (secondary) medical condition

1. DM/peripheral neuropathy
2. Iron deficiency
3. Pregnancy
4. Low magnesium
5. End-stage renal disease
6. Drug causes: lithium, anti-depressants (especially SSRI and TCA), antipsychotics, some CCB, anti-nauseants (domperidone and ondansetron may have least effect)

Differential Diagnoses

1. Nocturnal leg cramps
2. Peripheral neuropathy
3. Varicose veins
4. Akathisia
5. Intermittent claudication
6. Periodic limb movements of sleep (PLMS)
7. Positional discomfort
8. Leg pain (eg, from arthritis)
9. Fidgets or nervous leg shaking

Treatment

1. First-line treatment is non-pharmacologic
   Nutrition: avoid caffeine, alcohol, chocolate, smoking/nicotine
   Good sleep hygiene
   Stretching/exercise
2. Treat any underlying causes
3. Pharmacologic treatments
   Dopamine receptor agonists (eg, pramipexole, ropinirole)
   Anti-epileptics (eg, gabapentin, pregabalin)
   Dopamine precursors (eg, levodopa)
   Benzodiazepines
   Opioids

Bibliography

NIH. (2010). *Restless Legs Syndrome Fact Sheet.*. Bethesda, MD: National Institute of Neurological Disorders and Stroke; No. NIH Publication No. 10-4847.

Restless Legs Syndrome Foundation. *RLS Medical Bulletin: A Publication for Healthcare Providers.* 2005.

Rx Files. Restless legs syndrome: treatment options. *Drug Comparison Charts.* 8th ed. 2010:78.

Working Group on the Certification Process. Priority topics and key features with corresponding skill dimensions and phases of the encounter. The College of Family Physicians of Canada. 2010. http://www.cfpc.ca/uploadedFiles/Education/Certification_in_Family_Medicine_Examination/Definition%20of%20Competence%20Complete%20Document%20with%20skills%20and%20phases.pdf.

3
Infectious Diseases

Infections
Priority Topic 51

1. When investigating a patient with a possible infection:
   (a) Use a selective approach in ordering cultures before initiating antibiotic therapy (eg, cultures usually not required for pneumonia, UTI, abscess or uncomplicated cellulitis
      - Use throat swabs according to guidelines in acute pharyngitis.
      - Perform a culture in patients with history of unusual or resistant organisms on previous culture
      - Follow-up culture results to guide therapy when considering a broad infectious differential diagnosis (such as in immunocompromised patients)
   (b) Use the correct techniques and protocols for cultures
      - Selecting correct swabs and identification of appropriate culture and/or transport medium (eg, Diamond's medium for *Trichomonas vaginalis*)
      - Understanding and interpreting resistance and susceptibility patterns to influence choice of antimicrobial agent
2. If considering treatment for an infection, antibiotic use should be:
   (a) Judicious
      - Delayed treatment in otitis media (see Earache)
      - Treating acute bronchitis only if comorbid illness present
      - Avoiding screening for (or treating) asymptomatic bacteriuria in uncomplicated adult patients or those with indwelling catheters
   (b) Rational
      - Cost: taking into account the direct cost of the antimicrobial, as well as dispensing fees, and degree of coverage by provincial or private drug plans
      - Guidelines: following Canadian guidelines where applicable, and recognizing situations in which guidelines will not directly apply
      - Comorbidity: adjusting dose amount, frequency of dosing, length of treatment or choice of antimicrobial agent based upon individual patient factors (eg, presence of renal disease, severity of illness, or history of immunocompromise)

- Local resistance patterns: modifying antimicrobial selection and guidelines as needed
- Ease of treatment: considering the effect of dosing schedule and delivery route (eg, elixir vs tablet) on treatment adherence and outcomes

3. Use empiric treatment when appropriate, for example:
   - Life-threatening sepsis without culture report or confirmed diagnosis
   - Suspected meningitis
   - Acute otitis media in children <6 months
   - *Candida vaginitis* after antibiotic use
   - Uncomplicated cellulitis, pneumonia, UTIs, or abscesses

4. Consider infection as a possible cause of nonspecific signs and symptoms, such as:
   - Confusion in the elderly (eg, UTI, pneumonia)
   - Failure to thrive (eg, TB, HIV)
   - Unexplained pain (eg, necrotizing fasciitis, abdominal pain in children with pneumonia)
   - Fever of unknown origin (eg, endocarditis, intraabdominal abscess)
   - Chronic diarrhea (eg, *Giardia lamblia, Entamoeba histolytica*)

5. When a patient is deteriorating or is not responding to treatment after an original diagnosis of a simple infection, consider the possibility of a more complex infection
   - Look for a different type of organism (ie, viral vs fungal vs bacterial)
   - Consider a different dose, type, or route of antimicrobial
   - Perform an appropriate culture or conduct further investigations if the etiology is unclear
   - Reevaluate noninfectious causes (eg, neoplasm, autoimmune condition)

6. When using antibiotics to treat infections, employ other therapies as appropriate:
   - Fluid resuscitation in septic shock
   - Incision and drainage of abscesses
   - Tetanus booster as needed for lacerations and open wounds
   - Adequate analgesia

Bibliography

Working Group on the Certification Process. *Priority topics and key features with corresponding skill dimensions and phases of the encounter.* The College of Family Physicians of Canada; 2010. http://www.cfpc.ca/uploadedFiles/Education/Certification_in_Family_Medicine_Examination/ Definition%20of%20Competence%20Complete%20Document%20with%20skills%20and%20 phases.pdf.

Antibiotics
Priority Topic 5

1. When antibiotics are required, agents should be selected based on multiple factors, including:
   - Differences among first-line therapies for a specific indication
     - Considering evidence-based effectiveness, cost, and minimization of side effects
   - Local resistance patterns
     - Tailoring treatment based on epidemiological reporting and clinical experience
   - Clinical context
     - Choosing antibiotics based on previous bacterial infections and treatments, known immunodeficiencies, and to minimize interactions with critical medications (eg, warfarin)

- Patient's context
  - Simplifying dose schedules to improve adherence, or ensuring that pre-scribed medications are covered by provincial or private drug plans
2. Prescribe antibiotics only when the clinical presentation is likely to be caused by a bacterial infection, and when there is evidence for benefit from antibiotic treatment:
   - Avoiding antibiotics in non-severe cases of acute otitis media for children >6 months of age (see Earache)
   - Relying on decision rules to minimize the use of antibiotics in cases of acute pharyngitis (see Upper Respiratory Tract Infections)
   - Prescribing antibiotics in sinusitis only if signs or symptoms of bacterial infection present (see Upper Respiratory Tract Infections)
3. Be vigilant when evaluating reported allergies and reactions to antibiotics, and differentiate these from nonallergic events, such as:
   - Intolerance to known side effects
   - Nonallergic exanthem
   - Concurrent symptoms not related to drug administration
4. Use bacterial cultures in specific instances in which the result is likely to alter your choice of antibiotic therapy:
   - Performing bacterial cultures to assess community resistance patterns, as well as for patients with systemic symptoms, history of unusual or resistant organ-isms, and for those who are immunocompromised
5. Initiate antibiotics without delay before confirmation of the diagnosis in situa-tions in which:
   - The infection is life threatening (eg, sepsis)
   - Patient factors increase the likelihood of deterioration (eg, febrile neutropenia)
   - The infection has the potential for a rapid clinical course (eg, meningitis)

Bibliography

The College of Family Physicians Canada. http://www.cfpc.ca/uploadedFiles/Education/Priority%20 Topics%20and%20Key%20Features.pdf.

Fever

Priority Topic 39

IN CHILDREN

Recognize the potential for occult bacteremia and other serious infections in young children

- For ages up to 3 months:
  - Fever defined as a rectal temperature ≥38.0°C
  - Often a diagnostic challenge:
    - Usually caused by a self-limiting benign viral infection
      - A cause may not be obvious despite a careful history and physical examination
    - However, fever may be the only sign of a serious bacterial infection (eg, meningitis, pneumonia, UTI, bacteremia) or serious viral infection (eg, HSV) and should be further evaluated
  - Investigate with CBC and differential, blood culture, CSF analysis and culture, and urine culture
  - Admit to hospital in most cases for empiric antibiotics, and consider chest radiograph and antiviral therapy (eg, acyclovir) based on clinical appearance

as well as risk factors for serious infection (eg, prematurity, history of previous illness, prenatal complications, maternal history of HSV)

■ For ages 3 months to 3 years:

- Fever usually caused by a self-limiting viral infection, or a bacterial infection with a source identifiable on history and physical examination (eg, meningitis, UTI, pneumonia, skin infection, or osteomyelitis)
- Consider urinalysis and urine culture
- If child appears toxic, or has risk factors for infection (based on medical or immunization history):
  ○ Investigate with CBC and differential
  ○ Further work-up might include blood culture, urine culture, CSF analysis and culture, and chest radiograph

POSTOPERATIVE FEVER (5 W'S)
- Wind (atelectasis)
- Water (UTI)
- Walking (DVT, PE)
- Wound (infection)
- Wonder drugs (drug fever)

POSTPARTUM FEVER (TWO EXTRA W'S)
- Womb (endometrial infection)
- Weaning (mastitis)

FEVER OF UNKNOWN ORIGIN

Definition

■ Fever >38.3°C (oral)

- Lasting >3 weeks
- Or, diagnosis uncertain after 1 week of hospitalization or three outpatient visits

Symptoms

■ Enquire about past medical history, travel history, immunizations, sick contacts, fever onset/duration/pattern, occupational activities, sexual activity, drug use, and animal contacts

■ Investigate symptoms of systemic illness suggesting less benign course such as weight loss or night sweats

■ Ask about potentially localizing symptoms, including cough, dyspnea, abdominal pain, back pain, diarrhea, dysuria, headaches, neck stiffness, arthritides, and rashes

Physical Examination Findings

Complete examination, with particular attention paid to:

■ Eyes: redness, ulcers, retinal lesions

■ Skin: rashes, hemorrhagic/septic lesions, temporal artery tenderness

■ Lymph nodes and spleen: enlargement

■ Heart: new murmurs or extra sounds

■ Abdomen: focal tenderness or masses

■ Genitourinary: genital lesions or discharge, rectal/prostate abnormalities

■ Joints: inflammation, swelling

■ Neurological: cranial nerve palsies, focal signs

Differential Diagnosis

■ Infectious diseases (eventual diagnosis in 30-40% of initial FUO cases), including: meningitis, urinary tract infections, intra-abdominal abscess, hepatobiliary infection, endocarditis, osteomyelitis, or other systemic infections, such as:

- Viruses (eg, HIV, HAV, HBV, EBV, CMV)
- Bacteria (eg, TB, spirochetes, rickettsia)
- Funguses or parasites (eg, malaria)

■ Neoplasms (20%-30%) including lymphoma, leukemia, myelodysplastic syndromes, solid tumors

■ Collagen-vascular diseases (10%-20%) including lupus, rheumatoid arthritis, giant cell arteritis, rheumatic fever

- Other (15%-20%): drug fever (eg, antibiotics, methyldopa, phenytoin), pulmonary embolism, Crohn's disease
- Undiagnosed (5%-15%)

In special groups:

- Elderly: 30% of FUOs due to collagen-vascular diseases (eg, polymyalgia rheumatica, giant cell arteritis)
- HIV-positive: 75% due to infectious causes, 20% lymphoma, 5% HIV
- Patients with febrile neutropenia (temperature 38.3°C or >38°C for 1 hour, and ANC <500): high risk for infection

Investigations

Initial tests may include:

- CBC with differential
- Electrolytes and BUN/creatinine
- Urinalysis and urine culture
- Liver function tests
- ESR/CRP
- Chest x-ray
- Blood cultures

Additional tests to consider based on clinical scenario:

- Blood smear for parasites or spirochetes
- Cultures: CSF, sputum, and stool
- Infectious serological markers: HIV, EBV, CMV, HBV
- Other blood tests: TSH, ANA, RF, ACE
- Skin tests: PPD
- Biopsy: lymph nodes or blood vessels
- Cytology: urine

Imaging

- Abdominal ultrasound, CT, or endoscopy based on clinical signs and symptoms
- MRI or bone scans for osteomyelitis
- Ventilation-perfusion scans or CT pulmonary angiography for pulmonary embolus
- PET scans for occult neoplasms
- Echocardiography for endocarditis

INFECTIOUS ENDOCARDITIS

- Infection of the heart endothelium
- Risk factors: prosthetic valves, previous endocarditis, congenital heart disease, intravenous drug use (IVDU)
- Common pathogens:
  - Native valve endocarditis or IVDU: Streptococcus or Staphylococcus spp.
  - Prosthetic valve endocarditis: *S. epidermidis*, *S. aureus*, Enterococcus
- Mitral valve is most commonly affected, while tricuspid valve involvement is most common with IVDU
- Symptoms: fever, chills, dyspnea, chest pain
- Signs: clubbing, new murmur, Osler nodes, Roth spots, petechiae, splinter hemorrhages, Janeway lesions
- Immediate empiric IV antibiotics after blood cultures are drawn but before diagnosis is confirmed for those who are unwell with continued IV treatment for 4 to 6 weeks

Bibliography

Evans M. *Mosby's Family Practice Sourcebook*. 4th ed. Toronto: University of Toronto; 2006.

Roth AR, Basello GM. Approach to the adult patient with fever of unknown origin. *Am Fam Phy*. 2003;68(11):2223-2229.

Dysuria/Urinary Tract Infection
Priority Topic 32/95

Definitions

- Dysuria:
  - Pain, burning, or discomfort on urination
  - Differentiate:
    - "Internal": pain felt inside the body → more likely to be a UTI
    - "External": pain felt when urine passes over external genitalia → consider other diagnoses
- Uncomplicated UTI:
  - Otherwise healthy adult, premenopausal, nonpregnant women, without known urological abnormalities
- Complicated UTI:
  - Functional or anatomic abnormality of the urinary tract (eg, stones, strictures, reflux, neurogenic bladder)
  - History of urinary tract instrumentation (eg, catheters, ureteric stents, procedures, transplant)
  - Metabolic abnormalities (eg, renal failure)
  - Underlying disease (eg, poorly controlled diabetes, polycystic kidney disease, immunosuppression)
  - Pregnancy
  - Most infections in men

Recurrent infections: two or more UTIs within 6 months; or more than two positive urine cultures within 12 months

Reinfection: infection with a new organism >2 weeks after initial infection

Relapse: repeat or continued infection with the same organisms within 2 weeks of completing antibiotic course for a UTI

Symptoms/Clinical Manifestations

- Cystitis: dysuria, urinary urgency and frequency, suprapubic tenderness, cloudy urine, hematuria, absence of vaginal discharge or irritation, usually afebrile
- Pyelonephritis: fever, chills, nausea, vomiting, back pain, +/– cystitis symptoms
- Populations who may present with nonspecific symptoms:
  - Children: decreased appetite, irritability, fever, vomiting
  - Elderly: delirium, functional decline, abdominal pain, falls, incontinence

Differential Diagnosis of Dysuria

- Consider other diagnoses if external genital lesions, genital inflammation, or urethral discharge are present, or if the patient is experiencing scrotal, perineal, or rectal pain:
  - Infection (most common)
    - Includes cystitis, urethritis, prostatitis, epididymo-orchitis, and vulvovaginitis

○ Common organisms causing urethritis include *Neisseria gonorrhea*, *Chlamydia trachomatis*, *Trichomonas vaginalis*, and HSV
- Mechanical or chemical urethral irritation (eg, sexual activity, sensitivity to topical products)
- Hormonal (eg, endometriosis, hypoestrogenism)
- Trauma (eg, catheterization)
- Inflammatory disease (eg, Behçet syndrome, Reiter syndrome)
- Neoplasms
- Neurogenic and psychogenic conditions

UTI Risk Factors
- Previous UTIs
- Gender: higher incidence in women than men
- Age: higher rates among women aged 25 to 54; rates increase with increasing age in men
- Genitourinary tract abnormalities: BPH, strictures, renal cysts, diverticula, or bladder catheterization
- Other: increased rates among women who are sexually active (postcoital voiding can be preventative)

Physical Examination Findings
- Perform in everyone:
  - Temperature (usually normal in cystitis)
  - Blood pressure and heart rate (hypotension and tachycardia may be present in pyelonephritis)
  - Assess for CVA tenderness (suggestive of pyelonephritis)
  - Abdominal examination for suprapubic tenderness
- If vaginal signs or symptoms → perform a speculum and bimanual examination
- In males, consider digital rectal examination

Urine Dipstick Testing
- Appropriate investigation in most scenarios when UTI considered
- When to consider **not** performing:
  - Urine that is **not** cloudy: this alone has a 97% negative predictive value for a positive urine culture
  - Catheterized patients (very low predictive value)
  - Note: there are no studies on the predictive value of dipstick testing in men
- Nitrites: positive test has high specificity for UTI
- Leukocyte esterase: positive test has reasonable sensitivity for UTI
- If nitrites and leukocytes negative → UTI unlikely → explore other causes
- Red blood cells → may be present in UTI, but persistent hematuria post-UTI requires follow-up

Urine Cultures
- Do not wait for culture results before initiating treatment when UTI clinically suspected
- Consider cultures for:
  - All complicated UTIs (including all men)
  - Women >65 years
  - Pregnant women
  - Suspected pyelonephritis
  - Failed antibiotic treatment or persistent symptoms
  - Recurrent UTI (more likely to have a resistant strain)

Validated UTI Score for Uncomplicated Acute Cystitis
- One point each for: (a) dysuria; (b) positive leukocytes on urine dip; and (c) positive nitrites on urine dip
- For a score of 0 to 1: consider urine culture or another diagnosis; empirical treatment only if symptoms are severe
- For a score of 2 to 3: empirical antibiotics +/− culture

- Culture **not** usually required
  - Symptomatic women <65 years (first episode)
  - Do not send cultures (or treat) asymptomatic bacteriuria in the elderly or those with indwelling catheters

Further Investigations

- Anatomical and functional abnormalities should be ruled out (consider renal-bladder US +/– VCUG) for children in the following situations:
  - Diagnosis of pyelonephritis
  - Male child with first UTI
  - Female child with first UTI at <3 years of age
  - Female child with second UTI at >3 years
  - Family/personal history of urologic or renal abnormalities
- Ultrasound or CT may be used to investigate the presence of a complicating urolithiasis

Treatment

- Targeted at the most common organisms (*E. coli*, *S. saprophyticus*, *Proteus mirabilis*, *S. aureus*, Enterococcus spp., Klebsiella spp.) (see Table 3-1)

TABLE 3-1	UTI Antibiotic Treatment Choices	
	FIRST LINE	SECOND LINE
Uncomplicated UTI	TMP/SMX 1 DS tablet bid × 3 days Macrobid 100 mg bid × 5 days	Ciprofloxacin 250 mg bid × 3 days Amoxicillin 500 mg tid × 7 days
Complicated UTI	TMP/SMX 1 DS tablet bid × 7-14 days Macrobid 100 mg bid × 7-14 days	Amoxicillin/clavulanate 875 mg bid × 10-14 days
UTI in pregnancy	Cephalexin 250-500 qid × 7 days Amoxicillin 500 mg tid × 7 days Macrobid 100 mg bid × 5 days (do not use Macrobid at or near term)	TMP/SMX 1 DS tablet bid × 3 days (Do not use TMP/SMX in the first trimester or the last 6 weeks of gestation)
UTI in children	TMP/SMX, dosed as 5-10 mg/kg/day TMP, divided bid × 7-10 days Nitrofurantoin 5-7 mg/kg/day divided q6h × 7-10 days	Amoxicillin 40 mg/kg/day divided tid × 7-10 days
Pyelonephritis	Ciprofloxacin 500 mg bid x 10-14 days TMP/SMX 1 DS tablet bid x 10-14 days (if no underlying structural or functional abnormalities or underlying disease)	Amoxicillin/clavulanate 875 mg bid x 10-14 days
	• Outpatient treatment unless severe (eg, nausea/vomiting, hypotension)	

Key Points

- Query other diagnoses in addition to UTI when evaluating a patient with dysuria
- Identify factors that may make the infection "complicated"
- Consider UTI as a diagnosis in elderly or young patients with nonspecific history
- Use empiric antibiotic treatment before culture results are available in pregnant women, or in pyelonephritis or sepsis

Bibliography

Anti-infective Review Panel. *Anti-infective Guidelines for Community-Acquired Infections.* Toronto: MUMS Guideline Clearninghouse; 2012.

Bremnor JD, Sadovsky R. Evaluation of dysuria in adults. *Am Fam Phys.* 2002;65(8):1589-1597.

McIsaac WJ, Moineddin R, Ross S. Validation of a decision aid to assist physicians in reducing unnecessary antibiotic drug use for acute cystitis. *Arch Intern Med.* 2007;167(20):2201-2206.

Quick Reference Guide for Primary Care. http://www.hpa.org.uk/webc/HPAwebFile/HPAweb_C/1194947404720. Accessed April 4, 2012.

Woodford HJ, George J. Diagnosis and management of urinary tract infection in hospitalized older people. *J Am Geriatr Soc.* 2009 Jan;57(1):107.

Earache
Priority Topic 33

ACUTE OTITIS MEDIA

Definition
- Acute signs and symptoms of illness with:
  - Evidence of middle ear inflammation
  - Fluid in the middle ear

Symptoms
- Acute onset of ear pain (though may be absent in up to 40% of those with otitis media)
- Fever, irritability, nighttime awakening, decreased appetite, ear rubbing
- Usually presents with other symptoms of upper respiratory tract infection (eg, cough or rhinorrhea)

Risk Factors
- Exposure to cigarette smoke
- Attendance at large day care centers
- First Nations or Inuit ethnicity
- Formula feeding (especially supine bottle use)
- Use of a pacifier
- Household crowding
- Prematurity

Physical Examination Findings
- Note: the middle ear must be visualized for definitive diagnosis (ie, no wax occlusion)
- Not all red ears are infected: mobility, appearance, and position of the tympanic membrane are more important

Signs of Middle Ear Effusion
- Presence of liquid in the ear canal due to tympanic membrane rupture
- Opacification of the tympanic membrane with loss of bony landmarks
- Visible air-fluid level
- Decreased tympanic membrane motility on pneumatic otoscopy

Signs of Middle Ear Inflammation
- Bulging tympanic membrane with marked discoloration (ie, hemorrhagic, red, grey, yellow)
- No pain with pinna movement (unless coexisting otitis externa)

Differential Diagnosis of Ear Pain
- Eustachian tubule dysfunction
- Otitis externa
- Referred pain
- Cerumen impaction
- Foreign body
- Mastoiditis
- Basilar skull fracture
- Temporal arteritis
- Tumor

- Contact dermatitis
- Seborrheic dermatitis
- Herpes zoster oticus

Prevention
- Hand washing to minimize exposure to viral and bacterial agents (especially at day cares)
- Breastfeeding
- Minimize exposure to tobacco smoke
- Limit pacifier use
- Influenza vaccination

Management
- Immediate antibiotic therapy if:
  - Less than 6 months of age
  - Severe illness: severe pain, toxic appearance, temperature >39°C orally before antipyretics, bilateral otitis media, or perforation with purulent discharge
  - High-risk conditions: immunodeficiency, chronic cardiac or lung disease, anatomic abnormalities of the head or neck (eg, cleft palate), history of complicated otitis media, or Down syndrome
  - Uncertain follow-up: patients or parents who have difficulty recognizing worsening illness or recontacting care if child is not improving
- Watchful waiting (if >6 months of age):
  - Observe and provide analgesia, with reassessment at 48 to 72 hours for persistent or worsening illness
    - Acetaminophen 10 to 15 mg/kg/day q4h, maximum of 75 mg/kg/day
    - Ibuprofen: 5 to 10 mg/kg/day q6-8h, maximum of 40 mg/kg/day
  - If symptoms do not improve after 2 to 3 days, verify the diagnosis and start antibiotics

Antibiotics
- Ten-day course if less than 2 years or if frequent recurrent infections, 5-day course if greater than 2 years and uncomplicated
- No tympanic membrane perforation (*Streptococcus pneumoniae, Moraxella catarrhalis, Haemophilus influenzae*):
  - Amoxicillin 80 mg/kg/day divided bid or tid, up to 3 g/day maximum
  - Allergy to penicillin:
    - Non-anaphylactic:
      - Cefprozil 30 mg/kg/day divided bid
      - Cefuroxime axetil 30 mg/kg/day divided bid
    - Anaphylactic:
      - Clarithromycin 15 mg/kg/day divided bid
      - Azithromycin 10 mg/kg once and 5 mg/kg daily for 4 days
- Perforation or tubes in place (*Pseudomonas aeruginosa, S. aureus, S. viridans*):
  - Ciprofloxacin (Ciprodex) = 4 drops bid × 5 days

Follow-Up
- At 48 to 72 hours: if patient remains symptomatic, reassess for acute complications (eg, mastoiditis, meningitis), other diagnostic possibilities, and compliance with medications
- At 3 months: assess for persistent otitis media with effusion (see later)

- If recurrent: audiology and ENT referral if the patient has experienced >2 cases of acute otitis media in 6 months, or >3 cases in 12 months

Guideline Summary

- Immediate treatment for acute otitis media for those with severe illness and those less than 6 months of age
- Consider watchful waiting approach for those greater than 6 months of age with appropriate follow-up
- Use amoxicillin as the first-line antibiotic, with second- and third-line agents if the patient has a penicillin allergy

Key Points

- Always look for other causes of fever in a child presenting with fever and a red tympanic membrane
- Provide parent/patient education that viruses are often the cause of acute otitis media, and are not amenable to antibiotics, and that there is a high likelihood of resolution of acute otitis media without antibiotics in most cases
- Address modifiable risk factors
- Ensure appropriate follow-up

OTITIS MEDIA WITH EFFUSION

- Definition: fluid in the middle ear with ear discomfort, but without other signs or symptoms of infection, often following an episode of acute otitis media
- Ninety percent of effusions resolve spontaneously within 3 months of the acute infection
- Antibiotics are not required
- Refer for audiology and ENT assessment if the patient has persistent hearing loss or abnormalities of the tympanic membrane at 3 months

OTITIS EXTERNA

- Definition: infection of the external ear (*P. aeruginosa, S. aureus*)
- Signs and symptoms:
  - Pain and tenderness of the tragus and on movement of the pinna
  - Erythematous, edematous ear canal with pain on otoscopy
  - No fever, usually
- Treatment:
  - No perforation: Buro-Sol 2-3 drops tid-qid
  - Perforated TM: ciprofloxacin (Ciprodex) 4 drops tid
- Necrotizing/malignant otitis externa: spread of *P. aeruginosa* infection to the bone, leading to deep ear pain, systemic signs and symptoms, fever, elevated ESR/CRP, and evidence of osteomyelitis on CT or MRI
  - Ciprofloxacin 750 mg po bid and ciprofloxacin (Ciprodex) 4 drops bid for 4-8 weeks

Bibliography

Alberta CPG Working Group for Antibiotics. Guideline for the diagnosis and management of acute otitis media in children; 2008. http://www.topalbertadoctors.org/download/366/AOM_guideline.pdf Accessed November 2012.

Anti-infective Review Panel. Anti-infective guidelines for community-acquired infections. Toronto: MUMS Guideline Clearinghouse; 2012.

Evans M. *Mosby's Family Practice Sourcebook*. 4th ed. Toronto: University of Toronto; 2006.

Forgie S, Zhanel G, Robinson J. Management of acute otitis media. *Paediatr Child Health*. 2009;14(7): 457-460.

Cough

Priority Topic 17

ACUTE COUGH (<3 WEEKS DURATION)

Etiology:

- Virus—most common cause
- Rhinitis (allergic)/post-nasal drip—watery/itchy eyes, sneezing, afebrile, seasonal
- Sinusitis—fever, facial/tooth pain, purulent discharge
- Asthma—worse with activity and at night; triggers; +/− wheeze, atopy, seasonal, family hx
- Aspiration
- Exclude serious causes: pulmonary embolism (PE), pneumothorax, left heart failure, pneumonia, COPD exacerbation

Viral

- Low grade fever (<39°C); stable vitals; rhinorrhea; gradual onset; tend to get better over time

Bacterial

- High fever (>39°C); cough; more sudden onset; tend to get worse over time

PEDIATRIC PERSISTENT/RECURRENT COUGH (>8 WEEKS)

Differential Diagnosis

Infection, asthma, rhinitis, GERD, postnasal drip (PND), foreign body, Pertussis

- Most common cause in infants: infection, including otitis, bronchiolitis, bronchitis, *Bordetella pertussis*
- Most common cause in preschool child: infection (otitis, sinusitis, bronchitis), asthma, foreign body
- Most common cause in school-age child: asthma, infection, psychogenic

Treatment is based on suspected etiology. See specific sections for further details.

- **Do not** use cough suppressants and OTC medicines in children under 6 years old. Exceptions are drugs to treat fever (eg, ibuprofen, acetaminophen).
- Cough and cold medications are not recommended in the pediatric population

ADULT PERSISTENT/CHRONIC COUGH (>8 WEEKS)

Three most common causes of chronic cough in adults: PND, asthma, GERD

- Other common causes: rhinitis, smoking, COPD/chronic bronchitis, ACE inhibitors, congestive heart failure
- Less common causes: think of restrictive (eg, pulmonary fibrosis) or obstructive lung diseases (eg, lung cancer), infections (eg, TB), environmental factors (eg, workplace exposures)

History

- Onset, pattern/variations in cough, characteristics (eg, dry/productive, "barking," wheeze, nasal d/c), triggers and aggravating factors, occupation, smoking

Investigation

- CXR, CBC (WBC, Hgb), JVP, edema, %O_2 saturation, pulmonary function testing
  - Note: normal spirometry does **not** rule out cough-variant asthma
  - Assess for heart failure causing cough
  - Consider sinus imaging
  - Induced sputum after exclusion of common causes (cytology, infection, inflammatory cells)

- Consider upper endoscopy after treatment failure (eg, query hiatal hernia)
- Allergy testing if indicated by history
■ Physical examination: eye examination, ear, nasal, oropharynx, sinuses, mucosa, cardiovascular, respiratory, clubbing
■ Diagnosis may be in combination with trial of treatment for presumed cause:
  - For example, antibiotics, asthma, bronchodilation, and evaluation with spirometry, H2-blocker/PPI

Treatment

Depends on the presumed diagnosis, for example:
■ Encourage smoking cessation; d/c ACE inhibitor
■ Empiric treatment for PND, rhinosinus disease (including chronic sinusitis, allergic rhinitis) includes treatment with antihistamine/decongestant, nasal saline spray, intranasal steroids, and avoiding of allergens/triggers
■ Empiric treatment for asthma (inhaled corticosteroid and bronchodilator)
■ Empiric treatment for GERD with PPI or H2-blocker, diet/lifestyle modifications
■ Consider additional diagnostic testing if suboptimal response to treatment
■ See relevant topic heading for more information about treating these conditions, for example, asthma and COPD sections, smoking cessation

CHRONIC COUGH IN SMOKERS

■ Assess for COPD or chronic bronchitis
  - Chronic bronchitis = cough most days and increased sputum for 3 months in two consecutive years
  - COPD = spirometry = $FEV_1/FVC <0.7$ or $FEV_1 <80\%$ after bronchodilation
    ○ Dyspnea, decreased exercise tolerance, prolonged cough
  - Assess for lung cancer if suspected by history

Bibliography

Anti-infective Review Panel. *Anti-infective Guidelines for Community-Acquired Infections.* Toronto: MUMS Guideline Clearinghouse; 2010.

Dynamed. Chronic Cough. Accessed Feb 2, 2012.

Gahbauer M, Keane P. Chronic cough: Stepwise application in primary care practice of the ACCP guidelines for diagnosis and management of cough. *J Am Acad Nurse Prac.* August 2009;21(8):409-416.

Health Canada Releases Decision on the Labelling of Cough and Cold Products for Children. http://www.hc-sc.gc.ca/ahc-asc/media/advisories-avis/_2008/2008_184-eng.php. Accessed March 25, 2012.

Upper Respiratory Tract Infections

Priority Topic 94

LIFE-THREATENING URI'S

■ Epiglottitis
■ Retropharyngeal abscess

BACTERIAL SINUSITIS

Etiology

Most common is *Streptococcus pneumoniae, Haemophilus influenzae, Moraxella catarrhalis*

Usually preceded by viral URTI

Note: infants only born with ethmoid and maxillary sinus. By 5 years have sphenoid sinus; by 8 years have frontal sinus

Risk Factors

■ Smoking, anatomy (eg, deviated septum, polyps), allergic rhinitis, asthma

Signs/Symptoms

URI not improved in 7 to 10 days plus:

■ Purulent nasal drainage
■ Nasal congestion, hyposmia/anosmia
■ Facial pain/pressure/fullness; pain can be increased by leaning forward, diffuse or localized headache
■ PND
■ Fever
■ Cough
■ Maxillary dental pain
■ Ear fullness
■ Poor response to nasal decongestants

Diagnosis

Clinical assessment more accurate than any single sign/symptom

■ CDC (Centers for Disease Control and Prevention) criteria for clinical dx of acute bacterial rhinosinusitis:
  · Rhinosinusitis symptoms for ≥7 days (**7-10 day mark differentiates simple viral infection from bacterial sinusitis**)
  · Purulent nasal discharge
  · Maxillary tooth or facial (sinus) pain or tenderness (especially when unilateral)

Complications

■ Orbital cellulitis, venous sinus thrombosis, bacterial meningitis, brain abscess, osteomyelitis

Differential Diagnosis

■ Rule out migraine—many patients with "sinus headache" may have migraine

Investigations

■ Usually no tests
■ Rule out allergic sinusitis with allergy testing if suspected
■ CT only if suspect complications of infection

Treatment

■ Most cases resolve without treatment
■ Symptomatic: analgesics/antipyretics, intranasal corticosteroids
■ First line = amoxicillin 500 mg tid × 5 to 10 days (Peds: 40 mg/kg bid)

Note: successful treatment = good symptom improvement at 10 days but not complete resolution of symptoms

■ Other: hypertonic saline nasal rinse; nasal steroid (modest benefit)

PHARYNGITIS/TONSILLITIS

Etiology

■ Viruses—**cause 80% to 90% of pharyngitis cases**
  · Adenovirus, Epstein-Barr, parainfluenza, influenza, rhinoviruses, and more
  · In presentation of pharyngitis, always consider EBV/mononucleosis
■ Bacterial—group A beta-hemolytic streptococci

History and Physical

- Abrupt onset of sore throat—may have fever/chills/headache/myalgias
- Tonsillar swelling and/or exudate
- Sore throat score for *Streptococcus pyogenes*, aka GABHS (group A beta-hemolytic streptococcus) (see Table 3-2)

TABLE 3-2	Sore Throat Score Card	
POINTS	**CRITERIA**	**TOTAL POINTS: MANAGEMENT**
1	T >38	0–1: no culture or Abx
1	No cough	2–3: throat culture; Tx if (+)GAS
1	Ant. cervical nodes	≥ 3: start Abx; if culture (–) stop Abx.
1	Tonsils—swollen or exudate	
1	Age 3-14 years old	
0	15-44 years old	
−1	>45 years old	

Adapted with permission from Anti-infective Review Panel. *Anti-infective Guidelines for Community-Acquired Infections*. Toronto: MUMS Guideline Clearinghouse; 2012.

Diagnosis

- Clinical
- Rapid streptococcus test or throat culture

Differential Diagnosis

- Rule out mononucleosis/EBV pharyngitis

Treatment for Streptococcal Pharyngitis (Table 3-3)

- **Primary purpose—prevent acute rheumatic fever**
- Antibiotic choices:

TABLE 3-3	Treatment for Streptococcal Pharyngitis	
	ADULTS	**CHILDREN**
Penicillin V	600 mg bid x 10 days	20 mg/kg bid
Erythromycin	250 mg qid x 10 days	20 mg/kg bid
Cephalexin	250 mg qid x 10 days	25 mg/kg bid

- Note: if given beta-lactam Abx for suspected streptococcal pharyngititis, but the infection is actually caused by EBV, a urticarial and maculopapular rash will develop

MONONUCLEOSIS/EBV PHARYNGITIS

Etiology

- Caused by Epstein-Barr virus; transmitted by infected saliva

Symptoms

- **Classic triad = generalized LAD, moderate-high fever, pharyngitis**
- Fatigue/malaise
- Headache

History and Physical

- Generalized lymphadenopathy typically involves inguinal, axillary, posterior auricular/cervical nodes
- Splenomegaly
- Tonsillar swelling (+/− grayish exudate)
- Vaginal ulcers may be present

Mononucleosis symptom triad =
- Generalized lymphadenopathy
- Moderate-high fever
- Pharyngitis

Investigations
- Monospot test (+ heterophile Ab)
  - Negative result → order CBC with differential and EBV serology (anti-EBV titre)

Treatment
- **No antibiotics.** (Note: If given beta-lactam Abx, morbilliform rash will develop.)
- Avoid strenuous physical activity for 4 weeks, and avoid contact sports
- Hydration and pain relief
- Corticosteroids for acute airway obstruction or relief of sore throat; not for routine treatment

Complications
- Splenic rupture
- Tonsil hyperplasia → airway obstruction

Prognosis
- Most patients recover to normal activities by 2 to 3 months

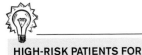

HIGH-RISK PATIENTS FOR COMPLICATIONS OF URTI
1. HIV, COPD, cancer with URI symptoms.
2. Consider:
   a. Antivirals (eg, Tamiflu).
   b. Flu vaccine every 1 year
   c. Pneumococcal vaccine 1 x /life if given after 65 years.

Bibliography

DynaMed [database online]. Acute sinusitis. EBSCO Publishing. http://web.ebscohost.com.cyber.usask.ca/dynamed/detail?vid=26&hid=9&sid=5fdbf4ec-bc94-440b-af64-b72b84140e48%40sessionmgr4&bdata=JnNpdGU9ZHluYW1lZC1saXZlJnNjb3BlPXNpdGU%3d#db=dme&AN=114974. Accessed December 5, 2012.

DynaMed [database online]. Infectious mononucleosis. EBSCO Publishing. http://web.ebscohost.com.cyber.usask.ca/dynamed/detail?vid=32&hid=9&sid=5fdbf4ec-bc94-440b-af64-b72b84140e48%40sessionmgr4&bdata=JnNpdGU9ZHluYW1lZC1saXZlJnNjb3BlPXNpdGU%3d#db=dme&AN=114945. Accessed December 5, 2012.

DynaMed [database online]. Streptococcal pharyngitis. EBSCO Publishing. http://web.ebscohost.com.cyber.usask.ca/dynamed/detail?vid=30&hid=9&sid=5fdbf4ec-bc94-440b-af64-b72b84140e48%40sessionmgr4&bdata=JnNpdGU9ZHluYW1lZC1saXZlJnNjb3BlPXNpdGU%3d#db=dme&AN=115782&anchor=anc-1428143566. Accessed December 5, 2012.

DynaMed [database online]. Upper respiratory infection. EBSCO Publishing. http://web.ebscohost.com.cyber.usask.ca/dynamed/detail?vid=28&hid=9&sid=5fdbf4ec-bc94-440b-af64-b72b84140e48%40sessionmgr4&bdata=JnNpdGU9ZHluYW1lZC1saXZlJnNjb3BlPXNpdGU%3d#db=dme&AN=114537. Accessed December 5, 2012.

Croup
Priority Topic 20

CROUP (LARYNGOTRACHEOBRONCHITIS [LTB])

Etiology
Parainfluenza virus is most common cause. Other causes: RSV, adeno/influenza/rhino-viruses, diphtheria, *Mycoplasma pneumoniae*
- Typically affects 6 month to 5 year olds during winter
- Transmitted by respiratory droplets
- Incubation period is 3 to 6 days

Differential Diagnosis
- Rule out acute epiglottitis, anaphylaxis, foreign body, retropharyngeal abscess

Signs/Symptoms
Upper airway (laryngeal or tracheal) obstruction leading to acute clinical syndrome with
- Barking cough
- Inspiratory stridor (90% of kids with stridor have croup!)
- Hoarse voice

- URTI prodrome
- Worse at night
- Improves with cold air/mist
- Fluctuating disease course
- May have 2 to 5 day prodrome of mild fever, rhinorrhea, sore throat
- Nasal flaring = severe croup +/− coexisting pneumonia

Investigations

- Assess ABCs!
- Clinical diagnosis
- Frontal neck x-ray shows steeple sign = subglottic narrowing—do only if unsure of diagnosis

Complications

- Rare! But can get severe airway obstruction + respiratory failure

Treatment

- PO dexamethasone 0.6 mg/kg (PO/IM) once (can repeat dose in 6-24 hours)
  - **Do not** undertreat mild to moderate croup
- Nebulized racemic epinephrine (for severe respiratory distress: marked sternal wall retractions and agitation)
  - 0.5 mL of 2.25% solution diluted in 3 mL NS or sterile water via nebulizer. Can repeat back-to-back if severe respiratory distress. Observe for 2 to 3 hours post tx (the effect of epinephrine does not last >2 hours)
- Explain fluctuating disease course that usually lasts 4 to 7 days to parents
- Consider hospitalization if:
  - Severe croup: cyanosis, decreased LOC, progressive/severe stridor and retractions, looks toxic
  - Dehydration
  - Relative indications for admission: social factors (inability to monitor child as outpatient); distance from hospital

BACTERIAL TRACHEITIS

It is also known as "acute bacterial laryngo tracheobronchitis." An invasive bacterial infection of the soft tissues of the trachea. Usually occurs in setting of prior airway mucosal damage, for example, antecedent viral infection

Etiology

- *Staphylococcus aureus* is most common cause. Other causes include *Haemophilus influenzae, Streptococcus pneumoniae, Moraxella catarrhalis, S. pyogenes.*

Epidemiology

- Rare, but is a pediatric airway emergency. Most occur in previously healthy children in setting of viral RTI. (Most common in 1-month to 6-year-olds in fall/winter.)

Differential Diagnosis

- Epiglottitis, croup, peritonsillar or retropharyngeal abscess or cellulitis. Severe bacterial pneumonia, foreign body aspiration, diphtheria (rare if immunized), inflammatory bowel disease.

Presentation

- Prodromal signs/symptoms of viral RTI for 1 to 3 days before more severe illness with stridor, dyspnea
- Onset fulminant with progression to acute respiratory distress <24 hours

Signs/Symptoms

- Stridor (inspiratory or expiratory)
- Cough (not painful; membranous exudates may be expectorated)
- Drooling—uncommon
- Preference to lie flat
- Fever may or may not be present
- Exudate can be minimal or extensive, sometimes forming pseudomembranes

Investigations

- Lateral neck or anteroposterior x-rays: steeple sign
- Pulmonary infiltrates common
- Labs: CBC + inflammatory markers are *not* helpful and do not correlate with illness severity
- Clinical diagnosis: poor response with nebulized epinephrine or glucocorticoids can help differentiate from croup
- Definitive diagnosis: direct endoscopy visualization of inflamed, exudate-covered trachea, normal epiglottis (best done in OR or ICU)
- Gram stain and culture (aerobic and anaerobic) during endoscopy; or sputum specimen in older patients

Treatment

- Admit to PICU
- Maintenance of airway (most children require endotracheal intubation for airway obstruction related to purulent secretions)
- Supplement O_2, +/− fluid resuscitation
- Endoscopy may be needed to remove pseudomembranous exudates
- Trial of inhaled bronchodilators, but stop if no clinical response
- Prevention:
  - Vaccination against pneumococci and virus (eg, measles, influenza) that can predispose to bacterial tracheitis

Suggested Intravenous Antimicrobial Treatment Regimens for Bacterial Tracheitis in Children

- Initial therapy for most common pathogens:
  - Anti-staphylococcal medicines (eg, vancomycin or clindamycin) + third-generation cephalosporin (eg, cefotaxime or ceftriaxone) or anti-staphylococcal medicines + ampicillin sulbactam
  - 10-day course
  - If influenza etiology, use antiviral if symptoms present for <72 hours

BRONCHIOLITIS

Etiology

RSV is the most common cause. Others: rhinovirus, parainfluenza, influenza, adenovirus.

- Typically affects 0 to 2 year olds (peak 2-6 months) from October to April

Differential Diagnosis

- Viral-triggered asthma, pneumonia, foreign body, GERD, congenital heart disease/heart failure—lack of preceding URT symptoms before onset of wheezing may help rule out bronchiolitis

Risk Factors for RSV

- Prematurity (<37 weeks GA), low birth weight, lung disease (eg, cystic fibrosis), congenital heart disease, congenital abnormalities of airway

- Environmental risk factors: older siblings, First Nations, passive smoke, household crowding, day care

Signs/Symptoms
- Expiratory wheeze
- URTI prodrome (eg, low grade fever, cough, nasal congestion/discharge, mild cough)
- Respiratory distress (apnea/tachypnea, grunting, nasal flaring, tachycardia), hypoxemia
- Factors associated with increased severity: look toxic, <95% O_2 saturation on room air, <3 months, respiratory rate $\geq$70, atelectasis on CXR

Associated Findings
- Atelectasis on CXR
- Acute otitis media
- UTI
- Dehydration

Investigations
- Clinical diagnosis!
- CBC and CXR if <3 months with fever and signs of LRTI or if diagnosis unsure. May see hyperinflation, peribronchial thickening, and patchy atelectasis with volume loss from airway narrowing and mucus plugging on CXR.
- Pulse oximetry; ABG in severe cases

Treatment
- Trial of inhaled bronchodilators; continue only if clinical response
- Glucocorticoids should **not** be used routinely
- Patients generally recover without treatment in 2 to 4 days. Wheezing can last for more than 7 days in some cases.
- Ribavirin may be beneficial in high-risk patients

Prevention
- Palivizumab prophylaxis if <24 months with chronic lung disease or history of prematurity <35 weeks gestational age or congenital heart disease

PERTUSSIS (AKA "WHOOPING COUGH")

Most commonly affected are <6 months olds (too young to be immunized); approx. 50% are adolescents/adults. Highly contagious! Acute tracheobronchitis caused by *Bordetella pertussis* bacteria; transmitted by respiratory droplets.

- Incubation period usually 7 to 10 days. Most contagious during catarrhal period (first 1-2 weeks) and first 2 weeks of paroxysmal phase.

Risk Factors
- Lack of/incomplete vaccination, exposure to infected person (household contact is most common source of infection in <6 month infant)

Signs/Symptoms
- Prolonged illness, cough >2 weeks
- Inspiratory "whoop" (in kids)
- Paroxysmal coughing
- Post-tussive vomiting
- Apnea (rather than cough)—young infants
- Low grade fever

- Stages:
  - Phase 1: catarrhal phase (1-2 weeks)
    - Nonspecific prodromal symptoms like URTI: coryza, rhinorrhea, mild cough, malaise, low grade fever
  - Phase 2: paroxysmal phase (4-6 weeks in children, 2-3 months in adults)
    - Spasmodic cough during day/night with minimal symptoms between coughing episodes
    - Inspiratory "whoop" (more common in younger due to small trachea)
    - May have post-tussive vomiting/syncope
  - Phase 3: convalescent phase (1-2 weeks)
    - Gradual decrease in cough frequency and severity
- In adolescents/adults: most have been vaccinated or had previous infection; present late with persistent cough (>4 weeks of coughing); cough may be only at night

Investigations

- Nasal swab (PCR). Report suspected cases.
- Diagnostic criteria for confirmed pertussis (≥1 of following):
  - Acute cough with culture(+) for *B. pertussis*
    - Culture from posterior nasopharynx is gold standard (not anterior nares or throat)
  - PCR(+) in patients meeting clinical diagnosis
  - Clinical diagnosis positive in patient in contact with verified *B. pertussis*

Treatment

- Supportive
- Erythromycin × 7days (decreases infectivity, but does not alter disease course or cough severity!)
  - If child <1 month: use azithromycin
- Patient remains contagious for 5 days after starting antibiotics
- Same antibiotic for close contacts and post-exposure prophylaxis
- Vaccination:
  - DTaP for incompletely immunized close contacts ≤7 year old
  - Consider booster (Tdap) after 10 year olds to 64 year olds are exposed
  - CDC recommendations for pregnant women and those having close contact with infant <12 months:
    - Tetanus toxoid, reduced diphtheria toxoid, and acellular pertussis vaccine (Tdap) in pregnant women and persons having close contact with an infant <12 months
    - Tdap should be given to pregnant women with no previous dose after the 20th week gestational age (third trimester preferred) or immediately postpartum
    - Pregnant women who have previously received Tdap and need tetanus or diphtheria vaccine while pregnant should get Td
  - The SOGC states: "Susceptible women to be vaccinated as per general guidelines for non-pregnant patients" and state there is no evidence of teratogenicity as diphtheria/tetanus is not a live virus

EPIGLOTTITIS (MEDICAL EMERGENCY!)

High airway inflammation (and obstruction) due to rapid infection and edema of epiglottis

Etiology

- *Haemophilus influenzae* type B, beta-hemolytic streptococci (groups A, B, C). Peaks at 2 to 8 years old, and 35 to 39 years old.

Signs/Symptoms

- Tripod position, stridor (late finding), hoarse/muffled voice, fever, sore throat, dysphagia, cervical adenopathy, drooling. Neck tenderness in adults.

Investigations

- Avoid inspection of airway and delay phlebotomy—can increase anxiety → complete obstruction!
- Lateral neck x-ray ("thumb sign," pencil-thin airway)
- Direct laryngoscopy—*done in OR! See "cherry-red" epiglottis
- Look for coexisting infections (otitis media, pneumonia, meningitis, cellulitis)
- CBC (increased neutrophils with left shift), blood culture

Treatment

- Intubation, admit to ICU, IV corticosteroids, IV ceftriaxone (drug of choice for *H. influenzae*), empiric broad-spectrum second- or third-generation for 7 to 10 days until culture and sensitivity result, IV fluids, O_2. (Avoid racemic epinephrine.)
- Alternative is ampicillin-sulbactam

Prevention: Vaccinate!

RETROPHARYNGEAL ABSCESS

Seventy-five percent of cases <5 year old. Unilateral presentation is more common in 15 to 30 year olds.

Etiology

GAS (50%) +/− aerobes/anaerobes of mouth flora

- Usually extension of pharyngeal infection (45%), foreign body (27%)

Signs/Symptoms

- Prodrome of sore throat + fever
- Odynophagia → decreased oral intake
- Torticollis
- Neck swelling/pain +/− mass, cervical lymphadenopathy

Investigations

- Aerobic and anaerobic culture and sensitivity of secretions/abscess
- Lateral neck x-ray (bulging posterior pharynx; >7 mm at C2, >14 mm at C6 is abnormal). Plain x-ray has limited use in evaluating deep neck space infections but can be helpful to detect retropharyngeal swelling or epiglottitis.
- U/S is tool for intra-operative aspiration and drainage; can distinguish between adenitis and abscess
- CT is imaging of choice for diagnosis of deep neck space infections

Treatment

- Secure airway
- Trans-oral approach for I&D
- Antibiotics: IV penicillin G × 10 days

PERITONSILLAR ABSCESS/QUINSY

Polymicrobial infection with collection of pus behind tonsil(s). Can be life-threatening! Usually unilateral.

Etiology

- More common in 20 to 40 year olds, more common from November to December and April to May (highest incidence of Streptococcal pharyngitis and exudative tonsillitis). Usually a complication of Streptococcal pharyngitis or tonsillitis → cellulitis → abscess formation due to salivary duct blockage.

Risk Factors

- Oropharynx/dental infection, periodontal disease, smoking

Signs/Symptoms

- Sore throat/neck, dysphagia, odynophagia, fever, "hot potato" voice, trismus, otalgia
- Drooling, halitosis
- Deviation of uvula, asymmetry of soft palate, ipsilateral palatal edema

Diagnosis

- Clinical

Investigations to Consider

- Needle aspiration
- Neck CT or MRI. U/S can differentiate peritonsillar abscess vs. cellulitis.

Treatment

- Aspiration or surgical drainage + antibiotics for 10 to 14 days
  - IV: ampicillin sulbactam; or penicillin G + metronidazole
    - Alternative is clindamycin
  - Oral: amox-clav or penicillin VK + metronidazole or clindamycin
- Hydration + pain control

Bibliography

CDC. http://www.cdc.gov/vaccines/pubs/vis/downloads/vis-td-tdap.pdf.

Chow AW, Calderwood SB, Thorner AR. Deep neck space infections. Up to Date.

DynaMed [database online]. Acute epiglottitis. EBSCO Publishing. http://web.ebscohost.com.cyber.usask.ca/dynamed/detail?vid=34&hid=9&sid=5fdbf4ec-bc94-440b-af64-b72b84140e48%40sessionmgr4&bdata=JnNpdGU9ZHluYW1lZC1saXZlJnNjb3BlPXNpdGU%3d#db=dme&AN=115468. Accessed February 3, 2012.

DynaMed [database online]. Croup. EBSCO Publishing. http://web.ebscohost.com.cyber.usask.ca/dynamed/detail?vid=41&hid=9&sid=5fdbf4ec-bc94-440b-af64-b72b84140e48%40sessionmgr4&bdata=JnNpdGU9ZHluYW1lZC1saXZlJnNjb3BlPXNpdGU%3d#db=dme&AN=114811. Accessed February 2, 2012.

DynaMed [database online]. Peritonsillar abscess. EBSCO Publishing. http://web.ebscohost.com.cyber.usask.ca/dynamed/detail?vid=43&hid=9&sid=5fdbf4ec-bc94-440b-af64-b72b84140e48%40sessionmgr4&bdata=JnNpdGU9ZHluYW1lZC1saXZlJnNjb3BlPXNpdGU%3d#db=dme&AN=115937. Accessed December 5, 2012.

DynaMed [database online]. Pertussis. EBSCO Publishing. http://web.ebscohost.com.cyber.usask.ca/dynamed/detail?vid=45&hid=9&sid=5fdbf4ec-bc94-440b-af64-b72b84140e48%40sessionmgr4&bdata=JnNpdGU9ZHluYW1lZC1saXZlJnNjb3BlPXNpdGU%3d#db=dme&AN=114591. Accessed December 5, 2012.

DynaMed [database online]. Respiratory syncytial virus (RSV) infection in infants and children. EBSCO Publishing. http://web.ebscohost.com.cyber.usask.ca/dynamed/detail?vid=38&hid=9&sid=5fdbf4ec-bc94-440b-af64-b72b84140e48%40sessionmgr4&bdata=JnNpdGU9ZHluYW1lZC1saXZlJnNjb3BlPXNpdGU%3d#db=dme&AN=115760. Accessed December 5, 2012.

DynaMed [database online]. Retropharyngeal abscess. EBSCO Publishing. http://web.ebscohost.com.cyber.usask.ca/dynamed/detail?vid=47&hid=9&sid=5fdbf4ec-bc94-440b-af64-b72b84140e48%40sessionmgr4&bdata=JnNpdGU9ZHluYW1lZC1saXZlJnNjb3BlPXNpdGU%3d#db=dme&AN=115742. Accessed February 3, 2012.

Guidelines for the diagnosis and management of croup. Towards Optimized Practice. 2008. http://www.topalbertadoctors.org/cpgs.php?sid=12&cpg_cats=35&cpg_info=7. Accessed on March 25, 2012.

SOCG Clinical Practice Guideline. Immunization in Pregnancy. December 2008; 220:1149-1154. http://www.sogc.org/guidelines/documents/gui220CPG0812.pdf.

Up to Date. Bacterial tracheitis in children: clinical features and diagnosis. Accessed Feb 3, 2012.

Up to Date. Bacterial tracheitis in children: treatment and prevention. Accessed Feb 3, 2012.

Up to Date. Bronchiolitis in infants and children: clinical features and diagnosis. Accessed Feb 12, 2012.

Up to Date. Bronchiolitis in infants and children: treatment; outcome; and prevention. Accessed Feb 12, 2012.

Pneumonia

Priority Topic 73

Definition

An inflammatory condition of the lung affecting the alveoli predominantly. It is associated with fever, chest symptoms, and a decrease in air space (consolidation) on a chest x-ray. Typically caused by an infection (bacteria, virus, fungi, or parasite).

ADULTS

1. Signs and symptoms
   - Dyspnea
   - Fever
   - Chest discomfort
   - Pleuritic pain
   - Productive cough
   - Increased heart rate and respiratory rate
   - Focal abnormal breath sounds
   - Atypical = insidious onset of fever, nonproductive cough, constitutional symptoms
   - Keep pneumonia on differential diagnosis in points with deterioration, delirium, and abdominal pain

2. Comorbidity includes
   - Chronic heart/lung disease
   - Liver disease
   - Renal disease
   - Diabetes mellitus
   - Alcohol abuse
   - Malignancy
   - Asplenia
   - Immunosuppressed
   - Hospital admission in past 3 months
   - Nursing home resident

3. Investigations
   - WBC, ABG, CXR, sputum culture and sensitivity, lytes if needed.
   - The CURB-65 score can be used to assess severity and guides decision if patient should be hospitalized.
   - **CURB-65** score (see Table 3-4):
     - **C**onfusion (based on specific mental test or new disorientation to person, place, or time)
     - **U**rea (BUN) >7 mmol/L (20 mg/dL)
     - **R**espiratory rate >30 breaths/minute
     - **B**lood pressure (systolic <90 mm Hg or diastolic <60 mm Hg)
     - Age >**65** years

TABLE 3-4	CURB-65 Score
SCORE	SUGGESTED MANAGEMENT
0-1 points	Low severity (risk of death <3%). Outpatient therapy is usually appropriate.
2 points	Moderate severity (risk of death 9%). Consider hospitalization.
3-5 points	High severity (risk of death 15%-40%). Hospitalization indicated. Assess patient for possible ICU admission, especially if the CURB-65 score is 4 or 5.

CHILDREN

1. Kids <5 years old and kids born at 24 to 28 weeks gestational age have increased risk of severe disease
2. Signs and symptoms
   - Cough, tachypnea, dyspnea, fever, wheezing, lethargy, irritability, poor feeding, signs of dehydration, vomiting, diarrhea, abdominal pain, and headache
3. Social history
   - Daycare; exposure to second-hand smoke
4. Physical
   - Temperature, respiratory rate, O_2 saturation, labored breathing, HEENT, chest, lungs, abdominal examination
5. Testing to consider
   - Pulse oximetry at triage to assess severity and then as needed
   - CXR, CBC, CRP/ESR
   - Bun/Cr, electrolytes
   - ABG if toxic
   - Blood culture
   - Nasopharyngeal specimen for rapid viral antigen testing for influenza and other viruses

PNEUMONIA IN ADULTS AND CHILDREN ETIOLOGY AND TREATMENT OVERVIEW

Etiology and Treatment (See Table 3-5)

TABLE 3-5 Etiology and Treatment of Pneumonia

	PEDIATRICS				ADULTS		
Age	0-4 weeks	4 weeks-3 months	3 months-5 years	5-18 years	CAP	Elderly/nursing home/comorbidities	HIV
Etiology	Escherichia coli GBS Listeria	Viral GAS E. coli Streptococcus Pneumonia	Viral (RSV, adeno, others) S. pneumonia Staphylococcus aureus GAS	Mycoplasma Chlamydia pneumoniae, S. pneumoniae Viruses	S. pneumoniae Mycoplasma. pneumoniae C. pneumoniae	Streptococcus Haemophilus influenzae Gram (−) rods Staphylococcus Legionella	PCP
Treatment	Ampicillin + Gentamicin	Second-generation cephalosporin	Amoxicillin or Macrolide *No antibiotic indicated if viral cause	Macrolide	Amoxicillin (>50 years old) or Macrolide or Quinolone	Amoxicillin + Macrolide or Quinolone	TMP-SMX

Use ciprofloxacin if pseudomonas is a concern.

Consider empyema if patient is not improving on antibiotics.

- Fluoroquinolones—reserved for treatment failures; recent antibiotic use; or allergy
- Aspiration—anaerobic coverage (amoxicillin-clavulanate or clindamycin)
- Duration of treatment: generally 7 to 14 days. If considering shorter course, patients should be treated for minimum of 5 days and be afebrile for 48 to 72 hours.
- Children 1-3 months → always admit and consult peds

Further Management Considerations

- Look for decompensation (need to ventilate, CPAP, BiPAP) before it happens
- Keep in mind to admit patients who may be at risk for complications
- Vaccinate those with comorbidities with influenza and pneumococcal infections

- Be aware of drug interactions (especially warfarin and antibiotics)
- Do contact tracing if needed
- Follow up is important
- Always rule out aspiration, tuberculosis, and HIV before choosing antibiotics (or reassess the diagnosis if patient not improving)

Bibliography

Anti-infective Review Panel. *Anti-infective Guidelines for Community-Acquired Infections.* Toronto: MUMS Guideline Clearinghouse; 2012.

Bauer T, et al. BRB-65 predicts death from community acquired pneumonia. *J Int Med.* 2006;260:93-101.

Chen AY, Tran C. Toronto Notes. Toronto, ON: Type & Graphics Inc; 2011.

CURB-65. http://www.mdcalc.com/curb-65-severity-score-community-acquired-pneumonia/. Accessed April 27, 2012.

Rx Files. Anti-infectives—oral. *Drug Comparison Charts.* 8th ed. 2010; 56-57.

Meningitis

Priority Topic 62

Definition

Inflammation of the meninges covering the brain and spinal cord.

Etiology

- Bacterial: *Escherichia coli*, GBS, *Haemophilus influenzae*, *Streptococcus pneumoniae*, *Neisseria meningitides*, *Listeria monocytogenes*, *Staphylococcus aureus*
- Viral: Enterovirus, HIV, HSV, West Nile
- Fungal: Cryptococcus, Coccidioidomycosis

Risk Factors

- Hematogenous spread (respiratory infection, bacterial endocarditis)
- Parameningeal focus (AOM, sinusitis)
- Head trauma (penetrating)
- Previous neurosurgery/shunts
- Immunocompromised/contact with infected person

Physical Examination

- Fever, vomiting, lethargy, irritability, poor feeding, headache, confusion, neck stiffness, seizure, meningismus
- Brudzinski sign: passive flexion of neck causes involuntary flexion of hip/knees
- Kernigs sign: resistance to knee extension when hip flexed to 90 degrees

TRIAD: fever, altered mental status, nuchal rigidity

Investigations

- Labs: blood culture, WBC with differential, LP/CSF
- CSF: See Table 3-6.

TABLE 3-6	CSF Profiles	
	BACTERIAL	VIRAL
Appearance	Normal or cloudy	Usually normal
Glucose	Low	Normal
Protein	High	Moderate increase
WBC count (cells/mm³)	>1000	<1000
Predominant WBC	Neutrophils (PMNs) predominant	Lymphocytes and monocytes

Treatment

- See Table 3-7

TABLE 3-7	Treatment				
	NEONATES (1-3 MONTHS)	**INFANTS/KIDS**	**TEENS/ADULTS**	**ELDERLY**	**SHUNT**
Bacterial	E. coli	H. influenzae	S. pneumoniae	S. pneumoniae	S. aureus
	GBS	S. pneumoniae	N. meningitis	N. meningitis	Gram (−)ve
	Listeria	N. meningitis		Listeria	
Treatment (empiric)	Ampicillin + Cefotaxime	Vancomycin + Ceftriaxone	Vancomycin + Ceftriaxone	Vancomycin + Ceftriaxone + Ampicillin (for listeria)	

Prevention

See "Immunizations" for further details

Note: Chemoprophylaxis of close contacts needed for HiB and meningococcus. Add Acyclovir if HSV on differential diagnosis.

Bibliography

Agabegi S, Agabegi E. Step-up to medicine. 2nd ed. Philadelphia, PA: Lippincott & Williams & Wilkins; 2008.

Chen YA, Tran C. *Toronto Notes–Comprehensive Medical Reference & Review for MCCQE I and USMLE II.* Toronto, Canada: Toronto Notes for Medical Students Inc; 2011.

4
Surgery

Abdominal Pain
Priority Topic 1

TABLE 4-1	Differential Diagnosis of Abdominal Pain by Quadrants	
Right hypochondrium • Gallbladder • Liver	**Epigastric** • Pancreatitis • Peptic ulcer	**Left hypochondrium** • Spleen
Right lumbar • Kidney stone • Renal	**Umbilical** • AAA	**Left lumbar** • Kidney stone • Renal
Right iliac • Appendicitis	**Hypogastric/suprapubic** • Urinary • Gynecological	**Left iliac** • Diverticulitis

ABDOMINAL PAIN–GENERAL CONSIDERATIONS

- Acute abdominal pain
  - Consider life-threatening causes, resuscitate and refer for definitive treatment
- Chronic abdominal pain
  - Ensure follow-up, manage symptoms with lifestyle modification and medication, consider malignancy
  - Consider extraintestinal manifestations of inflammatory bowel disease
- **Always consider pregnancy, pelvic examination, and rectal examination**

HEMORRHOIDS

- Arise from dilated vascular plexus in anal canal
- **Presentation**
  - Rectal bleeding, anal pruritus, prolapse, painful if thrombosed (especially external hemorrhoids)
  - Bleeding not mixed with stool, can lead to anemia if chronic, usually painless
- **Risk factors**
  - Pregnancy, obesity, heavy lifting, portal hypertension, prolonged sitting, pelvic tumors, straining, advanced age, diarrhea, chronic constipation

- **Physical examination**
  - Location (above/below dentate line), prolapse, thrombosis, strangulation if grade IV
  - External hemorrhoids arise from below dentate line
  - Classification of internal hemorrhoids:
    - ◦ Grade I—bleeding but no prolapse from anal canal
    - ◦ Grade II—prolapse with straining but reduce spontaneously
    - ◦ Grade III—prolapse with straining requiring manual reduction
    - ◦ Grade IV—permanently prolapsed, irreducible, may strangulate
- **Treatment**
  - Increase fibre, bulking agents, adequate fluid intake
  - Sitz baths, avoid straining
  - Steroid cream, hydrocortisone suppositories (short term only)
  - Surgery for internal hemorrhoids unresponsive to conservative treatment: banding, hemorrhoidectomy

ANAL FISSURE

- Tear in the lining of the anal canal distal to the dentate line—results in spasm of sphincter muscle causing further tearing
- **Presentation**
  - Very painful rectal bleeding, blood on paper not mixed in stool
- **Risk factors**
  - Local trauma (eg, passage of hard stool), Crohn's disease, tuberculosis, leukemia, tightening of anal canal due to nervousness or pain
- Physical examination: gentle examination; may be too painful for DRE; posterior midline is most frequent location, second is anterior midline
- Treatment
  - Increase fibre: bulking agents, for example, psyllium or polycarbophils, adequate fluid intake
  - Sitz baths, avoid straining
  - Topical nitroglycerin (increased local blood flow reduces pressure on sphincter to allow for healing)
  - Other: botulinum toxin, calcium channel blocker (nifedipine, diltiazem) to reduce sphincter pressure
  - Surgery if persistent and not responsive to above: lateral sphincterotomy
  - Consider endoscopy if persistent/recurrent to assess for possible Crohn's disease
  - Consider colonoscopy

RECTAL ABSCESS AND FISTULA

- Bacterial infection of blocked anal gland
- **Presentation**
  - Painful, may have systemic symptoms/signs
- **Physical examination**
  - Look for signs of spreading infection, may feel mass on DRE
- **Treatment**
  - Timely incision and drainage, take swab for culture and sensitivity (C&S)
  - Antibiotics if evidence of cellulitis, or if immunosuppressed, diabetes, valvular heart disease
- **Complications**
  - May develop chronic suppurative fistula which requires surgical treatment (except for patients with Crohn's disease)

APPENDICITIS

- Inflammation of appendiceal wall followed by localized ischemia, perforation, and generalized peritonitis +/– abscess formation
  - Appendiceal obstruction is primary cause.
- **Presentation**
  - Right lower quadrant pain, anorexia, **followed by** nausea and vomiting, and **then** fever
  - Pain starts periumbilical, then moves to McBurney point
- **Physical examination**
  - Rovsing sign: palpation of left iliac fossa causes pain in right iliac fossa
  - Psoas sign: extension of right hip exacerbates pain
  - Obturator sign: rotation of flexed right hip exacerbates pain
- **Investigations**
  - Elevated WCC with left shift
  - β-HCG to rule out pregnancy
  - Urinalysis
- Imaging is unnecessary with high clinical suspicion and timely appendectomy, useful if appendicitis is suspected but unclear
  - Ultrasound: can rule in but cannot rule out
  - Contrast CT: good sensitivity and specificity, and can provide alternate diagnosis
- **Complications**
  - Perforated appendix (especially with symptoms >24 hours duration), abscess, phlegmon
- **Treatment**
  - NPO
  - IV fluids
  - Antibiotics
  - Surgery

INFLAMMATORY BOWEL DISEASE

- Chronic disease
- Two major disorders: ulcerative colitis and Crohn's disease (see Table 4-2)

TABLE 4-2 Ulcerative Colitis Vs. Crohn's: Characteristics		
	ULCERATIVE COLITIS	CROHN'S DISEASE
Site of involvement	Only involves colon Rectum almost always involved	Any area of the gastrointestinal tract Rectum usually spared
Pattern of involvement	Continuous	Skip lesions
Diarrhea	Bloody	Usually non-bloody
Severe abdominal pain	Rare	Frequent
Perianal disease	No	In 30% of patients
Fistula	No	Yes
Endoscopic findings	Erythematous and friable Superficial ulceration	Aphthoid and deep ulcers Cobblestoning

TABLE 4-2	Ulcerative Colitis Vs. Crohn's: Characteristics (*Continued*)	
	ULCERATIVE COLITIS	CROHN'S DISEASE
Radiologic findings	Tubular appearance resulting from loss of haustral folds	String sign of terminal ileum, RLQ mass, fistulas, abscesses
Histologic features	Mucosa only	Transmural
	Crypt abscesses	Crypt abscesses, granulomas (<30%)
Smoking	Protective	Worsens course
Serology	p-ANCA more common	ASCA more common

ASCA, anti-Saccharomyces cerevisiae antibodies; p-ANCA, perinuclear antineutrophil cytoplasmic antibody; RLQ, right lower quadrant.

CROHN'S DISEASE

- Inflammatory bowel disease characterized by transmural inflammation
- "Gum to Bum": skip lesions affecting any part of GI tract from mouth to anus; cobblestoning
  - Transmural inflammation results in thickened, fibrotic, strictured gut
  - 80% have small bowel involvement, usually in distal ileum
  - 50% have ileocolitis
  - 20% have colitis, and half of these will have rectal sparing
  - 30% have perianal disease
- **Presentation**
  - Fatigue, diarrhea, abdominal pain (may be severe), weight loss, fever, bleeding less common
  - Gradual onset, chronic course with remission and relapses
  - Usually 16 to 30 years old, higher risk in smokers (and smoking worsens course of disease)
- **Investigations**
  - Endoscopy (45% have ileo-cecal disease) with biopsies
  - Bloods: CBC, CRP, LFT, electrolytes, renal panel
  - Rule out infectious causes of diarrhea
- **Complications**
  - Fistulas, strictures/stenosis, kidney stones, vitamin B_{12} deficiency if ileal disease, colonic adenocarcinoma if colonic disease
- **Extraintestinal manifestations**
  - Arthritis, uveitis, iritis, pyoderma gangrenosum, erythema nodosum, primary sclerosing cholangitis, renal stones, osteoporosis, vitamin B_{12} deficiency
- **Treatment**
  - Acute therapy: oral steroids, 5-ASA, sulfasalazine, antibiotics (metronidazole +/− ciprofloxacin), bowel rest with TPN
  - Maintenance therapy: elemental diet, 5-ASA (mild disease), azathioprine, 6MP, methotrexate, anti-TNF (infliximab), quit smoking
  - Surgery: not curative, usually reserved for complications

ULCERATIVE COLITIS

- Inflammatory bowel disease characterized by inflammation of mucosal layer of colon
- Typically affects rectum and extends proximally in a continuous fashion

- **Presentation**
  - Insidious or acute
  - Abdominal pain, diarrhea, urgency, rectal bleeding and mucous
- **Investigations**
  - Flexible sigmoidoscopy +/− colonoscopy
  - Bloods: CBC, CRP, LFT, electrolytes, renal panel
- **Complications**
  - Toxic megacolon, bowel perforation, anemia, colonic adenocarcinoma
- **Extraintestinal manifestations**
  - Arthritis, uveitis, iritis, pyoderma gangrenosum, erythema nodosum, primary sclerosing cholangitis, lung disease, osteoporosis, fatty liver
- **Treatment**
  - Acute therapy: 5-ASA or sulfasalazine, oral or IV steroids for severe disease
  - Maintenance therapy: 5-ASA, sulfasalazine, anti-TNF (infliximab), 6MP, azathioprine
  - Surgery: can be curative but associated with multiple postoperative complications, and should be reserved for complications or patients unresponsive to medical treatment

IRRITABLE BOWEL SYNDROME

- Chronic/recurrent abdominal pain/discomfort with associated change in bowel habits, etiology unknown
  - Also complain of bloating, mucus, nausea, lethargy
- May be diarrhea or constipation predominant
- **Diagnosis**
  - Rome III symptom-based criteria:
    - Recurrent abdominal pain or discomfort at least 3 days/month over the last 3 months. Symptoms must be present for 6 months and include two or more of the following:
    - (1) Improved with defecation
    - (2) Associated with change in stool frequency
    - (3) Associated with change in stool form
- **Rule out alarm features**
  - Acute onset, fever, nausea/vomiting, unintentional weight loss >10 lb, anemia, hematochezia, melena, positive fecal occult blood test, change in bowel habits, symptoms refractory to current therapy, family history of colon cancer or inflammatory bowel disease
- **Investigations**
  - Bloodwork: celiac antibodies, +/− CBC
  - No other investigations necessary unless alarm features are present
- **Treatment**
  - Chronic course so patient-doctor relationship, patient education, and reassurance are important
  - Diet: slow eating, eat regular meals, stool bulking (psyllium, polycarbophils), increased fluids, avoid insoluble fiber, trial lactose-free diet, reduce caffeine, alcohol and carbonated beverages
  - Anti-diarrheals (loperamide) or laxatives (PEG, milk of magnesia, lubiprostone) depending on stool composition
  - Antispasmodics: peppermint oil, hyoscine, pinaverium
  - Probiotics: bifidobacteria recommended, no evidence for lactobacillus, use minimum 4 weeks

- Rifaximin (2 week antibiotic course) for diarrhea-predominant IBS may reduce symptoms for up to 3 months
- Counseling, CBT, hypnotherapy, relaxation techniques
- Consider antidepressants (SSRI or TCA) in refractory disease

PANCREATITIS

I GET SMASHED
Idiopathic
Gallstones
ETOH
Trauma
Steroids
Mumps
Autoimmune
Scorpion venom
Hyperlipidemia/Hypercalcemia/Hypothermia
ERCP/Emboli
Drugs (thiazide diuretics, valproic acid, estrogen, azathioprine, didanosine)

- Acute inflammation of pancreas
- Causes: **IGETSMASHED**
  - Gallstones and alcohol the most common
- **Presentation**
  - Rapid-onset upper abdominal pain (epigastric)
  - Constant, not colicky, band-like radiation to back
  - Associated with nausea and vomiting, +/− shock
- **Diagnosis**
  - Typical history, tender epigastrium, elevated WCC, elevated lipase and/or amylase (usually two to three times normal), abnormal LFTs (may be typical of gallstones or ETOH)
- **Imaging**
  - US will show diffusely enlarged pancreas and imaging of biliary tree (ie, looking for gallstones/gallstone pancreatitis)
  - CT is good for intraabdominal complications (pseudocyst, pancreatic necrosis or hemorrhage, abscess formation)
- **Treatment**
  - IV fluids, analgesia, NPO, observation, investigation for cause
  - ICU may be required if cysts, abscesses, necrotizing pancreatitis

DIVERTICULITIS

- Inflammation of diverticula or pouch-like protrusions of the colon wall
  - Increased intraluminal pressure or stool can lead to erosion of the diverticular wall. This can lead to inflammation, followed by possible necrosis and perforation.
- **Presentation**
  - Left lower quadrant pain, usually present for a few days prior to presentation
  - May have painless rectal bleeding
  - Alternating diarrhea and constipation, +/− nausea and vomiting, low grade fever, may have cramping, bloating, flatulence
- **Risk factors**
  - Lack of exercise, obesity, possibly low dietary fiber
- **Physical examination**
  - LLQ tenderness, distention, may palpate LLQ mass, may see signs of generalized peritonitis
  - Asian population more likely to have right-sided disease so may see RLQ tenderness
- **Diagnosis**
  - Based on history and examination
  - Other investigations are typically to rule out other causes of acute presentation
  - CT scan with contrast will diagnose and assess for severity, can also assess for complications (perforation, abscess)

- **Treatment**
  - Uncomplicated
    - Bowel rest with clear fluids only for 2 to 3 days
    - Antibiotics for 10 to 14 days, need to cover gram-negative rods and anaerobes
    - High fiber diet—no need to avoid seeds and nuts
    - Admission decision based on comorbidities, ability to tolerate PO, severity of presentation
  - Complicated: resuscitation, broad spectrum antibiotics, and surgical intervention may be required if obstruction, perforation, abscess, or fistula are present
- **Follow-up**
  - Once acute episode has resolved, colonoscopy or barium enema and flexible sigmoidoscopy should be done to fully evaluate the colon

ABDOMINAL AORTIC ANEURYSM

- Degeneration of aortic wall leads to dilation of the aorta
  - Normal diameter approx. 2 cm
  - Aneurysmal ≥3 cm
- **Presentation**
  - Asymptomatic: found incidentally on abdominal examination or US/CT/MRI for other reason
  - Symptomatic: pain, may be abdominal, back, flank, groin; often mimics other disease presentations
    - May be described as ripping/tearing sensation
    - Pain unaffected by position or movement
  - Ruptured AAA:
    - Triad is pathognomonic: pain, pulsatile abdominal mass, hypotension
- **Risk factors**
  - Increased age, male gender (four to six times increased risk), atherosclerosis, hypertension, hypercholesterolemia, coronary artery disease, cerebrovascular disease, family history, Caucasian race
- **Physical examination**
  - Abdominal palpation: widened pulse/pulsatile abdominal mass
    - More common if located between xiphoid and umbilicus (infrarenal and above inferior mesenteric arteries)
    - Increased sensitivity with increasing aorta diameter
  - Peripheral vascular examination
- **Diagnosis**
  - Abdominal US is investigation of choice
  - CT can be used for monitoring of AAA size, however higher radiation doses and contrast required
- **Treatment**
  - Serial monitoring:
    - Unlikely to rupture if <5 cm
    - Aneurysm 4.0 to 5.5 cm: US or CT every 6 to 12 months
    - Aneurysm 3.0 to 4.0 cm: US every 2 to 3 years
  - Medical treatment:
    - Quit smoking
    - Risk factor reduction: statin, ASA, beta blocker are all recommended
    - Antibiotic therapy is under investigation

Ruptured AAA Triad
Pain
Pulsatile abdominal mass hypotension

- Elective surgical repair:
  - For asymptomatic aneurysms ≥5.5 cm
  - For asymptomatic aneurysms with rapid rate of expansion >0.5 cm in 6 months
  - For aneurysms greater than twice the size of the non-aneurysmal aorta

ACUTE MESENTERIC ISCHEMIA

- Caused by intestinal hypoperfusion due to an occlusive or non-occlusive obstruction affecting venous or arterial circulation
- **Four major causes**
  - Superior mesenteric artery embolism—50%
  - Superior mesenteric artery thrombosis—15% to 25%
  - Mesenteric venous thrombosis—5%
  - Non-occlusive ischemia—20% to 30%
- **Risk factors**
  - Coagulopathy, congestive heart failure, atrial fibrillation, peripheral vascular disease, aortic insufficiency, sepsis, cardiac arrhythmias, diuretics (reduce intestinal perfusion), digoxin, alpha-adrenergic agonists, history or family history of embolic events
- **Presentation**
  - Rapid onset of severe periumbilical pain
  - Nausea and vomiting
  - Hallmark is **pain out of proportion to physical findings**
- **Physical examination**
  - Abdominal examination may be normal
  - May see abdominal distention, signs of peripheral vasculitis
- **Imaging**
  - Dynamic CT scan if no peritoneal signs on examination
  - Mesenteric angiography if peritoneal signs present on examination
- **Diagnosis**
  - Clinical suspicion plus radiological evidence on dynamic CT or mesenteric angiography
- **Treatment**
  - Depends on imaging findings of embolus, thrombosis, or vasoconstriction, but may involve: anticoagulation, thrombolytics, surgical intervention

CONSTIPATION

- Rome III criteria for constipation requires the following criteria for 3 months, with symptoms present for at least 6 months:
  - Must include two or more of the following:
    - Straining during at least 25% of defecations
    - Lumpy or hard stools in at least 25% of defecations
    - Sensation of incomplete evacuation for at least 25% of defecations
    - Sensation of anorectal obstruction/blockage for at least 25% of defecations
    - Manual maneuvers to facilitate at least 25% of defecations (eg, digital evacuation, support of the pelvic floor)
    - Fewer than three defecations per week
  - Loose stools are rarely present without the use of laxatives
  - Insufficient criteria for IBS

- **Causes**
  - Most common cause is related to inadequate fiber intake, decreased fluid intake, physical inactivity
  - Primary constipation can be functional, due to slow transit, due to outlet dysfunction, or a combination
- **History**
  - Family history, comorbidities (secondary causes), diet, exercise, medications
- **Physical examination**
  - Rectal examination to assess for presence of mass, pathology causing pain during defecation, abnormal tone
  - Abdominal examination
- **Diagnosis**
  - In absence of alarm symptoms in patients <50 years old, the diagnosis is clinical
  - In presence of alarm symptoms, further investigations are required
- **Investigations**
  - None recommended routinely, investigation should be prompted by age and history/examination findings
  - If secondary cause suspected, or ≥50, consider:
    - CBC, electrolytes, calcium, blood sugar, thyroid
  - If alarm symptoms are present:
    - Fecal occult blood test and colon inspection (colonoscopy or flexible sigmoidoscopy with barium enema)
  - If refractory to treatment: further investigations of colon transit time and anorectal physiology are required, and specialist referral should be made
- **Treatment**
  - Dietary modifications
    - Increase fibre intake to 25 g/day, and ensure fluid intake of 1.5–2 L/day
  - Increased exercise
    - Laxatives
    - Surfactants—docusate sodium
    - Osmotic agents—polyethylene glycol, lactulose, milk of magnesia
    - Stimulants—bisacodyl, senna, sodium pico sulfate
  - Severe constipation
    - Manual disimpaction
    - Suppositories: glycerin or bisacodyl
    - Enema: mineral oil, saline, phosphate
    - Pharmacotherapy to increase colon transit may be trialed in refractory constipation, although evidence is not strong (misoprostol, colchicine)
  - Surgical treatment is rarely indicated

Secondary Constipation: DOPED
- **D**rugs: CCB, beta blocker, opioid, diuretic, antidepressant, anticonvulsant, antacid, anticholinergic, antispasmodic
- **O**bstruction: small bowel obstruction, colon cancer
- **P**ain
- **E**ndocrine: DM, hypothyroid, hypokalemia, hypercalcemia
- **D**epression
- also: Neurological (Parkinson, MS), Scleroderma, Ileus

CONSTIPATION ALARM FEATURES
Acute onset, fever, nausea/vomiting, unintentional weight loss >10 lb, anemia, hematochezia, melena, positive fecal occult blood test, change in bowel habits, symptoms refractory to current therapy, family history of colon cancer, or inflammatory bowel disease.

SMALL BOWEL OBSTRUCTION

- Obstruction is most often caused by mechanical obstruction of small bowel, but consider large bowel obstruction (usually due to malignancy) or nonmechanical obstruction secondary to ileus (see Table 4-3)
  - Low grade—partial obstruction
  - High grade—complete obstruction

TABLE 4-3	Obstruction: Type and Signs/Symptoms		
	SMALL BOWEL OBSTRUCTION	LARGE BOWEL OBSTRUCTION	PARALYTIC ILEUS
Nausea and vomiting	Early finding, may be bilious	Late finding, may be feculent	Present
Abdominal pain	Colicky	Colicky	Absent
Abdominal distention	+++	++	+
Bowel sounds	Normal or increased, may hear high-pitched BS	Normal or increased, may hear high-pitched BS	Decreased or absent
Abdominal x-ray findings	Air/fluid levels	Air/fluid levels	Air throughout colon

Adapted with permission from *Toronto Notes*.

- **Causes**
  - Hernia, adhesions (60%), neoplasm, gallstone ileus, intussusception, volvulus
  - Also: trauma, radiation, inflammatory bowel disease, foreign body
- **Presentation**
  - Crampy abdominal pain, abdominal distention, vomiting, inability to pass flatus
- **History**
  - Hematochezia, previous abdominal surgery, inflammatory bowel disease, history or family history of cancer, radiation
- **Physical examination**
  - Examine for abdominal masses, peritonism, hernias, and signs of shock
- **Diagnosis**
  - Typically diagnosed based on history and examination, with x-ray to confirm
  - Abdominal x-ray, three views: air/fluid levels, dilated bowel loops
  - Bloods: WCC, blood gas to assess for metabolic acidosis
  - CT with contrast may be considered for further information, for example, to identify a discrete transition point, or if x-ray is inconclusive
    - Useful for patients with a history of malignancy, those with no history of abdominal surgery or risk factors for SBO, or post-surgery
- **Complications**
  - Peritonitis, bowel necrosis, bowel perforation, sepsis
- **Treatment**
  - Conservative management if no signs of peritonitis, tachycardia, fever, leucocytosis, metabolic acidosis
    - More likely to be successful with partial SBO
    - NG tube on suction, IV fluids, strict bowel rest, serial abdominal examinations, foley catheter to monitor fluid status
    - If no improvement within 12 to 24 hours, consider contrast imaging studies and/or surgery

SBO Causes: HANG IV
- Hernia
- Adhesions
- Neoplasm
- Gallstone ileus
- Intussusception
- Volvulus

BILIARY TRACT AND CHOLELITHIASIS

- Cholelithiasis is the presence of stones (aka calculi) in the gallbladder
  - Stone composition: cholesterol, pigmented
- **Risk factors**
  - 4Fs: female, fat, forty, fertile
  - Also: pregnancy, cyclical weight loss, rapid weight loss, postmenopausal estrogen, ceftriaxone

4F's of Cholelithiasis
Female
Fat
Forty
Fertile

- Gallstones are typically asymptomatic
- Can precipitate biliary colic, acute cholecystitis, ascending cholangitis, acute pancreatitis
- **Diagnosis**
  - Abdominal ultrasound
  - May see elevated bilirubin, LFT abnormalities (elevated ALP)
- **Treatment**
  - No treatment required for asymptomatic cholelithiasis
  - See following sections for symptomatic gallstones

BILIARY COLIC

- This occurs when the gallbladder contracts, often due to a fatty meal resulting in hormonal or neural stimulation
  - Contraction forces a stone or sludge into the cystic duct opening, leading to increased pressure within the gallbladder, and resulting in pressure and pain
  - As the gallbladder relaxes, the pain subsides, usually lasting <8 hours
- **Presentation**
  - RUQ abdominal pain which is dull, intense, and constant (the term "colicky" is a misnomer)
  - May occur 1 to 2 hours following a fatty meal but often unrelated to meals
  - Pain lasts <8 hours
  - May complain of chest pain
  - May be associated with nausea, vomiting, diaphoresis
- **Diagnosis**
  - Known gallstones on abdominal ultrasound, typical history, no leucocytosis or fevers, clinically stable, pain settles with time
- **Treatment**
  - Analgesia
  - Elective cholecystectomy or conservative management depending on frequency of attacks

CHOLEDOCHOLITHIASIS

- Stones are present in the common bile duct
- Ductal stones can form in the absence of a gallbladder, but are usually formed in the gallbladder
- **Complications**
  - Ascending cholangitis, obstructive jaundice, secondary biliary cirrhosis
- **Presentation**
  - RUQ pain, may radiate to back, associated with fever/chills, jaundice
- **Diagnosis**
  - ERCP, endoscopic US, MRCP
- **Treatment**
  - Risk is stratified by visualization of CBD stone on abdominal US
    - "Very strong" predictors—treatment of choice is ERCP
      - CBD stone on transabdominal ultrasound
      - Clinical ascending cholangitis
      - Serum bilirubin >68 µmol/L

- "Strong" predictors—treatment is (1) laparoscopic cholecystectomy with intraoperative cholangiography, *or* (2) further imaging (MRCP/EUS) and reassessment
  - A dilated CBD on ultrasound (>6 mm)
  - Serum bilirubin 31-68 μmol/L
- "Moderate" predictors—treatment is laparoscopic cholecystectomy or look for alternate diagnosis
  - Abnormal liver biochemical test other than bilirubin
  - Age > 55 years
  - Clinical gallstone pancreatitis

ACUTE CHOLECYSTITIS

- Acute inflammation of the gallbladder with obstruction leading to gallbladder wall thickening and secondary infection
  - Calculous (>90%): obstruction of the cystic duct with a stone or sludge
  - Acalculous: no stones or sludge, difficult to diagnose, and high mortality rate
- **Common organisms**
  - *Escherichia coli* (40%), Enterococcus (12%), Klebsiella (11%), and Enterobacter (9%)
- **Risk factors**
  - Cholelithiasis, helminthic infection by ascariasis (common in Asia, Africa, Latin America)
- **Presentation**
  - Classic presentation is syndrome of fever, RUQ pain, and leucocytosis
  - Also anorexia, nausea and vomiting, change in mental status (especially in elderly)
- **Diagnosis & Physical Examination**
  - Clinical diagnosis requires at least one local sign/symptom and at least one systemic signs/symptoms
  - Local: Murphy's sign, RUQ tenderness or mass
  - Systemic: fever, leukocytosis, elevated C-reactive protein (CRP)
  - Confirm acute cholecystitis with US or HIDA scan
- **Treatment**
  - IV antibiotics, for example, ceftriaxone plus metronidazole
  - Early cholecystectomy

CHARCOT'S TRIAD
Fever
RUQ pain
Jaundice

RAYNAUD'S PENTAD
Fever
RUQ pain
Jaundice
Hypotension
Confusion

ACUTE CHOLANGITIS

- Clinical syndrome where stasis and infection of biliary tract lead to mild life-threatening disease
- **Risk factors**
  - Biliary obstruction, stasis (often due to calculus or stricture)
- **Presentation**
  - Charcot's triad occurs in 50% to 70%: fever, RUQ pain, and jaundice
  - Raynaud pentad: fever, RUQ pain, jaundice, hypotension/shock, and confusion

- **Diagnosis**
  - Bloodwork: elevated ALP, GGT, bilirubin, wbc's, neutrophil
    - May see aminotransferases around 1000 IU/L with abscess formation
  - Abdominal ultrasound
- **Treatment**
  - Antibiotics
  - ERCP (see "Choledocholithiasis") or surgical cholecystectomy

TABLE 4-4	Pediatric Abdominal Pain		
	DUODENAL ATRESIA	**PYLORIC STENOSIS**	**INTUSSUSCEPTION**
Definition	• Congenital defect of the duodenum • Leads to obstruction or complete atresia	• Thickened pylorus leads to gastric outflow obstruction	• Telescoping of proximal bowel segment into distal segment
Presentation	• Bile-stained vomit • Feed intolerance	• Nonbilious projectile vomiting post feeds • Good appetite • May present with dehydration or weight loss	• Triad: abdominal pain, sausage shaped mass in RUQ, red-currant jelly stools • Sudden onset of severe paroxysms of pain • Pain-free intervals
Physical examination	• No abdominal distention	• Palpable olive-shaped pylorus muscle • Visible peristalsis	• RUQ sausage-shaped mass
Risk factors	• Down syndrome	• 3-8 weeks of age • Males	• Cystic fibrosis • 3 months to 3 years old
Investigation	• Abdominal x-ray shows "double bubble" secondary to dilated stomach and duodenum • Consider upper GI series to rule out malrotation	• Abdominal ultrasound: pyloric muscle thickness >3 mm	• Abdominal x-ray with air or contrast enema • Abdominal ultrasound • Frequently at ileocecal junction
Treatment	• NPO and NG tube • Surgical correction	• Surgical pyloromyotomy	• Abdominal x-ray with air or contrast enema • Surgery for failed enema reduction

Bibliography

Afdhal NH. Acute cholangitis. In: Basow DS, ed., *UpToDate*. Waltham, MA; 2012. Retrieved from http://www.uptodate.com/. Accessed March 23, 2012.

Black CE, Martin RF. Acute appendicitis in adults: Clinical manifestations and diagnosis. In: Basow DS, ed. *UpToDate*. Waltham, MA; 2012. Retrieved from http://www.uptodate.com/. Accessed March 23, 2012.

Bleday R, Breen E. Overview of hemorrhoids. In: Basow DS, ed. *UpToDate*. Waltham, MA; 2012. Retrieved from http://www.uptodate.com/. Accessed March 23, 2012.

Bleday R, Breen E. Treatment of hemorrhoids. In: Basow DS, ed. *UpToDate*. Waltham, MA; 2012. Retrieved from http://www.uptodate.com/. Accessed March 23, 2012.

Breen E, Bleday R. Anal abscesses and fistulas. In: Basow DS, ed. *UpToDate*, Waltham, MA; 2012. Retrieved from http://www.uptodate.com/. Accessed March 23, 2012.

Breen E, Bleday R. Anal fissures. In: Basow DS, ed. *UpToDate*. Waltham, MA; 2012. Retrieved from http://www.uptodate.com/. Accessed March 23, 2012.

DynaMed. *Acute Cholecystitis*. Ipswich, MA: EBSCO Publishing; 2010. Retrieved from http://search.ebscohost.com.cyber.usask.ca/login.aspx?direct=true&site=DynaMed&id=113862.

DynaMed. *Cholangitis*. Ipswich, MA: EBSCO Publishing; 2010. Retrieved from http://search.ebscohost.com.cyber.usask.ca/login.aspx?direct=true&site=DynaMed&id=113862.

DynaMed. *Choledocholithiasis*. Ipswich, MA: EBSCO Publishing; 2011. Retrieved from http://search.ebscohost.com.cyber.usask.ca/login.aspx?direct=true&site=DynaMed&id=113862.

DynaMed. *Constipation in Adults*. Ipswich, MA: EBSCO Publishing; 2012. Retrieved from http://search.ebscohost.com.cyber.usask.ca/login.aspx?direct=true&site=DynaMed&id=113862.

DynaMed. *Duodenal Atresia or Stenosis*. Ipswich, MA: EBSCO Publishing; 2012. Retrieved from http://search.ebscohost.com.cyber.usask.ca/login.aspx?direct=true&site=DynaMed&id=113862.

DynaMed. *Gallstones*. Ipswich, MA: EBSCO Publishing; 2011. Retrieved from http://search.ebscohost.com.cyber.usask.ca/login.aspx?direct=true&site=DynaMed&id=113862.

DynaMed. *Intussusception*. Ipswich, MA: EBSCO Publishing; 2010. Retrieved from http://search.ebscohost.com.cyber.usask.ca/login.aspx?direct=true&site=DynaMed&id=113862.

Dynamed. *Irritable Bowel Syndrome (IBS)*. Ipswich, MA: EBSCO Publishing; 2011. Retrieved from http://search.ebscohost.com.cyber.usask.ca/login.aspx?direct=true&site=DynaMed&id=113862.

DynaMed. *Pyloric Stenosis*. Ipswich, MA: EBSCO Publishing; 2012. Retrieved from http://search.ebscohost.com.cyber.usask.ca/login.aspx?direct=true&site=DynaMed&id=113862.

DynaMed. *Small Bowel Obstruction*. Ipswich, MA: EBSCO Publishing; 2012. Retrieved from http://search.ebscohost.com.cyber.usask.ca/login.aspx?direct=true&site=DynaMed&id=113862.

Farrell RJ, Peppercorn MA. Overview of the medical management of mild to moderate Crohn's disease in adults. In: Basow DS, ed. *UpToDate*. Waltham, MA; 2012. Retrieved from http://www.uptodate.com/. Accessed March 23, 2012.

Freeman ML, Arain MA. Approach to the patient with suspected choledocholithiasis. In: Basow DS, ed. *UpToDate*. Waltham, MA; 2012. Retrieved from http://www.uptodate.com/. Accessed March 23, 2012.

Heppell J. Surgical management of inflammatory bowel disease. In: Basow DS, ed. *UpToDate*. Waltham, MA; 2012. Retrieved from http://www.uptodate.com/. Accessed March 23, 2012.

Hodin RA, Bordeianou L. Small bowel obstruction: Causes and management. In: Basow DS, ed. *UpToDate*. Waltham, MA; 2012. Retrieved from http://www.uptodate.com/. Accessed March 23, 2012.

Hodin RA, Bordeianou L. Small bowel obstruction: Clinical manifestations and diagnosis. In: Basow DS, ed. *UpToDate*. Waltham, MA; 2012. Retrieved from http://www.uptodate.com/. Accessed March 23, 2012.

Jim J, Thompson RW. Clinical evaluation of abdominal aortic aneurysm. In: Basow DS, ed. *UpToDate*. Waltham, MA; 2012. Retrieved from http://www.uptodate.com/. Accessed March 23, 2012.

Kolodziejak L, Schuster B, Regier L, Jensen B. Irritable bowel syndrome (IBS). *RxFiles Drug Comparison Charts*. 8th ed. Saskatoon, SK: Saskatoon Health Region; 2010; 43.

Peppercorn MA. Clinical manifestations, diagnosis and prognosis of Crohn's disease in adults. In: Basow DS, ed. *UpToDate*. Waltham, MA; 2012. Retrieved from http://www.uptodate.com/. Accessed March 23, 2012.

Peppercorn MA. Clinical manifestations, diagnosis, and prognosis of ulcerative colitis in adults. In: Basow DS, ed. *UpToDate*. Waltham, MA; 2012. Retrieved from http://www.uptodate.com/. Accessed March 23, 2012.

Peppercorn MA, Ferrell RJ. Medical management of ulcerative colitis. In: Basow DS, ed. *UpToDate*. Waltham, MA; 2012. Retrieved from http://www.uptodate.com/. Accessed March 23, 2012.

Smink D, Soybel DI. Acute appendicitis in adults: Management. In: Basow DS, ed. *UpToDate*. Waltham, MA; 2012. Retrieved from http://www.uptodate.com/. Accessed March 23, 2012.

Tendler DA, LaMont JT. Acute mesenteric ischemia. In: Basow DS, ed. *UpToDate*. Waltham, MA; 2012. Retrieved from http://www.uptodate.com/. Accessed March 23, 2012.

Vege SS. Clinical manifestations and diagnosis of acute pancreatitis. In: Basow DS, ed. *UpToDate*. Waltham, MA; 2012. Retrieved from http://www.uptodate.com/. Accessed March 23, 2012.

Vege SS. Etiology and pathogenesis of chronic pancreatitis in adults. In: Basow DS, ed. *UpToDate*. Waltham, MA; 2012. Retrieved from http://www.uptodate.com/. Accessed March 23, 2012.

Vege SS. Etiology of acute pancreatitis. In: Basow DS, ed. *UpToDate*. Waltham, MA; 2012. Retrieved from http://www.uptodate.com/. Accessed March 23, 2012.

Vege SS. Treatment of acute pancreatitis. In: Basow DS, ed. *UpToDate*, Waltham, MA; 2012. Retrieved from http://www.uptodate.com/. Accessed March 23, 2012.

Wald A. Clinical manifestations and diagnosis of irritable bowel syndrome. In: Basow DS, ed. *UpToDate*. Waltham, MA; 2012. Retrieved from http://www.uptodate.com/. Accessed March 23, 2012.

Wald A. Etiology and evaluation of chronic constipation in adults. In: Basow DS, ed. *UpToDate*. Waltham, MA; 2012. Retrieved from http://www.uptodate.com/. Accessed March 23, 2012.

Wald A. Treatment of irritable bowel syndrome. In: Basow DS, ed. *UpToDate*. Waltham, MA; 2012. Retrieved from http://www.uptodate.com/. Accessed March 23, 2012.

Young-Fadok T, Pemberton JH. Clinical manifestations and diagnosis of colonic diverticular disease. In: Basow DS, ed. *UpToDate*. Waltham, MA; 2012. Retrieved from http://www.uptodate.com/. Accessed March 23, 2012.

Young-Fadok T, Pemberton JH. Epidemiology and pathophysiology of colonic diverticular disease. In: Basow DS, ed. *UpToDate*. Waltham, MA; 2012. Retrieved from http://www.uptodate.com/. Accessed March 23, 2012.

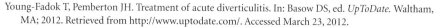

Young-Fadok T, Pemberton JH. Treatment of acute diverticulitis. In: Basow DS, ed. *UpToDate*. Waltham, MA; 2012. Retrieved from http://www.uptodate.com/. Accessed March 23, 2012.

Zakko SF, et al. Treatment of acute cholecystitis. In: Basow DS, ed. *UpToDate*. Waltham, MA: 2012. Retrieved from http://www.uptodate.com/. Accessed March 23, 2012.

Dehydration and Hypovolemia
Priority Topic 22

- Excessive intracellular fluid loss usually due to hypovolemia
  - Usually due to excess fluid loss from gastrointestinal tract, skin, and kidneys
- Highest morbidity and mortality in pediatric populations
- Types of hypovolemia:
  - Hypertonic/hypernatremic (GI losses, fever, diabetes, renal disease)
    - Net loss of extracellular water, or gain of sodium; Na > 145 mmol/L
  - Isotonic (hemorrhage, GI losses, trauma)
    - Loss of sodium is proportional to water; Na 135-145 mmol/L
  - Hypotonic/hyponatremic (GI losses, pancreatitis, heart failure, ascites, adrenal insufficiency, psychogenic polydipsia, salt wasting nephropathy)
    - Net loss of sodium relative to extracellular water; Na < 135 mmol/L
- **Signs and Symptoms**

  - Dry mucosa
  - Thirst
  - Concentrated urine
  - Decreased sweating
  - Dizzy

  - Flushed
  - Resting tachycardia/weak pulse
  - Hypotension
  - Delayed capillary refill
  - Coma

- **Risk Factors**
  - Extremes of age
  - Acute illness
  - Cognitive impairment—delirium, sedation, psychosis
  - Limited fluid intake—dysphagia, fear of incontinence, limited mobility
  - Increased fluid losses—illness (especially GI), environment, diuretics, hemorrhage, trauma
  - Altered thirst—CNS lesions, medications
- **Diagnosis**
  - History: consider vomiting, diarrhea, fluid intake, urine output, postural dizziness, medications
    - Pediatrics (see Table 4-5): number of wet diapers, crying tears, sunken eyes, recent weight when well
- **Physical examination**
  - Heart rate, blood pressure, capillary refill, skin turgor, sunken eyes, respiratory pattern, mucus membranes, overall appearance, and active/lethargic

TABLE 4-5 Degree of Dehydration Assessment in Pediatrics

CLINICAL EXAMINATION	MILD (3%-5%)	MODERATE (6%-9%)	SEVERE (≥10%)
Heart rate	Normal, good volume	Rapid	Rapid, weak
Systolic pressure	Normal	Normal to low	Low
Respirations	Normal	Deep, rate may be increased	Deep, tachypneic
Mucosa	Tacky or slightly dry	Dry	Parched
Anterior fontanelle	Normal	Sunken	Markedly sunken
Eyes	Normal	Sunken	Markedly sunken
Skin turgor	Normal	Reduced	Tenting
Skin	Normal	Cool	Cool, mottled, acrocyanosis
Urine output	Normal or mildly reduced	Markedly reduced	Anuria
Systemic signs	Increased thirst	Listlessness, irritability	Grunting, lethargy, coma

- **Investigations**
  - Serum
    - Electrolytes, urea, creatinine, glucose, calcium, osmolality
  - Urine
    - Increased urine specific gravity
    - Increased urine osmolality
- **Causes**
  - Gastrointestinal losses—nausea and vomiting
  - Dermal losses—sweating, burns
  - Vascular losses—trauma, hemorrhage
  - Diuretics
  - Pancreatitis
  - Heart failure
  - Cirrhosis with ascites
  - Renal disease
  - Diabetes
  - Psychogenic polydipsia
  - SIADH
  - Salt wasting nephropathy
  - Adrenal insufficiency
- **Treatment**
  - Fluid replacement
    - Oral fluids for mild to moderate dehydration
    - IV fluids for severe dehydration, shock, and if oral not possible (eg, vomiting, altered level of consciousness)
  - Need to (1) replace deficit, (2) provide maintenance fluids, and (3) replace ongoing losses
    - Deficit replacement can be calculated with various formulas:
      - Deficit = (pre-illness weight) − (post-illness weight)
      - Deficit = (% deficit) × (10ml/kg) × (pre-illness weight)
      - Deficit = (0.6 × weight) × (serum Na − 140)/140
  - Replace 1/2 the fluids (deficit + maintenance + ongoing losses) in the first 8 hours and the remaining over 16 hours

Hourly Maintenance Fluid—4-2-1 Rule

4 mL/kg/h for 0-10 kg (1st 10 kg of patient weight)

+

2 mL/kg/h for 10-20 kg (2nd 10 kg of patient weight)

+

1 mL/kg/h for each kg over 20 kg (eg, 60 kg person has a maintenance fluid rate of 100 mL/h)

ONGOING LOSSES

One large vomit or one large diarrhea = 8 mL/kg body weight

Diarrhea
Priority Topic 26

ACUTE DIARRHEA

- Defined as diarrhea of <14 days duration
- **Risk factors**
  - Food, travel, medications, outbreaks, malignancy, IBD, IBS
- **Diagnosis**
  - Do not over investigate if no red flags
- **Investigations**
  - Stool:
    - Viral studies: if no blood or mucus or systemic signs
    - Gram stain, culture, and sensitivity: if immunocompromised, IBD, bloody diarrhea, or persistent
    - Ova, cysts, and parasites: if travel history or persistent diarrhea
    - *Clostridium difficile: if recent antibiotic use or persistent diarrhea*
- **Treatment**
  - Rehydration and supportive care
  - Antibiotics should be considered if any of the following symptoms are present:
    - Severe traveler's diarrhea: >4 unformed stools/day, fever, and blood, pus or mucous in the stool
    - >8 stools per day
    - Symptoms for >1 week
    - Immunocompromised
    - Hospitalized patients
  - Probiotics
  - Loperamide (to reduce stool frequency)—consider if no fever or bloody stool
- **Complications**
  - Hemolytic-uremic syndrome
  - Clostridium difficile infection
  - Toxic shock syndrome
  - Toxic megacolon

CHRONIC DIARRHEA

- Loose stools with or without increased stool frequency lasting 4 or more weeks
- Associated with multiple medical conditions
  - Consider: malabsorption, inflammatory bowel disease, irritable bowel syndrome, infectious, maldigestion, laxative abuse, drugs, disordered motility, neuroendocrine tumours, colon cancer, HIV, recent cholecystectomy
- **Physical examination**
  - Signs of IBD (eg, mouth ulcers, skin rash, episcleritis)
  - DRE to assess for anal fissure or fistula (may indicate IBD), anal tone, and reflexes
  - Evidence of malabsorption (eg, wasting)
  - Abdominal masses
  - Lymphadenopathy
  - Thyroid

Consider public health notification, for example, if restaurant related, large outbreak, nursing home

DIARRHEA RED FLAGS
- Fever
- Unintentional weight loss >10 lb
- Anemia
- Hematochezia or melena
- Positive fecal occult blood test
- Pus in stool
- Nocturnal defecation
- Symptoms refractory to treatment
- Family history of colon cancer or inflammatory bowel disease

Fever and Diarrhea: associated with invasive bacteria (eg, Salmonella, Shigella, Campylobacter), enteric viruses, and cytotoxic bacteria (eg, *Clostridium difficile, Entamoeba histolytica*)

Bloody diarrhea: associated with *Escherichia coli, E. histolytica*, Shigella, Campylobacter, Salmonella

- **Investigations**
  - Bloodwork: CBC, TSH, electrolytes, albumin, creatinine, Vitamin B_{12}, folate
  - Stool:
    - Leukocytes, occult blood, gram stain, culture and sensitivity, ova/cysts/parasites, *C. difficile*, pH, fat content
  - Also consider as prompted by history:
    - Serologic testing for Celiac disease, endoscopy, HIV serology, further stool testing
- **Diagnosis**
  - In elderly, diarrhea is more likely to be due to underlying pathology
  - Consider inflammatory bowel disease, Celiac disease, malabsorption
- **Treatment**
  - Will be indicated by history, examination, and investigation findings
  - Probiotics
  - Loperamide
  - Consider empiric metronidazole

MALDIGESTION/MALABSORPTION

- Malabsorption refers to impaired nutrient absorption
- Maldigestion refers to impaired nutrient digestion
- Normal nutrient absorption relies on:
  - (1) processing by brush border, (2) absorption into intestinal mucosa, and (3) transport into circulation
- Global malabsorption:
  - Mucosa is diffusely involved; or there is a decrease in absorptive surface, for example, celiac disease
- Partial or isolated malabsorption:
  - Specific nutrient absorption is affected, for example, cobalamin malabsorption
- **Presentation**
  - Usually vague symptoms, may have abdominal distention, flatulence, anorexia
  - Global malabsorption: pale, greasy, foul-smelling stools, weight loss
  - Partial malabsorption: related to specific nutrient; for example, cobalamin malabsorption will lead to pernicious anemia
- **Diagnosis**
  - Bloodwork: CBC, electrolytes, iron studies, vitamin B_{12}, folate, calcium, magnesium, phosphate, albumin, liver function tests
  - Tests for specific malabsorption
    - Fat malabsorption: fecal fat
    - Carbohydrate malabsorption: D-xylose, lactose intolerance
    - Protein malabsorption: α1-antitrypsin clearance
    - Vitamin B_{12}: schilling test
  - Imaging: abdominal US and endoscopy
- **Treatment**
  - Will be based on diagnosis

CELIAC DISEASE

- A malabsorption syndrome due to gluten intolerance
  - Gliadin is a fraction of gluten mainly responsible for triggering an immune reaction

- Small bowel effects include villous atrophy, mucosal inflammation, crypt hyperplasia; these changes resolve on removal of gluten from the diet

■ **Risk factors**
- Family history, diabetes mellitus type II, persistent unexplained elevated AST and ALT on liver panel, HLA-DQ2, HLA-DQ8, possibly related to exposure to gluten in first 3 months of life

■ **Complications**
- Nutritional deficiencies (vitamin D, iron, calcium), intestinal ulcers or strictures, low bone mineral density, delayed puberty and menarche, decreased fertility until diagnosed and treated, low birth weight babies in untreated mothers
- Increased risk of autoimmune disorders, malignancy, and specifically of non-Hodgkin Lymphoma

■ **Presentation**
- Typically nonspecific with fatigue, change in bowel habit, bloating, weight loss, foul-smelling stool; may see skin or neurological symptoms
- Children often present with failure to thrive

■ **Extraintestinal manifestations**
- Skin: dermatitis herpetiformis; CNS: cerebellar ataxia, peripheral neuropathy

■ **Diagnosis**
- Clinical diagnosis is made based on history and positive serology; for confirmation, endoscopic biopsy is required
- Serology:
  - IgA tissue transglutaminase (tTG)—best single serological test
  - IgA antiendomysial antibody (EMA)
  - Both tTG and EMA have high sensitivity (89%-94%) and specificity (98%-99%)
- If serology is positive, refer to gastroenterology for biopsy

■ **Treatment**
- Avoid gluten-containing foods lifelong: barley, wheat, and rye
- Treat nutritional deficiencies: iron, folate, vitamin B_{12}
- Dietician referral
- Bone mineral density testing
- Level 2 evidence for budesonide in addition to gluten-free diet resulting in decreased symptoms

Bibliography

Bonis PAL, LaMont JT. Approach to the adult with chronic diarrhea in developed countries. In: Basow DS, ed. *UpToDate*. Waltham, MA; 2012. Retrieved from http://www.uptodate.com/. Accessed March 23, 2012.

DynaMed. *Acute Diarrhea in Adults*. Ipswich, MA: EBSCO Publishing; 2011. Retrieved from http://search. ebscohost.com.cyber.usask.ca/login.aspx?direct=true&site=DynaMed&id=113862. Accessed March 23, 2012.

DynaMed. *Chronic Diarrhea*. Ipswich, MA: EBSCO Publishing; 2011. Retrieved from http://search. ebscohost.com.cyber.usask.ca/login.aspx?direct=true&site=DynaMed&id=113862. Accessed March 23, 2012.

DynaMed. *Celiac Disease*. Ipswich, MA: EBSCO Publishing; 2012. Retrieved from http://search.ebscohost. com.cyber.usask.ca/login.aspx?direct=true&site=DynaMed&id=113862. Accessed March 23, 2012.

Kelly CP. Diagnosis of celiac disease. In: Basow DS, ed. *UpToDate*. Waltham, MA; 2012. Retrieved from http://www.uptodate.com/. Accessed March 23, 2012.

Schuppan D, Dieterich W. Pathogenesis, epidemiology, and clinical manifestations of celiac disease in adults. In: Basow DS, ed. *UpToDate*. Waltham, MA; 2012. Retrieved from http://www.uptodate.com/. Accessed March 23, 2012.

Wanke CA. Approach to the adult with acute diarrhea in developed countries. In: Basow DS, ed. *UpToDate*. Waltham, MA; 2012. Retrieved from http://www.uptodate.com/. Accessed March 23, 2012.

Dyspepsia
Priority Topic 31

Intermittent epigastric discomfort, early satiety, or bothersome post-prandial fullness

- Dyspepsia is a symptom and **not** a diagnosis
- Differential diagnosis of patients presenting with dyspepsia includes:
  - Functional dyspepsia (ie, no organic pathology): up to 60% of pts with typical symptoms
  - Peptic ulcer disease: up to 25% of dyspepsia
  - Gastroesophageal reflux disease
  - Medications: steroids, NSAIDs, bisphosphonates, calcium channel blockers, digoxin
  - Irritable bowel syndrome
  - Pancreatitis
  - Biliary disease
  - Malignancy
  - Consider cardiac chest pain!
- **Presentation**
  - 3 common patterns (with a lot of overlap)
    - Ulcer-type/acid dyspepsia
      - Burning epigastric pain, relieved with antacids, food
      - Obtain history of NSAID use
    - Dysmotility type
      - Nausea, bloating, anorexia
    - Unspecified
- **Physical examination**
  - Should be normal, although may have epigastric tenderness
  - Look for abdominal masses, signs of anemia, signs of weight loss
  - Rectal examination or fecal occult blood if suggested by history
- **Investigations**
  - Will be based on age and presence of alarm symptoms
  - Routine bloods should be considered for all patients
    - CBC, LFTs (to rule out hepatobiliary disease, add on lipase/amylase if concerned about pancreatic disease)
  - No investigations:
    - In patients with no alarm symptoms, no NSAID use, and a classic history of GERD-type symptoms
    - In patients with NSAID use and no alarm symptoms
  - *Helicobacter pylori* testing:
    - In patients with no alarm symptoms, and symptoms are not typical of GERD, and in patients with failed trial of acid supression therapy
      - If testing is positive, treat with *H. pylori* eradication
      - If testing is negative, trial PPI for 4 to 6 weeks
  - Endoscopy:
    - For any patient over 50, alarm symptoms, family history of cancer, or not responding to therapy
- **Treatment**
  - See discussion under GERD and PUD sections
  - Lifestyle modifications are number 1!

Dyspepsia Alarm Symptoms: VBAD
V—vomit
B—blood (hematemesis or melena)
A—Abdominal mass/ Anemia / Age>50
D—Dysphagia

Others: weight loss, early satiety, refractory to treatment

- Exercise, decrease alcohol, quit smoking, avoid spicy foods, decrease caffeine, avoid overeating especially in the evenings.
- Discontinue NSAIDs, or combine with acid suppression as discussed later if unable to discontinue
- Acid suppression
  - Histamine type 2 receptor blockers (H2 blockers)
    - Standard dose PPI is more efficacious than H2 blocker
  - Proton pump inhibitors
  - Good evidence in heartburn and epigastric pain predominant dyspepsia
  - Standard dose PPI is more efficacious than H2 blocker
  - Ineffective in patients with dysmotility (belching, bloating) type symptoms
  - Bismuth salts
  - Antacids: often used as self-medication; provide rapid, but less sustained symptom relief
- Prokinetics: some evidence in functional and non-ulcer dyspepsia
- Herbals: peppermint, caraway, turmeric

PEPTIC ULCER DISEASE

- Includes gastric and duodenal ulcers
  - An increase in gastric acid secretion and a weakening of the mucosal barrier can result in ulcer formation
- **Risk factors**
  - *Helicobacter pylori* infection, and NSAID use are most common risk factors
    - Note that most individuals infected with *H. pylori* do not develop ulcers
  - Other: smoking, steroids, bisphosphonates, tumors, Crohn's disease, gastritis (can be secondary to alcohol), radiation damage, CMV infection
- **Complications**
  - Bleeding
  - Penetration: retroperitoneal
  - Perforation: more common with duodenal ulcers
  - Gastric outlet obstruction
- **Presentation**
  - Episodic epigastric pain
  - Symptom relief with eating, antacids, or acid suppression medications
  - Gastric ulcers more likely to have pain soon after eating
  - Duodenal ulcers—pain relieved with food, pain during sleep, pain 3 hours after eating
  - Chronic ulcers—asymptomatic, especially if NSAID induced
- **Investigations**
  - CBC
  - *Helicobacter pylori* testing
    - Urea breath test—for active infection, useful for pre- and post-treatment
    - Serology (antibody testing)—not useful if have been treated previously
    - Fecal antigen testing—for active infection, less well-validated than breath test
  - Endoscopy
    - Required if any family history of cancer, alarm symptoms, or if over 50 years old
    - For failed *H. pylori* eradication or not responding to treatment

- Biopsy
  - ○ Recommended for all gastric ulcers; duodenal ulcers are less likely to be malignant
- **Treatment**
  - Lifestyle modifications
    - ○ Exercise, decrease alcohol, quit smoking, avoid spicy foods, decrease caffeine, avoid overeating especially in the evenings
    - ○ Discontinue NSAIDs, or combine with acid suppression as discussed later if unable to discontinue
  - *Helicobacter pylori* eradication
    - ○ First line: triple therapy for 7 to 14 days
      - □ Proton pump inhibitor
      - □ Clarithromycin
      - □ Amoxicillin or metronidazole
    - ○ Second line: Quadruple therapy for 10 to 14 days
      - □ Proton pump inhibitor
      - □ Bismuth
      - □ Metronidazole
      - □ Tetracycline
    - ○ Patients with gastric ulcer may benefit from 3 weeks of PPI following eradication, however evidence is lacking
  - For *H. pylori* negative ulcers: treat with PPI for 4 to 8 weeks
  - Surgical treatment may be necessary in patients in whom medical therapy fails

Helicobacter pylori serology can be positive for 1 to 2 years after treatment.

GASTROESOPHAGEAL REFLUX DISEASE

- Occurs when stomach contents reflux into the esophagus due to an inappropriate relaxation of the lower esophageal sphincter
  - May result in extraesophageal disease with symptoms of cough, laryngitis, asthma, and dental erosions
  - Reflux contents may be gastric or bile (duodenogastroesophageal reflux)
- **Risk factors**
  - Increased intraabdominal pressure, pregnancy, obesity
  - Medications that decrease LES pressure:
    - ○ Calcium channel blockers, anticholinergics, theophylline, nitrates, sildenafil, albuterol
  - *Helicobacter pylori* infection is not associated with GERD, in fact there is a lower prevalence of *H. pylori* in patients with GERD
- **Complications**
  - Barrett esophagus, esophageal adenocarcinoma, chronic laryngitis
- **Presentation**
  - Heartburn sensation (aka acid brash or water brash)—burning or discomfort behind sternum, rising into neck, worse after meals, worse when lying flat, relieved with antacids
  - Regurgitation—flow of acid secretions into mouth
  - Atypical presentations include: cough, laryngitis, hoarse voice, halitosis, chest pain
- **Physical examination**
  - Typically normal
  - May see evidence of dental erosions, nasopharyngeal sinusitis, nasal or pharyngeal polyps
- **Alarm symptoms**
  - See list given earlier

- **Diagnosis**
  - Presumptive diagnosis based on history, lack of alarm symptoms, and <50 years old
    - Confirmed with symptomatic improvement with 4 to 6 week trial of acid suppression treatment
  - If no symptomatic relief, consider alternate diagnosis, may require endoscopy (see "Dyspepsia")

> Must use urea breath test if testing for cure. Do test 4 weeks after treatment completed, if indicated.

- **Treatment**
  - Lifestyle modifications
    - Elevate head of bed, avoid acidic foods, avoid large meals
    - Exercise, decrease alcohol, quit smoking, avoid spicy foods, decrease caffeine, avoid overeating especially in the evenings
  - Proton pump inhibitor or H2 receptor blocker
    - Standard dose PPI is more efficacious than H2 blocker
  - Reassess therapy at **4 to 8 weeks**
    - If no response, consider increased dose, or change to PPI if on H2 blocker
    - If no symptomatic relief still, consider alternate diagnosis, may require endoscopy (see "Dyspepsia")
  - Reassess need for long-term therapy periodically and wean to minimum effective dose (or discontinue if symptoms do not recur)
  - May consider on-demand PPI use in patients who have had good response to PPI therapy

Bibliography

Canadian Agency for Drugs and Technologies in Health. Screening and diagnostic tests before endoscopy: clinical evidence and guidelines. 2011. Retrieved from http://www.cadth.ca/media/pdf/htis/oct-2011/RB0434-000%20Endoscopy%20Guidelines.pdf. Accessed March 23, 2012.

DynaMed. *Functional Dyspepsia*. Ipswich, MA: EBSCO Publishing; 2012. Retrieved from http://search.ebscohost.com.cyber.usask.ca/login.aspx?direct=true&site=DynaMed&id=113862. Accessed March 23, 2012.

DynaMed. *Peptic Ulcer Disease*. Ipswich, MA: EBSCO Publishing; 2012. Retrieved from http://search.ebscohost.com.cyber.usask.ca/login.aspx?direct=true&site=DynaMed&id=113862. Accessed March 23, 2012.

Longstreth GF. Approach to the patient with dyspepsia. In: Basow DS, ed. *UpToDate*. Waltham, MA; 2012. Retrieved from http://www.uptodate.com/. Accessed March 23, 2012.

Schuster B. Gastrointestinal-acid suppression drugs: evidence, tips and pearls. *RxFiles Drug Comparison Charts*. 8th ed. Saskatoon, SK: Saskatoon Health Region; 2010: 40.

Gastrointestinal Bleeding

Priority Topic 41

TABLE 4-6	Upper and Lower GI Bleed	
	UPPER GI BLEED	**LOWER GI BLEED**
Definition	• Bleeding from the gastrointestinal tract proximal to the ligament of Treitz	• Bleeding from the gastrointestinal tract distal to the ligament of Treitz

Etiology	• Peptic ulcer disease
	• Varices
	• Gastritis (eg, NSAID/ETOH induced)
	• Esophagitis
	• Mallory-Weiss tear
	• Vascular anomalies
	• Malignancy
		• Hemorrhoids
		• Anal fissure
		• Diverticular bleeding
		• Ischemic bowel disease
		• Inflammatory bowel disease
		• Colonic ulcer
		• Malignancy
		• Vascular lesions
		• Paediatric
		  • Intussusception
		  • Meckel diverticulum

TABLE 4-6 Upper and Lower GI Bleed (*Continued*)

	UPPER GI BLEED	LOWER GI BLEED
Presentation	• Melena—black tarry stool indicates digested upper GI blood • Hematochezia—bright rectal bleed indicates profuse upper GI bleed • Hematemesis—bright red indicates fresh bleed • Coffee ground emesis—indicates digested blood	• Hematochezia • Melena
Investigations	• CBC • INR and PTT • Electrolytes, renal panel, LFTs • ECG • Type and crossmatch • Esophagoduodenoscopy	• CBC • INR and PTT • Electrolytes, renal panel, LFTs • ECG • Type and crossmatch • Sigmoidoscopy and/or colonoscopy (may start with sigmoid in unprepared bowel) • Angiography if bleeding >0.5 mL/min
Treatment	• Proton pump inhibitor • NPO +/− NG tube • Esophagoduodenoscopy (both diagnostic and therapeutic) • For suspected varices: somatostatin analog (eg, octreotide), and continue for 3-5 days post confirmation • *Helicobacter pylori* testing and treatment if peptic ulcers diagnosed • Antibiotics in patients with cirrhosis	• NPO +/− NG tube (rule out upper GI cause) • Identify and treat source of bleeding • Consider risks/benefits of anticoagulants, NSAIDs, aspirin, steroids, SSRIs

- **Risk factors**
  - Alcohol, anticoagulant therapy, NSAIDs, smoking, liver cirrhosis, *H. pylori* infection, chronic renal insufficiency
  - ICU admission, previous GI bleed
  - Medications: steroids, calcium channel blockers, SSRIs
- Be sure to inquire about diet and medications which can cause red or black stool
  - Beets, iron, Pepto-Bismol
- **Presentation**
  - Depends on degree of bleeding
    - Consider risk factors, previous GI bleeds
    - Differentiate between upper and lower GI bleed if possible
    - Resuscitate as needed

ESOPHAGEAL VARICEAL BLEEDING

- Consider in all patients with upper GI bleeding and a history of liver cirrhosis
- **Risk factors**
  - Cirrhosis with portal hypertension and development of gastric or esophageal varices, ascites, active alcohol use
- Regular endoscopies to monitor varices and prevent bleeds
- Consider antibiotic prophylaxis if upper GI bleed and cirrhosis to prevent spontaneous bacterial peritonitis
- **Treatment**
  - Acute: somatostatin analogue, for example, octreotide
  - Chronic: non-selective β-blocker, for example, propranolol to decrease heart rate by 25% and prevent rebleeding

TABLE 4-7	Degree of Blood Loss in Adults			
FIT MALE, 70 KG (5 L OF BLOOD WHEN WELL)	CLASS I	CLASS II	CLASS III	CLASS IV
Blood loss	750 mL	750-1000 mL	1500-2000 mL	>2000 mL
HR	N	100-120	>120	>140
BP	N	N, postural hypotension	Often N, may see narrow pulse pressure	↓↓
CNS	N	Anxious	Agitated	↓Consciousness
Respiratory rate	N	↑	↑↑	↑↑↑
Urine output	↓	↓↓	Minimal	None
Replacement fluid	NS	NS/Hartmann	Mix—crystalloid, colloid, plasma	Blood ± colloid

Bibliography

DynaMed. *Acute Lower Gastrointestinal Bleeding.* Ipswich, MA: EBSCO Publishing; 2012. Retrieved from http://search.ebscohost.com.cyber.usask.ca/login.aspx?direct=true&site=DynaMed&id=113862. Accessed March 23, 2012.

DynaMed. Acute Upper Gastrointestinal Bleeding. Ipswich, MA: EBSCO Publishing; 2012. Retrieved from http://search.ebscohost.com.cyber.usask.ca/login.aspx?direct=true&site=DynaMed&id=113862. Accessed March 23, 2012.

Leddin DJ, Enns R, Hilsden R, et al. Canadian Association of Gastroenterology position statement on screening individuals at risk for developing colorectal cancer: 2010. *Can J Gastroenterol.* 2010;24(12):705-714.

5
Pediatrics

In Newborns
Priority Topic 67

IMPORTANT POINTS

- Always look for subtle physical anomalies (eg, low-set ears, sacral dimples) that may hint toward an association with other anomalies or syndromes.
- When assessing newborns with nonspecific concerns from the caregiver, **always** think of sepsis as a differential and look for signs as it may not present as in adults (eg, feeding difficulties, respiratory changes, irritability).
- Stay up to date with neonatal resuscitation guidelines if you have newborns in your practice.
- Encourage breast feeding for newborn babies, but do not criticize a parent's decision to bottle feed.
- Continually monitor for abnormalities such as hip abnormalities, hearing difficulties, heart murmurs, as they may not be immediately obvious.
- Educate parents on signs and symptoms of impending illness when discharging newborns from hospital and ensure that they are aware of how to access care.

Bibliography

Working Group on the Certification Process. *Priority Topics and Key Features with Corresponding Skill Dimensions and Phases of the Encounter.* The College of Family Physicians of Canada.

Well Baby Care
Priority Topic 99

IMPORTANT POINTS

- Assess development, weight, height, and head circumference at every visit and chart on growth scale (WHO Canadian Growth Chart).
- Provide anticipatory information for milestones.
- Always ask about family adjustment, include mood disorders.
- Discuss importance of vaccination.

- Be aware of cultural factors and resources available (eg, circumcision).
- Screen for anemia at 6 to 12 months in at-risk populations (eg, lower socioeconomic status, Asians, First Nations, low birth weight babies, infants fed with whole cow's milk in first year of life).
- Tylenol can be used as anti-pyretic—10 to 15 mg/kg every 4 to 6 hours.

ROUTINE VISITS

Address all of following at each visit:

A. General questions
- Note risk factors, family history, pregnancy history, delivery history (including resuscitation)
- Address parental concerns at every visit

B. Feeding
- No honey
- No beets, carrots, spinach, or turnips before 6 months (contain nitrates)
- Avoid dry, solid, round, smooth, or sticky foods that can cause choking and sugary foods and drinks
- Introduce new foods one at a time with 3 to 5 days in between to monitor for reactions
- Avoid potential allergens—carefully introduce citrus fruits, cow's milk, corn, egg whites, wheat after 1 year, and chocolate, nuts, peanuts, shellfish after 3 years especially if there is a family history of allergies
- Many pediatricians advise not giving eggs and fish in baby's first year due to the risk of developing an allergy, but there is limited evidence for this

C. Developmental milestones
- Should be monitored closely
- Delay in achieving age-appropriate milestones may unmask an underlying developmental/learning disorder

Use ROURKE in clinical practice http://www.rourkebabyrecord.ca/.

Well baby checks are required at 1 week, 2 months, 4 months, 6 months, 12 months, 18 months, 2 to 3 years, and 4 to 5 years. Add additional visits if the child is unwell or needs closer monitoring.

TABLE 5-1	Baby's First Foods
0-6 months	Recommend exclusive breast feeding for the first 6 months of life with 400 IU of vitamin D supplementation • Can express breast milk, can freeze for up to 6 months, and refrigerate for up to 3 days • Warm milk by placing in hot water (microwaving can destroy vitamins) If feeding with formula, use iron-fortified formulas, 5 oz/kg/day for first 2 weeks then increase
6-9 months	Start with iron-fortified infant cereals, grain products such as dry toast or crackers pureed cooked yellow, green, orange vegetables, pureed cooked fruits, ripe mashed fruits pureed cooked meat, fish, chicken, tofu, mashed beans, egg yolk
9-12 months	Plain cereals, whole grain bread, rice, pasta soft mashed, cooked vegetables, soft fresh fruits, peeled, seeded, diced, canned fruits (in water or juice) minced/diced meat, fish, chicken, tofu At 9 months, offer high fat yogurt, cottage cheese, grated hard cheese, **introduce whole milk from 9-12 months**, limit milk products to 720 mL/day (risk of iron deficiency anemia)
http://www.caringforkids.cps.ca/handouts/feeding_your_baby_in_the_first_year. See introducing solid foods.	

TABLE 5-2	Developmental Milestones			
AGE	**GROSS MOTOR**	**FINE MOTOR**	**LANGUAGE**	**SOCIAL/COGNITION**
2 months	Lifts head/chest when lying on stomach	**Vision tracks past midline**	Coos, reacts to sounds	**Recognizes parent, smiles**
6 months	**Sits alone**	Transfers between hands	Babbles	**Stranger anxiety**
9-10 months	Crawls, pulls to stand up	Three finger pincer grasp	Mama/dada	Waves, plays pat-a-cake
12 months	Cruises, **walks**	Two finger pincer grasp	Mama/dada specifically	**One step command**
18 months	Runs, kicks ball	Builds tower of 2-4 cubes	Names common things	Copies parents
2 years	Jumps, **walks up/down stairs** with help	Builds tower of 6 cubes	**Two word phrases**	**Obeys two step commands,** removes clothes alone

Chart adapted from Le T, et al. *First Aid for the USMLE Step 2 CK.*

D. Education
- Car seat, helmets
- Bath safety
- Second-hand smoke
- Sleeping position, crib safety, safe toys
- Fever advice
- Child proofing, keep OTC meds and poisons out of reach

E. Physical examination
- Measure height, weight, and head circumference at every visit (WHO Canadian Growth Chart)
- Correct percentiles if born at <37 weeks, until 24 to 36 months
- Check skin, fontanelles, red reflex, heart, lungs, abdomen, umbilicus, hips, tone, testicles, foreskin

Bibliography

American Academy of Pediatrics. *Ages & stages—switching to solid foods.* 2008. Last updated 2012. http://www.healthychildren.org/English/ages-stages/baby/feeding-nutrition/Pages/Switching-To-Solid-Foods.aspx.

Health Canada—Food and Nutrition. *Nutrition for healthy term infants—statement of the Joint Working Group: Canadian Paediatric Society, Dieticians of Canada and Health Canada.* 2007. http://www.hc-sc.gc.ca/fn-an/pubs/infant-nourrisson/nut_infant_nourrisson_term-eng.php.

Le T, et al. Developmental milestones. *First Aid for the USMLE Step 2 CK.* 5th ed. McGraw-Hill; 2005:302.

Leslie R, Denis L, James R, *Rourke Baby Record—Evidence-based infant/child health maintenance guide.* 2011. http://www.rourkebabyrecord.ca/.

The Canadian Pediatric Society. *Pregnancy and babies—feeding your baby in the first year.* 2006. http://www.caringforkids.cps.ca/handouts/feeding_your_baby_in_the_first_year.

In Children
Priority Topic 50

IMPORTANT POINTS

- Always keep your differential broad to include common medical problems such as UTIs, pneumonia, depression, appendicitis, even though they may present differently in children.
- At every visit, try to ask about other aspects of their lives—school performance, relationships, friends, home life, bullying, modifiable risk factors such as exercise or diet, and practicing preventative measures such as wearing helmets and seatbelts.

- Ask directly about risky behaviours such as drug use, smoking, driving, and sex.
- Advise adolescents that their visits are confidential but try to encourage them to openly discuss issues with their parents/guardians such as sex, bullying, drugs, pregnancy, suicide, depression.
- Always use age appropriate language, and try to talk to children and adolescents directly, rather than just to their parents.
- When communicating with children, come to their eye level.
- Do not limit investigations if they are needed just because they make cause distress for the patient or parents.

Bibliography

Chen YA, Tran C. Chapters 23 (Pediatrics) and 26 (Psychiatry). *Toronto Notes—Comprehensive Medical Reference & Review for MCCQE I and USMLE II.* Toronto, Canada: Toronto Notes for Medical Students Inc; 2011.

Working Group on the Certification Process. Priority topics and key features with corresponding skill dimensions and phases of the encounter. The College of Family Physicians of Canada; 2010.

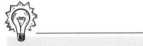

HEADSS mnemonic—cover these points when assessing children and adolescents
- **H**ome life
- **E**ducation
- **A**ctivities/Social
- **D**rugs
- **S**ex
- **S**moking

Learning
Priority Topic 57

IMPORTANT POINTS

- Early detection improves outcome.
- Always consider hearing and visual difficulties and psychiatric disease when children present with learning difficulties.
- Try to always ask about learning difficulties at routine visits.
- Five areas of potential difficulty: intelligence, academic achievement, attention/concentration, perceptual (visual/motor) function, and behaviour.
- Can also have difficulty with listening, speaking, writing, reasoning, or computing.
- Always assess the impact of disability on family and child.
- Use history, examination, and investigations to identify/exclude medical causes (eg, otitis media, iron deficiency, hearing difficulty), detect trauma, perinatal events, pregnancy history, school performance, hobbies, family history of similar problems, behavioural problems, substance, verbal, physical abuse, developmental delay.
- Educate parents to their level of understanding about their child's condition.
- Try to organize community resources for family.
  - Multidisciplinary team members can include family doctors, pediatricians, parents, psychologist, teachers, nurses, educators, counselors, administrators, social workers, occupational therapists, physiotherapy, speech and language specialist.

PERVASIVE DEVELOPMENTAL DISORDERS

Include autism, childhood disintegrative disorder, Rett disorder, Asperger syndrome, and PDD not otherwise specified

Autism

Two-thirds of patients present with lack of communication skills.
   Deficits in three main areas:

1. **Social interaction**—impaired nonverbal behaviour (eye contact, gestures, expressions), failure to make appropriate peer relationships, lack of sharing interests, achievements, and lack of emotional reciprocity

2. **Communication**—delayed or absent verbal speech or ability to converse, repetitive use of language, absence of age-appropriate imaginary play

3. **Restricted and repetitive behaviours, interests, and activities**—inflexible stereotypical hand or body movements (eg, rocking), routines, mannerisms, and preoccupations

Before the age of 3, six features should be present (at least two from social interaction category).

Asperger Syndrome

- Atypical social interaction skills with extreme behavioural rigidity and rituals
- No cognitive or milestone delays except **social interaction**
  - Impaired nonverbal behaviours (expressions, eye contact, postures, gestures), impaired ability to make peer relationships, lack of emotional reciprocity
  - Restricted repetitive behaviours, interests, and activities
  - May not respect social boundaries, one-sided conversations about a topic obsessively, lack of interest in other activities, disregards how interested the listener is, avoidant or intense gaze, or abnormal facial expressions
- Patients with Asperger syndrome have a better knowledge of language, higher cognitive functioning, and more interest in social activities

Bibliography

Augustyn M, et al. Clinical features of autism spectrum disorders. 2011. http://www.uptodate.com/contents/clinical-features-of-autism-spectrum-disorders?view=print.

Chen YA, Tran C. Chapters 23 (Pediatrics) and 26 (Psychiatry). *Toronto Notes—Comprehensive Medical Reference & Review for MCCQE I and USMLE II*. Toronto, Canada: Toronto Notes for Medical Students Inc; 2011.

Phillips DM, Longlett SK, Mulrine C, Kruse J, Kewney R. School problems and the family physician. *Am Fam Physician*. 1999;59(10):2816-2824. http://www.aafp.org/afp/1999/0515/p2816.html.

Von Hahn L, et al. Specific learning disabilities in children: Evaluation. 2010. http://www.uptodate.com/contents/specific-learning-disabilities-in-children-evaluation?

Von Hahn L, et al. Specific learning disabilities in children: Role of the primary care provider. 2011. http://www.uptodate.com/contents/specific-learning-disabilities-in-children-role-of-the-primary-care-provider?

Immunizations

Priority Topic 49

IMPORTANT POINTS

- Document **all** vaccinations.
- Inquire about immunization status if presenting with infectious disease as treatment options might be different if unvaccinated.
- Vaccination is not a guarantee of protection!
- Should **not** be delayed in mild acute illness, concurrent antibiotic use, or seizure.
- Vaccines and autism—most recent research suggests **no** link between development of autism and vaccines (2006 Immunization Guide—*Health Canada*).

TABLE 5-3	Specific Groups Benefitting from Vaccination
GROUP	**RECOMMENDED VACCINATIONS**
>65 years	Pneumococcal × 1 (or more often if at high risk), yearly influenza vaccine
Sickle cell/β-thalassemia	Pneumococcal (both polysaccharide and conjugated), Haemophilus influenza B, meningococcal, influenza (yearly)

TABLE 5-3 Specific Groups Benefitting from Vaccination (*Continued*)

GROUP	RECOMMENDED VACCINATIONS
Chronic liver disease	Hepatitis A and B, +/− pneumococcal, influenza
Health-care workers	Hepatitis A and B, yearly influenza
HIV	No live vaccinations (MMR, varicella, yellow fever, oral typhoid, rotavirus, FluMist, BCG, zoster, smallpox) Pneumococcal, influenza (yearly), meningococcal
Chronic disease (COPD, DM, CKD)	Pneumococcal, yearly influenza
G or C−females 9-26 years, may be given to females >26 years G−males 9-26 years, males >9 years who have sex with men	HPV (Gardasil [G])−HPV types 6,11,16, 18, Cervarix (C)−HPV types 16 and 18
Travelers	Yellow fever, typhoid, Japanese encephalitis, Dukoral (*Vibrio cholerae* and ETEC), RotaTeq (rotavirus), hepatitis (Twinrix), measles, mumps, rubella, pertussis, typhoid, tetanus, diphtheria, meningococcal (Saudi Arabia), rabies, malaria oral prophylaxis

Egg allergy is no longer a contraindication to influenza vaccine. Please see www. publichealth.gc.ca. for details.

Rules for Vaccinating Certain Populations

(1) Allergy—thimerosal, egg, latex, preservatives
   - Eggs—do not give yellow fever vaccinations
   - Streptomycin/neomycin—do not give IPV, MMR
(2) Live vaccines—give 1 month apart, or at separate sites
(3) Pregnancy—no live vaccinations (MMR, Varicella)
(4) Breastfeeding—safe to vaccinate except smallpox and yellow fever
(5) Preterm infants:
   - Vaccinate based on chronological age, not from birth date
   - Must be >2 kg for first Hepatitis B vaccination
(6) Anaphylaxis/encephalopathy/CNS complication with DTaP—can give only DT (no pertussis)
(7) Previous vaccination reaction—there are **no** contraindications for further vaccinations. Note vaccination reaction:
   - Temperature <40.5°
   - Redness, swelling, sore at injection sit

TABLE 5-4 Routine Adult Vaccines

RECOMMENDED VACCINE	DOSAGE
Tetanus, diphtheria, pertussis	Td every 10 years, Tdap if not given before × 1
Measles, mumps, rubella	Once in adulthood if born after 1970
Varicella	Not if history of chickenpox, two doses in adulthood if not immune (especially immigrants, females of childbearing age, immunocompromised, cystic fibrosis)

TABLE 5-5 Vaccine Classifications

Live attenuated	MMR, oral polio, typhoid, yellow fever, anthrax, intranasal influenza, varicella
Killed	Salk polio (IPV)
Inactivated	Hepatitis B vaccine, DTaP (DT-inactivated toxin, P is inactivated cells)
Capsular polysaccharide	Pneumococcal, *H. influenza*

The immunization schedule details vary in each province in Canada. Please see provincial guidelines.

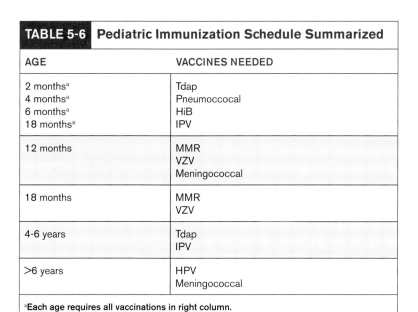

TABLE 5-6	Pediatric Immunization Schedule Summarized
AGE	**VACCINES NEEDED**
2 months[a] 4 months[a] 6 months[a] 18 months[a]	Tdap Pneumoccocal HiB IPV
12 months	MMR VZV Meningococcal
18 months	MMR VZV
4-6 years	Tdap IPV
>6 years	HPV Meningococcal

[a]**Each age requires all vaccinations in right column.**

Bibliography

Public Health Agency of Canada. *Canadian Immunization Guide.* 7th ed. 2006. http://www.phac-aspc. gc.ca/publicat/cig-gci/.

Public Health Agency of Canada. Travel vaccines. 2007. http://www.phac-aspc.gc.ca/im/travelvaccines-eng.php.

Public Health Agency of Canada. Canada communicable disease report—Volume 38, ACS-1—update on human papillomavirus virus (HPV) Vaccines. Jan 2012. http://www.phac-aspc.gc.ca/publicat/ccdr-rmtc/12vol38/acs-dcc-1/index-eng.php#a3-3.

Rx Files Academic Detailing Program. *Rx Files—Objective Comparisons for Optimal Drug Therapy: Vaccinations.* 8th ed. 50.

6
Psychiatry

Depression
Priority Topic 24

MAJOR DEPRESSIVE EPISODE

The patient should have at least five symptoms from the mnemonic MSIGECAPS (with one being depressed mood or decreased interest) lasting for at least 2 weeks to be diagnosed with major depressive episode (MDE).

DYSTHYMIA

Depressed mood for most of the day, on most days, for at least 2 years. No MDE is present in this 2 year period.

Risk Factors for MDE

- Chronic insomnia or fatigue
- Chronic pain
- Multiple or unexplained somatic complaints
- Chronic medical illnesses
- Acute cardiovascular events
- Recent psychological or physical trauma
- Other psychiatric disorders
- Family history of mood disorder

Treatment

- Start with a comprehensive evaluation of the patient
- Assess suicide risk at every evaluation
- Aim for full remission of symptoms and return to baseline psychological function [eg, Patient Health Questionnaire 9 (PHQ-9) score of <5]
- Plan two phases of treatment:
  - Acute phase (8-12 weeks) to achieve remission of symptoms
  - Maintenance phase (at least 6 months, but often longer) to prevent relapse/recurrence
- Monitor response using validated outcome measures, such as Patient Health Questionnaire 9 (PHQ-9).

Depression Symptoms (M SIGECAPS)
M–Depressed mood
S–Sleep disturbance
I–Interest reduced
G–Guilt and self blame
E–Energy loss and fatigue
C–Concentration problems
A–Appetite change
P–Psychomotor changes
S–Suicidal thoughts

Common SSRI Side Effects
(1) Nausea
(2) Anxiety
(3) Insomnia
(4) Agitation
(5) Tremor
(6) Headache
(7) Sexual dysfunction

- Follow-up patients weekly or biweekly, depending on severity, until they show clear improvement. After that, visits can be reduced to monthly and then less often.

First-Line Treatments

- Cognitive therapy (CT)* or cognitive behavioural therapy (CBT)* (Level 1 evidence)
- Interpersonal therapy (IPT)* (Level 1 evidence)

*At mild-to-moderate levels of severity, these treatments have efficacy comparable with medications, but they may be less effective in severe depression.

- Selective serotonin reuptake inhibitors (SSRIs) (Level 1 evidence)
- Venlafaxine (SNRI) may have higher remission rates than SSRIs (Level 1 evidence)

Second-Line Treatments

- Behaviour therapy (BT) (Level 1 evidence)

Third-Line Treatments

- Brief dynamic psychotherapy (BDP) (Level 2 evidence)
- Amitriptyline and clomipramine have greater efficacy than SSRIs in hospitalized patients with depression (Level 2 evidence). Safety and tolerability issues, however, need to be considered.
- Tricyclic antidepressants (TCAs) and monoamine oxidase inhibitors (MAOIs) are third-line treatments because of safety and tolerability issues (Level 2 evidence)

Maintenance Pharmacotherapy

- All patients should be maintained on antidepressants for at least 6 months after clinical remission (Level 1 evidence)
- Patients with the following risk factors should be maintained on antidepressants for at least 2 years: older age, psychotic features, chronic episodes, recurrent episodes (three or more in lifetime), frequent episodes (two or more in 5 years), difficult-to-treat episodes, and severe episodes (Level 2 evidence)
- The antidepressant dosage in the maintenance phase should be the same as in the acute phase (Level 2 evidence)
- Antidepressants should be tapered slowly to avoid discontinuation. Education about early signs of relapse should continue, and patient should have regular follow-up every 2 to 3 months for the first 6 months. Psychotherapy is helpful to prevent relapse.

Managing Nonresponse to Antidepressant Therapy

- MDD is a chronic condition that requires close monitoring until symptoms are eliminated. After this periodic monitoring can be done to ensure no signs of recurrence occur. Using the PHQ-9 is crucial to monitoring treatment response.
- For antidepressant treatment, expect the usual trajectory of response:
  - Initial mild symptom improvement (eg, >20% improvement in PHQ-9) within 2 to 4 weeks
  - Good clinical response (eg, >50% improvement in PHQ-9) within 4 to 8 weeks
  - Remission of symptoms (eg, PHQ-9 <5) by 8 to 12 weeks
  - Once an antidepressant is selected, an initial improvement (at least 20% reduction in depression scores) should be seen within 2 to 4 weeks. Otherwise, the following interventions are indicated in order listed:
    - Optimize the antidepressant by increasing the dose as tolerated (Level 2 evidence)
    - Switch to an antidepressant with a different neurochemical action (Level 2 evidence)

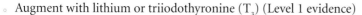

- ○ Augment with lithium or triiodothyronine (T_3) (Level 1 evidence)
- ○ Switch to an antidepressant with a similar neurochemical action (Level 2 evidence)
- ○ Augment with buspirone or an atypical antipsychotic such as olanzapine (Level 2 evidence)
- ○ Combine with another antidepressant (Level 3 evidence)

BIPOLAR DISORDER (SUPPLEMENTARY TOPIC)

Definitions

Manic Episode

- ■ Elevated mood lasting for at least 1 week with at least three symptoms listed in DIG FAST

Hypomania

- ■ Hypomania is defined the same as mania, but has a shorter duration of symptoms (4-6 days)

Bipolar Type I

- ■ At least one manic episode with or without an episode of major depression

Bipolar Type II

- ■ At least one hypomanic episode and one major depressive episode

Differential Diagnosis

- ■ Cyclothymia: hypomania and depressive symptoms (but not meeting criteria for MDE) with symptoms lasting for at least 2 years
- ■ ADHD
- ■ Schizophrenia
- ■ Substance abuse
- ■ Medical condition (thyroid, MS, epilepsy)

Treatment

- ■ Mood stabilizers (lithium, valproic acid, carbamazepine), anticonvulsants, antipsychotics, antidepressants, lamotrigine, ECT
- ■ Before starting on lithium, one must screen for pregnancy, order TSH, electrolytes, lipids, BUN, Cr, and complete an ECG
- ■ Monotherapy with antidepressants should be avoided
- ■ Send for CBT, psychotherapy
- ■ Patient may need vocational help, substance abuse help, time off work, education for themselves and their family

Mania symptoms (DIGFAST)
Distractibility
Impulsivity
Grandiosity
Flight of ideas
Activities
Sleep, decreased need
Talkative

Long term lithium use can lead to diabetes insipidus (DI) and hypothyroidism.

Bibliography

American Psychiatric Association. *Diagnostic and Statistical Manual of Mental Disorders*. 4th ed. Washington DC: American Psychiatric Publishing Inc; 2000.

Chen YA, Tran C. *Toronto Notes–Comprehensive Medical Reference & Review for MCCQE I and USMLE II*. Toronto, Canada: Toronto Notes for Medical Students Inc; 2011.

Kaplan HI, Sadock BJ, Sadock VA. *Kaplan and Sadock's Synopsis of Psychiatry: Behavioural Sciences/Clinical Psychiatry*. 10th ed. New York, NY: Lippincott Williams and Wilkins; 2007.

RxFiles. Antidepressant comparison chart. *Drug Comparsion Charts*. 8th ed. Saskatoon, SK. Saskatoon Health Region; 2010;105.

Anxiety Disorder
Priority Topic 6

DEFINITIONS/SYMPTOMS

Generalized Anxiety Disorder

Excessive worry that is difficult to control. The symptoms persist for at least 6 months and include at least three symptoms from the mnemonic BE SKIM:

Agoraphobia

A fear of being somewhere when escape might be difficult. The patient will often avoid the situations that bring on this fear.

Post-Traumatic Stress Disorder

Avoidance, hyperarousal, and reexperiencing of a traumatic, life-threatening event. Patient often relives the experience through hallucinations or flash backs and they often avoid stimuli that they associate with the trauma. These symptoms persist for at least 1 month.

Obsessive-Compulsive Disorder

A compilation of obsessions (intrusive, recurrent, undesired thoughts), and/or compulsions (repetitive behaviours or rituals). These symptoms cause significant distress in a patient's life and at some point the patient recognizes that their obsessions/compulsions are excessive.

Specific Phobias

Marked fear of a specific thing or situation. This involves high levels of anxiety and avoidance of the feared object, to the point that it affects the patient's life.

Common phobias:

- Animals (snake, spider)
- Natural environments (heights, water)
- Medicine (injections, blood)

Panic Disorder

Involves recurrent and unexpected panic attacks. There is a significant fear that these panic attacks will recur and this fear has persisted for at least 1 month.

Symptoms of panic attacks can be remembered with the mnemonic STUDENTS.

RISK FACTORS (ANXIETY DISORDERS)

- Family history of anxiety (or other mental disorder)
- Personal history of anxiety in childhood or adolescence, including marked shyness
- Stressful life event and/or traumatic event, including abuse
- Female
- Comorbid psychiatric disorder (particularly depression)

DIAGNOSIS

- Based on DSM-IV criteria (see definition section)
- Use baseline laboratory investigations to rule out organic causes of anxiety
  - CBC
  - Fasting glucose
  - Electrolytes

Generalized Anxiety Disorder Symptoms (BE SKIM)
- **B**lank mind
- **E**asily fatigued
- **S**leep disturbance
- **K**eyed up
- **I**rritability
- **M**uscle tension

Panic Attack Symptoms (STUDENTS)
Sweating
Trembling
Unsteadiness
Derealization
Excessive heart rate
Nausea
Tingling
Shortness of breath
Symptoms usually peak within 10 minutes.

- U/A
- TSH
- Urine toxicology for substance use

GENERAL MANAGEMENT OF ANXIETY DISORDERS

1. Identify anxiety symptoms
   - Determine whether anxiety is causing distress or functional impairment
   - Assess suicidality
2. Determine differential diagnosis
   - Is anxiety due to another medical or psychiatric condition?
   - Is anxiety medication-induced or drug-related?
   - Perform physical examination and baseline laboratory assessment.
3. Identify specific anxiety disorder
4. Consider psychological (CBT, desensitization techniques, relaxation therapies) and pharmacological treatment. Specific treatment will depend on diagnosis.

PHARMACOLOGICAL TREATMENT OF GAD

- Pharmacological treatments include SSRIs, SNRIs, TCAs, anticonvulsants, benzodiazepines, and Buspirone.
- **First-line agents** include escitalopram, paroxetine, sertraline, or venlafaxine XR. Antidepressants have the additional benefit of being effective against depressive symptoms and they treat ruminative worry (the core feature of GAD) much more effectively than do benzodiazepines.
- If an SSRI was chosen initially, and was ineffective after optimization, a switch to a second SSRI, or an agent with a different mechanism of action (an SNRI) would a reasonable.
- **Second-line choices** include benzodiazepines, bupropion extended release, buspirone, imipramine, and pregabalin.
- **Acute anxiety:** Benzodiazepines may be used if symptoms are severe. Usually recommended for short-term use, due to side effects (including sedation), potential cognitive impairment in the elderly, dependence, and withdrawal issues.

Medical Conditions That May Mimic or Aggravate Anxiety Symptoms
- Hypothyroidism, Hyperthyroidism
- CHF
- PE
- Arrhythmia
- Angina
- Asthma
- Adrenal insufficiency
- COPD
- Pneumonia
- Migraines
- IBS
- UIT (in elderly)
- Caffeine, nicotine, alcohol

SSRIs may increase anxiety in first 2 weeks of treatment.

Bibliography

American Psychiatric Association. *Diagnostic and Statistical Manual of Mental Disorders.* 4th ed. Washington DC: American Psychiatric Publishing Inc; 2000.

Chen AY, Tran C. *Toronto Notes.* Toronto, ON: Type & Graphics Inc; 2011.

Kaplan HI, Sadock BJ, Sadock VA. *Kaplan and Sadock's Synopsis of Psychiatry: Behavioural Sciences/Clinical Psychiatry.* 10th ed. New York, NY: Lippincott Williams and Wilkins; 2007.

Rx Files. Anxiety disorder medication chart. *Drug Comparison Charts.* 8th ed. Saskatoon, SK: Saskatoon Health Region; 2010:100.

Suicide

Priority Topic 90

- Always ask about suicidal ideation in **all** patients presenting with **any** mental illness.
- Know your community resources (eg, suicide hotline, local mental health clinic).
- If the patient is suicidal, assess the need for admission (voluntary or involuntary).
- If the patient is suicidal, but has a low risk of completing the act, you can treat as an outpatient. However, create a **safety plan** with the patient and provide very close follow-up.

Suicide Risk Factors (SAD PERSONS)

Sex—male
Age >60 or <18
Depression
Previous attempts
Ethanol abuse
Rational thinking loss
Suicide in family
Organized plan
No spouse/lack of support system
Serious illness/intractable pain

Transference—unconscious redirection of feelings from one person to another

Counter-transference—redirection of a therapist's feelings towards a client

Use SAD PERSONS mnemonic to remember the risk factors for suicide. The more risk factors a patient has, the more likely you are going to treat them as an inpatient.

Bibliography

Filate W, Ng D, Leung R, Sinyor M. *Essentials of Clinical Examination Handbook.* 5th ed. University of Toronto: The Medical Society Faculty of Medicine; 2005.

Yingming A. Chen. *Toronto Notes 2011: Comprehensive Medical Reference Review for MCCQE I USMLE II.* 27th ed. Toronto, ON: Toronto Review Notes; 2011.

Counseling
Priority Topic 18

Key Points

- Counseling should be explored when examining patients with mental and physical illness
- Allow adequate time when counseling patients
- Physician must recognize his/her own beliefs may interfere with counseling
- Must identify the patient's understanding of his/her problem before beginning counseling
- Clinicians must recognize when they are exceeding boundaries (eg, transference, counter-transference) or limits (problem is more complex than initially thought) and refer appropriately

Bibliography

Working Group on the Certification Process. Priority topics and key features with corresponding skill dimensions and phases of the encounter. The College of Family Physicians of Canada; 2010. http://www.cfpc.ca/uploadedFiles/Education/Certification_in_Family_Medicine_Examination/Definition%20of%20Competence%20Complete%20Document%20with%20skills%20and%20phases.pdf.

Eating Disorders
Priority Topic 34

TABLE 6-1　Anorexia vs. Bulimia: Characteristics, Diagnosis, and Treatment

	ANOREXIA NERVOSA	BULIMIA
Definition	An obsession with controlling food intake.	A binge eating disorder characterized by repeated cycles of binging followed by purging.
Symptoms	Fear of gaining weight and/or obsession with becoming thinner. Signs of starvation = decreased blood pressure, decreased HR, amenorrhea, constipation, dry skin, brittle nails, lanugo hair, osteoporosis, pre-renal failure.	Repeated cycles of binging followed by purging. A feeling of loss of control over eating behaviour. Russel sign = calloused knuckles. Dental issues, renal failure, Mallory –Weiss tear, abnormal lab values (metabolic alkalosis, hypokalemia, decreased sodium, decreased chloride).
Risk factors	Most commonly seen in women between the ages of 15-19. Obesity, concurrent mental illness, competitive athlete, history of sexual abuse, family history of mood or eating disorder, societal pressures.	90% of cases occur in women. Other risk factors include mood disorders, history of sexual or physical abuse, drug use, and parental obesity.
Diagnosis	Four following criteria must be met: • Resistance to maintaining proper body weight • Great fear of gaining weight • Unrealistic evaluation of body image • Amenorrhea for at least three consecutive cycles	The five following criteria must be met: • Eat large quantities of food in discrete intervals of time and lack of control over eating (binge eating) • Repetitive behaviour to prevent weight gain (laxatives, exercise) • Binge/purge at least two times/week for 3 months • Self worth influenced by body shape and weight • Symptoms do not occur during episodes of anorexia

TABLE 6-1	Anorexia vs. Bulimia: Characteristics, Diagnosis, and Treatment (*Continued*)	
	ANOREXIA NERVOSA	BULIMIA
Treatment	• Establish a therapeutic relationship • Monitor for low bone density	• Relapses are very common in bulimic patients. • Monitor closely for relapse. • Cognitive behavioural therapy is useful. • The combination of CBT + antidepressants is more effective than antidepressants alone.
	• Use multidisciplinary approach (psychologist, dietician, psychiatrist). • Monitor lab values for complications of eating disorder. • Provide close follow up. • Consider admission to hospital if low body weight, abnormal lab values, abnormal vitals, or actively suicidal. • Early intervention is proven more effective for both anorexia and bulimia. • Pharmacotherapy can include SSRIs or TCAs. SSRIs are more effective in anorexia.	

KEY POINTS

- Disorders of self-image
- Must rule out coexisting psychiatric conditions
- Anorexia has a better prognosis than bulimia
- Multidisciplinary approach is required for treatment
- Therapeutic relationship with patient is essential

Bibliography

American Psychiatric Association. *Diagnostic and Statistical Manual of Mental Disorders*. 4th ed. Washington, DC: American Psychiatric Publishing Inc; 2000.

BMJ Clinical Evidence. http://clinicalevidence.bmj.com.cyber.usask.ca/x/systematic-review/1009/overview.html. Accessed March 30, 2012.

Cochrane Database. Antidepressants versus psychological treatments and their combination for bulimia nervosa. 2001;(4)CD003385.

Dynamed [database online]. Anorexia Nervosa. EBSCO Publishing. http://web.ebscohost.com/dynamed/detail?sid=4a423eb2-9470-4d0e-886f-fc25c5e74c61%40sessionmgr114&vid=4&hid=108&bdata=JnNpdGU9ZHluYW1lZC1saXZl JnNjb3BlPXNpdGU%3d#db=dme&AN=114614. Accessed March 30, 2012.

Dynamed [database online]. Bulimia Nervosa. EBSCO Publishing. http://web.ebscohost.com/dynamed/detail?vid=3&hid=108&sid=4a423eb2-9470-4d0e-886f-fc25c5e74c61%40sessionmgr114&bdata=JnNpdGU9ZHluYW1lZC1saXZl JnNjb3BlPXNpdGU%3d#db=dme&AN=114924. Accessed March 30, 2012.

Kaplan HI, Sadock BJ, Sadock VA (2007). *Kaplan and Sadock's Synopsis of Psychiatry: Behavioural Sciences/Clinical Psychiatry*. 10th ed. New York, NY: Lippincott Williams and Wilkins.

National Eating Disorder Information Centre. nedic.ca. Accessed March 29, 2012.

National Guideline Clearinghouse. Practice guideline for the treatment of patients with eating disorders. http://www.guideline.gov/content.aspx?id=9318. Accessed on March 30, 2012.

Personality Disorders

Priority Topic 72

Definitions

- Axis II disorders
- Persistent pattern of behaviour that is not consistent with the norm's of the individual's culture[i]
- Results in impairment of social or occupational functioning
- Patients have intact reality testing and abstract abilities without any thought disorder

CLUSTER A–WEIRD

- Odd, eccentric. The patient does not see behaviours as a problem (see Table 6-2).

TABLE 6-2   Cluster A Personality Disorders

	PARANOID	SCHIZOID	SCHIZOTYPAL
Mnemonic	SUSPECT **S**pousal infidelity suspected **U**nforgiving (bears grudges) **S**uspicious **P**erceives attacks (and reacts quickly) **E**nemy or friend? (suspicious) **C**onfiding in others is feared **T**hreats perceived in benign events	DISTANT **D**etached or flattened affect **I**ndifferent to criticism or praise **S**exual experiences of little interest **T**asks done solitarily **A**bsence of close friends **N**either desires nor enjoys close relationships **T**akes pleasure in few activities	ME PECULIAR **M**agical thinking **E**xperiences unusual perceptions **P**aranoid ideation **E**ccentric behaviour or appearance **C**onstricted or inappropriate affect **U**nusual thinking or speech **L**acks close friends **I**deas of reference **A**nxiety in social situations **R**ule out psychotic or pervasive developmental d/o
Description	-Distrustful and suspicious nature -Emotionally cold and odd -Social isolation -Brief episodes of psychosis with persecutory delusion -Causes distress/impairment in daily functioning	-Detached and emotionally restricted -"Happy loners" -Disinterested in others, praise, or criticism -Social drifters -Dysphoria	-Eccentric -Odd behaviour, appearance, speech, and perceptions -Odd and magical thinking -Discomfort with social relationships
Risk factors	-Family h/o schizophrenia and delusional d/o, paranoid type. -Childhood abuse, minority, immigrant, deaf	-Male -Family h/o schizophrenia; troubled family relationships	-Relative with schizophrenia -Genetic: monozygotic twin > dizygotic twins
Management	-Cognitive behavioural therapy (CBT) and insight-oriented counseling -Meds: low dose antipsychotics. SSRI if comorbid depression, OCD, or agoraphobia	-Tx of choice = insight psychotherapy -Supportive therapy, eg, ID emotions -Meds: antipsychotics, antidepressants, psychostimulants	-Tx like residual schizophrenia -Insight-oriented, supportive therapy, milieu therapy -Meds: low dose neuroleptic (eg, pimozide). Haloperidol for eccentric thoughts

CLUSTER B–WILD

- Dramatic, emotional, erratic, attention seeking (see Table 6-3)
- Associated with substance abuse/dependence
- Prognosis: hard to treat, no cure; usually stable or deteriorating

TABLE 6-3   Cluster B Personality Disorders

	BORDERLINE	HISTRIONIC	NARCISSISTIC	ANTISOCIAL
Mnemonic	DESPAIRER **D**isturbance of identity **E**motionally labile **S**uicidal behaviour **P**aranoia or dissociation **A**bandonment (fear of) **I**mpulsive **R**elationships (unstable) **E**mptiness (feelings of) **R**age (inappropriate)	ACTRESSS **A**ppearance focused **C**enter of attention **T**heatrical (exaggerated behaviour) **R**elationships (believed to be more intimate than they are) **E**asily influenced **S**eductive behaviour **S**hallow emotions **S**peech (impressionistic and vague)	GRANDIOSE **G**randiose **R**equires attention **A**rrogant **N**eed to be special **D**reams of success and power **O**thers (unable to recognize feelings/needs of; lacks empathy) **S**ense of entitlement **E**nvious	CORRUPT **C**annot conform to law **O**bligations ignored **R**eckless disregard for safety **R**emorseless **U**nderhanded (deceitful) **P**lanning insufficient (impulsive) **T**emper (irritable and aggressive)
Description	-Unstable relationships and self-image -Causes significant distress and impaired functioning -Uses splitting defense mechanisms to manipulate **Red flags**: doctor shopping/legal suits against doctor; suicide attempts	-Pervasive pattern of excessive emotionality and attention-seeking behaviour that generally begins in early adulthood	-Begins by early adulthood and causes significant distress or impairment in multiple domains of functioning -Rage with criticism	-Onset <15 years old (conduct d/o); but called antisocial PD when ≥18 years old.

TABLE 6-3	Cluster B Personality Disorders (*Continued*)			
	BORDERLINE	HISTRIONIC	NARCISSISTIC	ANTISOCIAL
Risk factors	-Childhood abuse and neglect; abandonment. -5× more likely if d/o present in first degree relative	Note: this patient (unlike other PD) will often seek treatment, but are emotionally needy and hesitant to stop therapy	-Childhood abuse and neglect	-Familial -Maternal depression -Lower SES; abandonment or abuse; repeated harsh punishments -100% conduct d/o as child
Management	-CBT -Meds: SSRIs (aggression/anger)[ii] Low-dose antipsychotics (impulsivity and psychotic episodes) -Psychiatric consult -Assess suicide risk often	-Insight-oriented psycho-therapy -Meds: SSRIs can be helpful, but be aware they can use it for self-harm -Assess suicide risk	-CBT -Meds: SSRI (impulsivity or depression), mood stabilizers (impulse ctrl or bipolar)	-CBT -Assess for associated conditions: spousal/child abuse, drunk driving

CLUSTER C–WORRIED AND WIMPY

- Anxious, fearful (see Table 6-4)
- Causes significant impairment and distress in daily functioning
- Begins by early adulthood

TABLE 6-4	Cluster C Personality Disorders		
	OBSESSIVE-COMPULSIVE	AVOIDANT	DEPENDENT
Mnemonic	SCRIMPER **S**tubborn **C**annot discard worthless objects **R**ule obsessed **I**nflexible **M**iserly **P**erfectionistic **E**xcludes leisure due to devotion to work **R**eluctant to delegate to others	CRINGES **C**riticism or rejection preoccupies thoughts in social situations **R**estraint in relationships due to fear of shame **I**nhibited in new relationships **N**eeds to be sure of being liked before engaging socially **G**ets around occupational activities with need for interpersonal contact **E**mbarrassment prevents new activity or taking risks **S**elf viewed as unappealing or inferior	RELIANCE **R**eassurance required **E**xpressing disagreement difficult **L**ife responsibilities assumed by others **I**nitiating projects difficult **A**lone (feels helpless and uncomfortable when alone) **N**urturance (goes to excessive lengths to obtain) **C**ompanionship sought urgently when a relationship ends **E**xaggerated fears of being left to care for self
Description	-Maladaptive personality style defined by excessive rigidity, need for order and control, preoccupation with details, and excessive perfectionism -Symptoms increase with stress	-Social inhibition -Sensitive to criticism and rejection -Feelings of inadequacy -Fear of being disliked and avoid social situations yet lonely Similar to schizoid personality disorder but *wants* relationships	-Excessive need to be taken care of -Begins by early adulthood -Submissive and clingy -Difficulty making decisions -Avoids disagreements -At risk for spousal abuse
Risk factors	-Genetic: monozygotic > dizygotic twins, first degree relative with OCD or Tourette syndrome	-Childhood abuse or neglect	-Chronic physical illness in childhood or separation anxiety d/o -Early childhood parental loss
Management	-CBT—improves up to 70% of patients. -R/o coexisting Tourette syndrome -Meds: SSRI or clomipramine[iii]	-Tx of choice is individual psychotherapy (improve self-esteem) -Behaviour therapy—systematic desensitization, social skills, assertiveness training -Meds: MAOI, beta-blocker, stimulant	-Tx of choice is insight-oriented CBT -Anxiety management, assertive training -Set limits -Meds: TCA, MAOI, BDZ for sx -Relatively favorable prognosis

Obsessions: intrusive and inappropriate thoughts, impulses, or images.
Compulsions: behaviours or mental acts performed in response to obsessions or rigid application of rules.

KEY POINTS

- Personality disorders often coexist with Axis I disorders (medical) and substance abuse.[iv]
- These are chronic disorders with no cure and difficult to treat—clearly establish limits (time, drugs, accessibility), and try to reduce the impact of your personal feelings when dealing with personality disorder patients.
- Also see Table 6-5

TABLE 6-5	Personality Disorders–Cluster-Specific Key Points		
	CLUSTER A (WEIRD)	**CLUSTER B (WILD)**	**CLUSTER C (WORRIED AND WIMPY)**
Axis II disorder	Paranoid, schizoid, schizotypal	Antisocial, borderline, histrionic, narcissistic	Avoidant, dependent, obsessive-compulsive
Key points	-Odd, eccentric	-Dramatic, emotional, erratic, attention seeking -Associated with substance abuse/dependence -Prognosis: hard to treat, no cure; usually stable or deteriorating	-Anxious, fearful -Causes significant impairment and distress in daily functioning
Treatment	Psychotherapy	Psychotherapy and medications (mood stabilizers/antidepressants)	Psychotherapy and medications for associated symptoms

Bibliography

Caplan JP, Stern TA. *Current Psychiatry*. 2008;7(10):27-33.

DynaMed [database online]. Antisocial personality disorder. EBSCO Publishing. http://web.ebscohost.com.cyber.usask.ca/dynamed/detail?vid=16&hid=9&sid=5fdbf4ec-bc94-440b-af64-b72b84140e48%40session mgr4&bdata=JnNpdGU9ZHluYW1lZC1saXZlJnNjb3BlPXNpdGU%3d#db=dme&AN=114962. Accessed March 24, 2012.

DynaMed [database online]. Avoidant personality disorder. EBSCO Publishing. http://web.ebscohost.com.cyber.usask.ca/dynamed/detail?vid=20&hid=9&sid=5fdbf4ec-bc94-440b-af64-b72b84140e48%40session mgr4&bdata=JnNpdGU9ZHluYW1lZC1saXZlJnNjb3BlPXNpdGU%3d#db=dme&AN=114108. Accessed March 24, 2012.

DynaMed [database online]. Borderline personality disorder. EBSCO Publishing. http://web.ebscohost.com.cyber.usask.ca/dynamed/detail?vid=9&hid=9&sid=5fdbf4ec-bc94-440b-af64-b72b84140e48%40s essionmgr4&bdata=JnNpdGU9ZHluYW1lZC1saXZlJnNjb3BlPXNpdGU%3d#db=dme&AN=116319. Accessed December 5, 2012.

DynaMed [database online]. Dependent personality disorder. EBSCO Publishing. http://web.ebscohost.com.cyber.usask.ca/dynamed/detail?vid=22&hid=9&sid=5fdbf4ec-bc94-440b-af64-b72b84140e48%40 sessionmgr4&bdata=JnNpdGU9ZHluYW1lZC1saXZlJnNjb3BlPXNpdGU%3d#db=dme&AN=114240. Accessed March 24, 2012.

DynaMed [database online]. Histrionic personality disorder. EBSCO Publishing. http://web.ebscohost.com.cyber.usask.ca/dynamed/detail?vid=18&hid=9&sid=5fdbf4ec-bc94-440b-af64-b72b84140e48%40ses sionmgr4&bdata=JnNpdGU9ZHluYW1lZC1saXZlJnNjb3BlPXNpdGU%3d#db=dme&AN=114862. Accessed March 13, 2012.

DynaMed [database online]. Narcissistic personality disorder. EBSCO Publishing. http://web.ebscohost.com.cyber.usask.ca/dynamed/detail?vid=14&hid=9&sid=5fdbf4ec-bc94-440b-af64-b72b84140e48%40 sessionmgr4&bdata=JnNpdGU9ZHluYW1lZC1saXZlJnNjb3BlPXNpdGU%3d#db=dme&AN=116855. Accessed March 13, 2012.

DynaMed [database online]. Paranoid personality disorder. EBSCO Publishing. http://web.ebscohost.com.cyber.usask.ca/dynamed/detail?vid=3&hid=9&sid=5fdbf4ec-bc94-440b-af64-b72b84140e48%40sess ionmgr4&bdata=JnNpdGU9ZHluYW1lZC1saXZlJnNjb3BlPXNpdGU%3d#db=dme&AN=114532. Accessed March 15, 2012.

DynaMed [database online]. Schizoid personality disorder. EBSCO Publishing. http://web.ebscohost.com.cyber.usask.ca/dynamed/detail?vid=7&hid=9&sid=5fdbf4ec-bc94-440b-af64-b72b84140e48%40sess ionmgr4&bdata=JnNpdGU9ZHluYW1lZC1saXZlJnNjb3BlPXNpdGU%3d#db=dme&AN=114747. Accessed March 15, 2012.

DynaMed [database online]. Schizotypal personality disorder. EBSCO Publishing. http://web.ebscohost.com.cyber.usask.ca/dynamed/detail?vid=5&hid=9&sid=5fdbf4ec-bc94-440b-af64-b72b84140e48%40s essionmgr4&bdata=JnNpdGU9ZHluYW1lZC1saXZlJnNjb3BlPXNpdGU%3d#db=dme&AN=116517. Accessed March 15, 2012.

Ferri F. *Ferri's Clinical Advisor*. 1st ed. 2011 (5 books in 1).

Endnotes

i Angstman KB, Rasmussen NH. Personality disorder: Review and clinical application in daily practice. *Am Fam Physician.* 2011;84(11):1253-1260.

ii Paris J. Pharmacological treatments for personality disorders. *Int Rev Psychiatr.* June 2011;23:303-309.

iii Stein DJ, Denys D, Gloster AT, et al. Obsessive-compulsive disorder: Diagnostic and treatment issues. *Psychiatr Clin N Am.* 2009;2:665-685.

iv Devens M. Personality disorders. *Prim Care Clin Office Prac.* 2007;34:623-640.

Substance Abuse
Priority Topic 89

Definition

- Abuse: maladaptive pattern of use leading to impairment with one of the following in a 12-month period:
  - Failure to fulfill major obligation
  - Recurrent use in hazardous situations
  - Substance-related legal problems
  - Use despite interference in social or interpersonal function
- Dependence: maladaptive pattern of use with three or more of the following in a 12-month period
  - Tolerance
  - Withdrawal
  - Consuming larger amounts
  - Unsuccessful efforts to cut down
  - Excessive time spent to obtain the substance in question
  - Decreased interest in activities as a result of drug use
  - Use despite physical/psychological problems caused by use

Risk Factors

- Mental illness, chronic disability, lower socioeconomic class
- Comorbid conditions = poverty, sexually transmitted infections, mental illness, cirrhosis, HIV, hepatitis C

Diagnosis

- CAGE questionnaire:
  - Validated screening questionnaire for alcohol problems

> **C** = Have you ever felt you needed to **cut down** your drinking?
> **A** = Are you **annoyed** by people criticizing your drinking?
> **G** = Do you feel **guilty** about your drinking?
> **E** = Do you ever need a drink in the **morning** to steady your nerves? (**eye opener**)

  - Score ≥ 2 = further investigation indicated!(Some sources suggest that in women ≥ 1 = further investigation indicated)[i]

Some sources suggest that one or more positive responses should be used for women

Management of Alcohol Dependence

- Assess stage of change
- Offer behaviour modification/psychotherapy
- Offer services such as Alcoholics Anonymous, detoxification center, halfway house
- Schedule regular follow-up appointments
- Pharmacotherapy can include SSRI, naltrexone, disulfiram

Wernicke Encephalopathy
- Thiamine deficiency
- Symptoms of ataxia and tremor
- Double vision
- Nystagmus

Korsakoff Syndrome
- Tends to develop as Wernicke symptoms go away
- Thiamine deficiency
- Hallucinations
- Confabulation
- Loss of memory
- Inability to form new memory

Stages of Change
Stage 1: Precontemplation
Stage 2: Contemplation
Stage 3: Preparation
Stage 4: Action
Stage 5: Maintenance

Alcohol Withdrawal

Stage 1: tremor, sweating, anorexia, diarrhea, agitation

Stage 2: hallucinations

Stage 3: seizures

Stage 4: delirium tremens, autonomic hyperactivity

- Most likely to occur in those who routinely consume more than four to five drinks per day[ii]
- Treat alcohol withdrawal with supportive care, benzodiazepines, and thiamine

Canadian Safe Drinking Guidelines[iii]

- Women—10 drinks per week, no more than 2 drinks per day
- Men—15 drinks per week, no more than 3 drinks per day

Key Points

- Maintain a high index of suspicion for substance abuse in adolescents, adults, and the elderly
- Must also screen for and treat comorbid conditions

Five A's

Ask about substance use.

Assess their willingness to quit.

Advice to quit.

Assist in quitting.

Arrange follow-up.

Bibliography

American Psychiatric Association. *Diagnostic and Statistical Manual of Mental Disorders.* 4th ed. Washington, DC: American Psychiatric Publishing Inc; 2000.

Chen AY, Tran C. *Toronto Notes.* Toronto, ON: Type & Graphics Inc; 2011.

Kaplan HI, Sadock BJ, Sadock VA. *Kaplan and Sadock's Synopsis of Psychiatry: Behavioural Sciences/ Clinical Psychiatry.* 10th ed. New York, NY: Lippincott Williams and Wilkins; 2007.

Endnotes

i   Dhalla S, Kopec JA. The CAGE questionnaire for alcohol misuse: a review of reliability and validity studies. *Clin Invest Med.* 2007;30(1):33-41.

ii *Dynamed* [database online]. Alcohol Withdrawal. EBSCO Publishing. http://web.ebscohost.com/ dynamed/detail?vid=3&hid=118&sid=6d7eb159-b513-4455-a850-7f34b384dc23%40sessionmgr104 &bdata=JnNpdGU9ZHluYW1lZC1saXZlJnNjb3BlPXNpdGU%3d#db=dme&AN=114807. Accessed April 4, 2012.

iii Centre for Addiction and Mental Health. Canada's Low-Risk Alcohol Drinking Guidelines. http:// www.camh.net/About_Addiction_Mental_Health/Drug_and_Addiction_Information/low_risk_ drinking_guidelines.html. Accessed April 4, 2012.

Somatoform Disorders

Priority Topic 86

- Somatoform disorders are conditions involving multiple somatic complaints in multiple organ systems that cannot be explained by a general medical condition
- Symptoms are produced unconsciously and they cause significant distress or impairment in functioning

SOMATIZATION DISORDER

Definition

- Recurring, multiple complaints not explained by a medical etiology
- Onset of symptoms prior to 30 years of age[i]

Symptoms

- Common symptoms include (but not limited to) headache, abdominal pain, back pain, pelvic pain, dizziness, numbness, weakness, fatigue, shortness of breath, vomiting, dysphagia, sexual symptoms[ii]

Diagnosis

- At least eight or more physical symptoms that involve four body systems

Management

- See later
- CBT and SSRI medications may be helpful

Key Points

- Tends to be chronic in nature
- Somatization can be present in a patient who has a diagnosed medical condition[i]

CONVERSION DISORDER

Definition

- Symptoms affecting voluntary motor (weakness) or sensory systems (loss of sensation)[iii]

Symptoms

- Picture often suggests neurologic disease, but mix of symptoms does not fit any neurologic disorder
- Stress is trigger for symptoms[iv]

Diagnosis

- Diagnosis depends on four features:[iii]
  - Symptoms involving motor or sensory systems and may include loss of consciousness
  - No findings on examination to support the diagnosis of a neurologic condition
  - Symptoms are triggered by stressors
  - The possibility of intentional display of fictitious symptoms has been ruled out

Management

- See later

Key Points

- Spontaneous remission in most cases

HYPOCHONDRIASIS

Diagnosis

- Preoccupation with or fear of having a serious illness or belief that a serious illness is present based on misinterpretation of symptoms

Symptoms

- Expression of fear that a serious illness is present
- Usually a single symptom is the trigger for fear (ie, tachycardia)[i]

Diagnosis

- No evidence to support a diagnosis of a medical disorder
- Fear persists despite medical reassurance
- Duration >6 months

Management

- See later

Key Points

- Belief is not delusional. The patient realizes they have an unrealistic thought.

Need to rule out anorexia and bulimia when considering diagnosis of body dysmorphic disorder.

BODY DYSMORPHIC DISORDER

Definition

- Preoccupation with perceived defect in physical appearance

Symptoms

- Expression of dissatisfaction with physical appearance
- Usually related to face but can also involve penis, breasts, skin (wrinkles, spots), hair
- May lead to avoidance of social situations[v]
- Individuals may spend several hours per day involved in activities such as checking their appearance in a mirror, grooming, or seeking reassurance in regards to their appearance[vi]

Diagnosis

- History of concern about physical appearance
- Physical examination shows little if any actual defect to support the chief complaint

Management

- See later
- There is some limited evidence for CBT and SSRI drugs[vi]

MANAGEMENT PRINCIPLES FOR SOMATOFORM DISORDERS

- Create strong doctor–patient relationship
- Attempt to avoid multiple physicians being involved
- Set limits on number of visits, encourage regular scheduled visits
- Attempt to focus on psychosocial, not physical, symptoms
- Avoid unnecessary testing
- Use multidisciplinary approach (biofeedback, acupuncture, psychotherapy, group therapy)
- Treat comorbid psychiatric illnesses if present
- Avoid anxiolytics (if needed use only in short term)
- Help patients develop their problem-solving skills

KEY POINTS

- Empathy is important when working with patients with somatoform disorders
- Somatoform disorders can lead to many unnecessary tests, surgeries, and drug dependence
- Need to rule out depression and substance abuse

Bibliography

American Psychiatric Association. *Diagnostic and Statistical Manual of Mental Disorders*. 4th ed. Washington, DC: American Psychiatric Publishing Inc; 2000.

Chen AY, Tran C. *Toronto Notes*. Toronto, ON: Type & Graphics Inc; 2011.

Kaplan HI, Sadock BJ, Sadock VA. *Kaplan and Sadock's Synopsis of Psychiatry: Behavioural Sciences/Clinical Psychiatry*. 10th ed. New York: Lippincott Williams and Wilkins; 2007.

Endnotes

i   MD Consult. Search for Somatization Disorder. http://home.mdconsult.com/das/book/63108090-5/view/1353. Accessed April 2, 2012.

ii *Dynamed* [database online]. Somatization Disorder. EBSCO Publishing. http://web.ebscohost.com/dynamed/detail?vid=6&hid=108&sid=4a423eb2-9470-4d0e-886f-fc25c5e74c61%40sessionmgr114

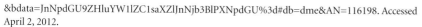

&bdata=JnNpdGU9ZHluYW1lZC1saXZlJnNjb3BlPXNpdGU%3d#db=dme&AN=116198. Accessed April 2, 2012.

iii Conversion disorder: a problematic diagnosis. *J Neurol Neurosurg Psychiatry*. 2011;82:1267-1273.

iv Conversion disorder: advanced in our understanding. *CMAJ*. 2011 May 17;183(8).

v *Dynamed* [database online]. Body Dysmorphic Disorder. EBSCO Publishing. http://web.ebscohost.com/dynamed/detail?vid=8&hid=108&sid=4a423eb2-9470-4d0e-886f-fc25c5e74c61%40sessionmgr114&bdata=JnNpdGU9ZHluYW1lZC1saXZlJnNjb3BlPXNpdGU%3d#db=dme&AN=116253. Accessed April 2, 2012.

vi Perceived ugliness: an update of treatment-relevant aspects of body dysmorphic disorder. *Curr Psychiatry Rep*. 2011;13:283-288.

Schizophrenia
Priority Topic 80

Definition

Two or more of the following symptoms for ≥1 month with continuous **disturbance in functioning** for ≥ 6 months

- Delusions
- Hallucinations
- Disorganized speech/behaviour
- Negative symptoms: flat affect, anhedonia, poverty of speech, avolition (inability to complete goal-directed activities)

Must exclude mood disorders, substance abuse, and general medical conditions as cause of psychosis.

Subtypes include: paranoid, disorganized, catatonic, or undifferentiated

Delusion: fixed false belief that is out of keeping with a person's cultural background and is firmly held despite proof to the contrary

Hallucinations: sensory perception in the absence of external stimuli, most often **auditory**

Symptoms

- Delusions—usually persecutory or grandiose
- Hallucinations—usually auditory
- Disordered speech—looseness of association, word salad, perseverations
- Disordered thoughts—fast or slow, thought blocking, loss of initiative
- Disordered social functioning—social withdrawal, poor functioning at work/school
- Substance use is common
- Suicidal ideation is common

Treatment: Non-pharmacological

- Encourage abstinence from drugs and alcohol
- Psychosocial supports—housing, family support, disability issues, vocational retraining
- For stable patients with schizophrenia (not floridly psychotic) assess at every visit:
  - Positive and negative symptoms
  - Suicidal, homicidal ideation
  - Performance of activities of daily living
  - Level of social functioning
  - Medication compliance and side effects

In teens with problem behaviours—consider schizophrenia!

Schizophrenia Risk Factors
- Strong genetic component
- First-degree relative affected by bipolar depression
- Increasing paternal age
- Cannabis use
- Birth in winter or early spring

- For decompensating patients determine if related to:
  - Substance use/abuse
  - Medication compliance and side effects
  - Change in psychosocial supports

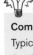

Common Antipsychotic Drug Side Effects
Typical—extrapyramidal side effects
Atypical—increased cardio-metabolic risk

Typical Antipsychotics (eg, Haloperidol, Chlorpromazine):

Goal of antipsychotic treatment is to increase functioning, minimize side effects, maximize compliance, and prevent relapse

Typical antipsychotics (eg, haloperidol, chlorpromazine)
- Mechanism of action: dopaminergic blockade
- Side effects are due to low dopamine; **extrapyramidal side effects** are more common

Atypical antipsychotics (eg, risperidone, olanzapine, quetiapine, clozapine)
- Mechanism of action: more complex, act on dopamine and serotonin receptors
- Treats negative symptoms more effectively
- Side effects: cardiometabolic more common

Side Effects

1. Extrapyramidal side effects: more common with typical antipsychotics or high dose atypical (risperidone >8 mg/day)
   - Dystonia: sustained muscle spasm, often involves neck, eyes-oculogyric crisis
   - Akathisia: feeling of internal restlessness; increased risk of suicide
   - Pseudoparkinsonism: TRAP-tremor, rigidity, akinesia, postural instability
   - **Tardive dyskinesia:**
     - Caused by long-term usage (≥6 months); often irreversible
     - Hyperkinetic disorder, involuntary irregular choreoathetoid movement
     - Most commonly face and mouth including chewing, sticking out tongue, and grimacing
     - Lifetime risk: 25% with typical; 10% with atypical antipsychotics
2. Increased prolactin (more common with typical)
   - Men: gynecomastia, decreased libido
   - Women: lactation, amenorrhea, infertility
3. Increased cardio-metabolic risk (more common with atypical medications)
   - Weight gain, insulin resistance and diabetes, dyslipidemia
4. Anticholinergic side effects
5. Antihistamine side effects:
   - Sedation
6. Antiadrenergic side effects (alpha 1):
   - Orthostatic hypotension
7. **Neuroleptic malignant syndrome**[ii]:
   - **FARM = f**ever, **a**utonomic (↑HR, ↑BP, sweating), **r**igidity, **m**ental status changes
   - It is a *life-threatening* complication that can occur *at any time* during treatment
   - Cause: massive dopamine blockade, develops over 24 to 72 hours
   - Lab result:
     - ↑ WBC, ↑ CK, ↑liver enzymes, ↑ plasma myoglobin, myoglobinuria
   - Risk factors:
     - Sudden increase in dosage or starting a new drug
     - Patient: young, male, medical illness, dehydration, poor nutrition
     - External heat load (hot summer days)

Anticholinergic Toxidrome/Side Effects
- Hot as a hare—fever/sweating.
- Blind as a bat—visual disturbance.
- Mad as a hatter—confusion.
- Dry as a bone.
- Bowel and bladder lose their tone.
- Heart goes off alone.

Neuroleptic Malignant Syndrome
FARM
Fever
Autonomic (↑HR, ↑BP, sweating)
Rigidity
Mental status changes

- Treatment:
  - Admit to ICU
  - **Stop** antipsychotic immediately (and any other DA blockers, ie, antiemetics)
  - Treat fever, hydrate, use cooling blankets
  - Dantrolene: a muscle relaxant, or benzodiazepines
  - Bromocriptine: a dopamine agonist

Key Points

- Schizophrenia is a **chronic disease** that involves one or more psychotic episodes.
- There is often a **prodromal period** of decline lasting months to years: increasing impairment in work, school, or home life followed by social withdrawal and finally overt psychosis.
- Generally patients with schizophrenia have **poor insight**. This can lead to the patients stopping their medicines. It is important to discuss the disease and the rationale behind the treatment plan with the patient.
- Consider schizophrenia in adolescents presenting with behavioural problems.
- Get collateral history from family, social workers.
- Screen for alcohol and drug use.
- Mental illnesses are highly prevalent in this population and increase morbidity and early mortality[iii]

Bibliography

American Psychiatric Association. *Diagnostic and Statistical Manual of Mental Disorders.* 4th ed. (text rev.) Washington, DC: American Psychiatric Publishing Inc; 2000.

Chen AY, Tran C. *Toronto Notes.* Toronto, ON: Type & Graphics Inc; 2011.

McPhee SJ, Papadakis MA, eds. *Current Medical Diagnosis and Treatment.* 49th ed. New York: McGraw Hill Medical; 2010.

Endnotes

i *Dynamed* [database online]. Schizophrenia. EBSCO Publishing. http://web.ebscohost.com/dynamed/detail?vid=3&hid=111&sid=23399d76-7182-4457-97ed-f542627c53a8%40sessionmgr110&bdata=JnNpdGU9ZHluYW1lZC1saXZlJnNjb3BlPXNpdGU%3d#db=dme&AN=115234. Accessed April 5, 2012.

ii Ables AZ, Nagubilli R. Prevention, recognition, and management of serotonin syndrome. *Am Fam Physician.* 2010 May 1;81(9):1139-1142.

iii Viron M, Baggett T, Hill M, Freudenreich O. Schizophrenia for primary care providers: How to contribute to the care of a vulnerable patient population. *Am J Med.* 2012;125:223-230.

Grief

Priority Topic 43

Key Points

- Prepare patients for emotional and physical responses they will be having when experiencing the loss of a loved one.
- Assess what stage of grief the patient is in.
- Inquire about depression and suicidal ideation in grieving patients, especially in those with prolonged grief reactions.
- Very young or elderly may have atypical grief reactions.
- Diagnosis of major depressive episode (MDE) is usually withheld until at least 2 months after a loss as normal bereavement can last this long. However, there is no concrete definition as to how long a "normal" grief reaction can last.
- Patients may present with a grief reaction, without an obvious trigger. Look for triggers that are unique to the patient including things such as death of pets, loss of a job.

Five Stages of Grief
(1) Denial
(2) Anger
(3) Bargaining
(4) Depression
(5) Acceptance

Bibliography

Kaplan HI, Sadock BJ, Sadock VA (2007). *Kaplan and Sadock's Synopsis of Psychiatry: Behavioural Sciences/Clinical Psychiatry.* 10th ed. New York, NY: Lippincott Williams and Wilkins.

Kübler-Ross E. *On Death and Dying.* Routledge: Simon and Schuster;1969.

Working Group on the Certification Process. Priority topics and key features with corresponding skill dimensions and phases of the encounter. The College of Family Physicians of Canada; 2010. http://www.cfpc.ca/uploadedFiles/Education/Certification_in_Family_Medicine_Examination/Definition%20of%20Competence%20Complete%20Document%20with%20skills%20and%20phases.pdf.

Behavioural Problems

Priority Topic 10

ATTENTION DEFICIT/HYPERACTIVITY DISORDER

- Affects 5% to 12% of school-aged kids. Male to female ratio is 4:1
- Associated higher risk for conduct disorder, oppositional defiant disorder, and substance abuse
- Seventy to eighty percent continue into adolescence, and 65% into adulthood

Definition

- Requires ≥6 symptoms of inattention, hyperactivity or impulsivity
- Symptoms must meet the following criteria:
  - Onset before age 7
  - Present for ≥ 6 months
  - Present in ≥2 environments (eg, school and home)

Can have teachers and parents fill out Swanson, Nolan, and Pelham IV Form (SNAP-IV Form) to assist in diagnosis.

Treatment

- Parent management
- Anger control
- Positive reinforcement
- Tutors
- Exercise
- Routine social skills training
- Medications (stimulants)—methylphenidate (>3 years of age), dextroamphetamine (<3 years of age)

Recommended that all children/adolescents on stimulants should have their height, weight, BP, and HR checked four times/year and have an annual physical examination.

CONDUCT DISORDER

Definition

Pattern of behaviour that violates rights of others and age-appropriate social norms. Behaviours include aggression to people and animals, destruction of property, deceitfulness or theft, and violation of rules. Patient must demonstrate ≥3 behaviours in past 12 months, and ≥1 in past 6 months. The behaviours must cause a significant impairment in the patient's life.

Conduct Disorder–if diagnosed before age 18
Antisocial Personality Disorder–if diagnosed after age 18

Treatment

- Early intervention with aid of CBT, parenting skills, anger management, family therapy, employment programs, and social skills training
- Drugs mostly used for comorbid conditions

OPPOSITIONAL DEFIANT DISORDER

Definition

Pattern of negative/hostile and defiant behaviour for ≥6 months with significant impairment in the patient's life

Treatment

- Parenting skills, psychoeducation, individual/family therapy, establish generational boundaries
- Drugs mostly used for comorbid conditions

KEY POINTS

- Keep broad differential diagnosis, as behavioural issues are often multifactorial, including medical conditions (eg, hearing problems, depression, abuse, drug use)
- Use multiple resources when gathering data on behaviour concerns
- Use multidisciplinary approach
- Never assume behaviour problems in the elderly are secondary to dementia. Must consider medication interactions/side effects, depression, infection.

Bibliography

American Psychiatric Association. *Diagnostic and Statistical Manual of Mental Disorders.* 4th ed. Washington DC: American Psychiatric Publishing Inc; 2000.

Kaplan HI, Sadock BJ, Sadock VA. *Kaplan and Sadock's Synopsis of Psychiatry: Behavioural Sciences/ Clinical Psychiatry.* 10th ed. New York, NY: Lippincott Williams and Wilkins; 2007.

Tao L, Dehlendorf C, Mendoza M, Ohata C. *First Aid for the Family Medicine Boards.* New York, NY: McGraw Hill; 2008.

Working Group on the Certification Process. Priority topics and key features with corresponding skill dimensions and phases of the encounter. The College of Family Physicians of Canada; 2010. http:// www.cfpc.ca/uploadedFiles/Education/Certification_in_Family_Medicine_Examination/Definition%20of%20Competence%20Complete%20Document%20with%20skills%20and%20phases.pdf.

Yingming A. Chen. *Toronto Notes 2011: Comprehensive Medical Reference Review for MCCQE I USMLE II.* 27th ed. Toronto, ON: Toronto Review; 2008.

7
Chronic Disease

Chronic Disease
Priority Topic 14

- Chronic diseases are illnesses that are prolonged in duration and are rarely cured completely.
- Chronic diseases, such as heart disease, stroke, cancer, chronic respiratory diseases, and diabetes, are the leading causes of mortality in the world, representing 63% of all deaths.
- Inquire about: (a) psychological impact of their diagnosis and treatment, (b) functional impairment, (c) depression or risk of suicide, and (d) underlying substance abuse, as these patients are at greater risk.
- Patients may seek medical attention for acute symptoms of their chronic disease such as:
  - (a) Acute complications of chronic disease (eg, DKA in DM or compression fracture in osteoporosis)
  - (b) Acute exacerbations of the disease (eg, asthma exacerbation, acute arthritis, AECOPD)
  - (c) A new, unrelated condition (eg, MI in a patient with underlying panic attacks with chest pain as a symptom)
- Pain is often a predominant symptom in chronic disease. Actively inquire about pain and treat it appropriately by titrating medication to the patient's pain. Consider non-pharmacologic treatment and adjuvant therapies (eg, cognitive behavioural therapy, physiotherapy, acetaminophen combined with opioids for synergistic effects).
- Regularly reassess adherence to the treatment plan (including medication) and in a nonadherent patient, explore the reasons why, with a view to improving future adherence to the treatment plan. Some example questions to ask are: "Do you sometimes forget to take your medication?", "Have you been regularly attending your physiotherapy/counselling appointments?"

Strategies to Improve Adherence Include
- Regularly scheduled visits (eg, DMII visits every 3 months)
- Bubble packing medications
- Two-in-one drug combinations
- Long-acting drug formulations

Bibliography

The College of Family Physicians of Canada. http://www.cfpc.ca/uploadedFiles/Education/Priority%20 Topics%20and%20Key%20Features.pdf.

World Health Organization. http://www.who.int/topics/chronic_diseases/en/.

Asthma

Priority Topic 7

Definition

Chronic inflammatory disease of the airways characterized by reversible airflow limitation and a variable degree of hyperresponsiveness of airways to stimuli.

Symptoms

- Wheeze, cough, difficulty breathing, chest tightness
- Symptoms are frequent, recurrent, and worse at night and in the early morning
- These are exacerbated by exercise, allergen exposure (house dust mites, pets, pollens, moulds, spores, cockroaches), viral infections, cigarette smoke, cold or damp air, or with emotions
- History of improvement in symptoms or lung function in response to trial of beta-agonists or inhaled corticosteroids

Risk Factors

- Personal history of atopic disorder
- Family history of atopic disorder and/or asthma

Diagnosis in younger children is based on history, symptoms, physical findings such as more than three episodes of wheezing/chronic cough at night or with exercise, a family history of atopy, and response to short-acting beta-agonists (SABA) and inhaled corticosteroids (ICS).

Diagnosis/Investigation

- Rule out other disorders, for example, tumors in adults, foreign body in children
- Spirometry in adults and children >6 years (measures presence and severity of airflow obstruction): improvement in FEV_1 >12% and >200 mL from the baseline 15 minutes after an inhaled short-acting beta$_2$-agonist in adults
- If spirometry results are non-diagnostic, but there is still some probability of asthma consider methacholine challenge test performed in pulmonary function laboratory, exercise challenge, and/or inhaled corticosteroid trial for 4 to 6 weeks
- Chest x-ray is not required and is normal (unless other disease process is present, eg, pneumonia)

General Management

- Most people with asthma should have minimal to no impact on their quality of life
- Good asthma control defined as: daytime symptoms less than four per week, no limitation of activities, no nocturnal symptoms/awakening, require reliever/rescue treatment less than four per week except one per day for exercise induced asthma, lung function (PEF or FEV1> 80% personal best), no exacerbations in the last year
- Evaluate and assess impact and exposure to allergens and irritants in individual patients
- Recommend complete cessation of smoking and avoidance of environmental tobacco smoke
- Recommend annual influenza vaccination for patients and their families

Asthma Severity Index Based on Medications

- Mild—well-controlled symptoms, treated with short-acting beta$_2$-agonist occasionally and low-dose inhaled corticosteroid
- Moderate—well-controlled symptoms, treated with short-acting beta$_2$-agonist and low to moderate dose of inhaled glucocorticosteroid
- Severe—well-controlled symptoms, treated with short-acting beta$_2$-agonist, high-dose inhaled corticosteroid, and additional therapy, for example, LTRA, LABA
- Very severe—symptoms not controlled, treated with short acting beta$_2$-agonist and high-dose inhaled glucocorticosteroids, additional therapy, and oral glucocorticosteroid

Pharmacological Management

- With normal expiratory flows and controlled symptoms, employ an inhaled short-acting beta$_2$-agonist prn
- If a rescue beta$_2$-agonist is needed more than two times per week (excluding pre-exercise), or if lung function is abnormal, the next step is an inhaled glucocorticosteroid
- Devices: For children, first line is a metered dose inhaler (MDI) and spacing device. In adults a dry powdered device (DPI) is efficacious and often more convenient (second line in children)

Stepwise Approach to Management of Chronic Asthma

Patients should start treatment at the step most appropriate to the initial severity of their asthma

- At each step, review medication adherence, inhaler technique, and patient education
- Use an action plan in concert with patient education (http://www.Asthma-ActionPlan.com)
- Reconsider diagnosis if no or poor response to therapy
- Modify the environment to reduce exposure to triggers, for example, smoking cessation, avoidance of second-hand smoke, pet removal, prevention of house dust mites, and mould
- If symptom control maintained over 3 months, step down to the least medication necessary to maintain control
  - **Step 1**—inhaled short-acting beta$_2$-agonist (SABA, eg, salbutamol) prn
  - **Step 2**—add inhaled corticosteroid (ICS, eg, fluticasone, budesonide). In children age 6 to 11 years, start at a low dose
    - Adults: budesonide 400 to 2400 mcg/day, fluticasone 250 to 2000 mcg/day
    - Children: budesonide 200 to 400 mcg/day, fluticasone 100 to 400 mcg/day
  - **Step 3**—Add inhaled long-acting beta$_2$-agonist (LABA, eg, salmeterol, formoterol in combination with an ICS

    Note: Assess control of asthma. If good response to LABA/ICS combination, continue; if benefit from LABA/ICS combination but control still inadequate, continue LABA and increase steroid dose to high-dose ICS; if no response to LABA/ICS combination, stop LABA combination and continue high-dose inhaled steroid. LABAs are contraindicated as monotherapy, but can be used in combination with an appropriate dose of ICS.
  - **Step 4:** Consider the following:
    - Short course of oral corticosteroids in adults to stabilize the patient, for example, prednisone 0.6 mg/kg/day for 5 days
    - Referring patient for specialist care
    - Adding a third drug (eg, leukotriene receptor antagonist, eg, montelukast, SR theophylline, or low-dose steroids) (Figure 7-1).

Acute ER Treatment

- Supplemental oxygen to keep sats >90%
- Salbutamol by mask q20 mins × 3
- Add ipratropium to first three doses of salbutamol
- Give prednisone or dexamethasone asap since it takes 4 hours to work
- If glucocorticosteroid required in the ED, discharge home with 30 to 60 mg prednisone po × 7 to 10 days in adults or 1 to 2 mg/kg/day × 3 to 5 days in children

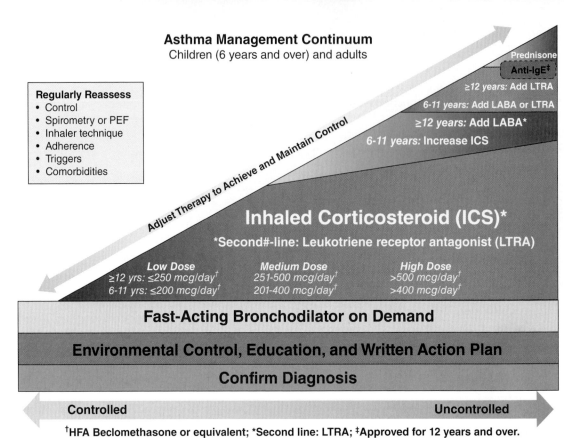

Asthma Management Continuum
Children (6 years and over) and adults

FIGURE 7-1:   Asthma management continuum. Printed with permission from the Canadian Thoracic Society.

Bibliography

Evans M, Meuser J. *Mosby's Family Practice Sourcebook*. 4th ed. Ontario, Canada: University of Toronto; 2005.

Lougheed MD, Lemière C, Dell SD, et al. Canadian Thoracic Society asthma management continuum—2010 consensus summary for children six years of age and over, and adults: *Can Resp J*. 2010;17(1):15-24. http://www.respiratoryguidelines.ca/canadian-thoracic-society-asthma-management-continuum-%E2%80%93-2010-consensus-summary-for-children-six-year. Accessed February 20, 2012

Chronic Obstructive Pulmonary Disease

Priority Topic 15

Definition

Chronic obstructive pulmonary disease (COPD) encompasses both chronic bronchitis and emphysema. It is a chronic, slowly progressive disease characterized by airway obstruction that is largely fixed but may be partially reversible with bronchodilators.

Symptoms

Frequent respiratory infections, dyspnea, and chronic/recurrent cough

Risk Factors

- Smoking (90% of cases)—most important cause of and contributing factor for COPD progression
- α-1 antitrypsin deficiency (1%)

Diagnosis

- Definitive diagnosis requires spirometry. (Post bronchodilator spirometry: FEV_1 <80% and FEV_1/FVC <0.7)

- Indications for spirometry include:
  - Smokers/ex-smokers ≥40 years of age plus one of the following:
    - Frequent respiratory infections
    - Dyspnea
    - Chronic cough
    - Wheeze
    - Sputum production
    - Nonsmokers with occupational exposures or α-1 antitrypsin deficiency
    - Early childhood lung infections
    - Exposure to air pollutants
- Mass screening of asymptomatic people with spirometry not recommended
- Chest x-ray useful if comorbidities need to be excluded

TABLE 7-1 COPD Stages and Drug Treatments

STAGE	SIGNS/SYMPTOMS	FEV$_1$	FEV$_1$/FVC	DRUG MANAGEMENT
At risk	Asymptomatic smoker or ex-smoker with chronic cough/sputum	>80%	0.7	
Mild	Dyspnea with strenuous exercise, hurrying on the level, or walking up a slight hill	60%-79%	<0.7	SABA or anticholinergic prn
Mild persistent				SABA prn + LABA or anticholinergic—regular use
Moderate	Dyspnea causing patient to walk slower than others of the same age or to stop walking after 100 m	40%-59%	<0.7	SABA prn + LABA + anticholinergic—regular use
Severe	Patient too breathless to leave the house, breathless on dressing, or presence of chronic respiratory failure or clinical signs of right heart failure	<40%	<0.7	*If >one exacerbation per year or asthma:* add inhaled corticosteroid Theophylline may be used if persistent symptoms despite optimal inhaled therapy

SABA, short-acting beta$_2$-agonist (salbutamol); LABA, long-acting beta$_2$-agonist (salmeterol); anticholinergic (ipratropium, tiotropium).

Management

Drug and nondrug strategies can improve symptoms, activity levels, and quality of life

Goals: prevent progression, alleviate symptoms, improve exercise tolerance, reduce exacerbations, treat complications, improve health status, and reduce mortality

(a) **Smoking cessation**
  - Most effective intervention for preventing COPD progression, even in long-term smokers
  - Offer help to all smokers/families and reinforce at every contact

(b) **Education and self-management**
  - Focus on improving coping skills and quality of life
  - Encourage exercise—if activities are limited by symptoms, refer to an exercise training program
  - Refer to a pulmonary rehabilitation program/community respiratory services. Early participation has been shown to improve QOL

(c) **Drug management** (refer to Table 7-1)
  - Consider a combination product if using long-acting beta$_2$-agonist + inhaled corticosteroid
  - Evaluate inhaler technique regularly and consider a spacer for metered dose inhalers
  - Avoid long-term oral steroid use (use only in acute exacerbations of COPD [AECOPD])

Ipratropium is associated with increased risk of cardiovascular death and myocardial infarction in patients with chronic obstructive pulmonary disease (COPD), whereas tiotropium does not appear to be associated with increased cardiovascular risk.

(d) Ongoing care
- Vaccinations:
  - Influenza—annually
  - Pneumococcal—once per lifetime (repeat in 5-10 years if high risk)
- O$_2$ may be a useful addition to exercise therapy
- In severe disease, discuss end of life issues, and patient's wishes on aggressive treatments

Acute Exacerbations of COPD

- Characterized by ≥48 hours of worsening dyspnea and cough, with or without sputum
- Triggers:
  - Viral or bacterial upper respiratory infection—most common cause
  - Others: irritants, PE, MI, anemia, CHF, systemic infection
- Severe AECOPD can be a medical emergency; develop an exacerbation plan with the patient
- Therapies include:
  - Short-acting beta$_2$-agonists and anticholinergic bronchodilators
  - Oral corticosteroids (eg, prednisone 25-50 mg/day) for <2 weeks in moderate to severe COPD
  - Use antibiotics if two of the following are present:
    - Increased dyspnea or cough
    - Increased sputum
    - Increased sputum purulence
- Choose antibiotics based on risk factors:
  - **Low risk:**
    - Amoxicillin 1 g tid, (2) doxycycline 100 mg od, or (3) TMP/SMX 1 DS tab bid, (4) azithromycin
  - **High risk**
    - Definition: patient with comorbidities (including ischemic heart disease or CHF) and/or greater than three exacerbations/year: (1) amoxicillin-clavulanate 875 mg bid, (2) levofloxacin 500-750 od, or (3) moxifloxacin 400 mg od. (Figure 7-2)

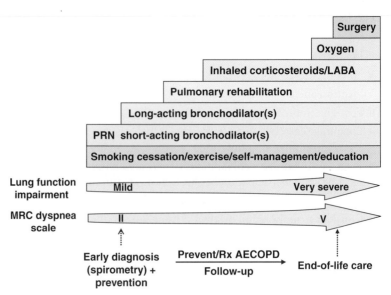

FIGURE 7-2: COPD management continuum. Printed with permission from Canadian Thoracic Society.

Bibliography

Evans M, Meuser J. *Mosby's Family Practice Sourcebook*. 4th ed. University of Toronto: Ontario, Canada; 2005.

O'Donnell DE, Hernandez P, Kaplan A, et al. Canadian Thoracic Recommendations for management of chronic obstructive pulmonary disease—2008—a primary care update. *Can Resp J.* 2008;15(supplement A):1A-8A.

Singh S, Loke Y, Furberg C. Inhaled anticholinergics and risk of major adverse cardiovascular events in patients with chronic obstructive pulmonary disease: a systematic review and meta-analysis. *JAMA* 2008;300(12):1439-1450.

Diabetes

Priority Topic 25

Prevention: Reduction of Risk Factors

- Healthy diet and lifestyle with optimal BMI (target 18.5-24.9)
- Waist circumference (M <94 cm; F <80 cm)
- Encourage aerobic activity (30 minutes) most days of the week and resistance training three times per week
- Encourage smoking cessation

TABLE 7-2	Symptoms/Characteristics
DM TYPE 1	**DM TYPE 2**
• Polyuria • Polydipsia • Polyphagia • Weight loss • Blurry vision • Dehydration • Neuropathy (late sign)	• Commonly asymptomatic • Acanthosis nigrans (sign of insulin resistance)

TABLE 7-3	Risk Factors for DM type 2	
• Dyslipidemia • Overweight • Abdominal obesity • Age 40-70 • HTN • 1st-degree relative with DM • Hx of IGT or IFG	• Schizophrenia • Steroid use • 2nd-generation antipsychotic use: (olanzapine, risperidone, clozapine, quetiapine) • High-risk population (Aboriginal, Hispanic, South Asian, African)	• Hx GDM • Delivery of a macrosomic infant • Acanthosis nigrans • Vascular Dz • DM-associated complications • PCOS

TABLE 7-4	Screening
DM TYPE 2	**GDM**
Fasting Plasma Glucose (FPG) • Q 3 years if >40 years • Q 1 year if risk factors	50 g OGTT (screen at 24-28 weeks) • <7.8 mmol/L = normal • 7.8-10.2 = do 75 g OGTT • >10.3 = GDM

Use acarbose to reduce risk of developing DM.

Frequency of Glucose Self-Monitoring
DM Type 1
  Minimum 3×/day
DM Type 2
  Insulin+/− oral: >1×/day
  Oral only: 1-2×/week
  Diet only: occasional testing

TABLE 7-5	Diagnosis of Diabetes and Glucose Impairment		
		GLUCOSE TEST	
DIAGNOSIS		FPG (MMOL/L)	75G OGTT
Normal		<6.1	<7.8
DM		>7.0 on two occasions or Random glucose >11.1 with DM symptoms	>11.1
IFG (impaired fasting glucose)		6.1-6.9	
IGT (impaired glucose tolerance)			7.8-11.0

TABLE 7-6	Type 2 Diabetes Medications		
CLASS	**ADVANTAGES**	**DISADVANTAGES**	
Biguanide • Metformin	• Weight neutral • ↓ hypoglycemia	• GI side effects • CI: CrCL/eGFR <30 mL/min • Caution if liver failure or CrCL/eGFR <60 mL/min • Risk of lactic acidosis in HF, renal or liver disease, or hypoxemia	
Insulin secretagogues: Sulfonylureas • Gliclazide • Glyburide	• Newer agents (Gliclazide) associated with ↓ hypoglycemia	• Weight gain (Glyburide) • CI: sulfa allergy—rash, photosensitivity	
Insulin secretagogues: Meglitinides • Repaglinide	• ↓ hypoglycemia with missed meals • Better postprandial control	• TID to QID dosing	
Insulin sensitizers: TZDs • Rosiglitazone	• ↓ hypoglycemia • Good monotherapy	• 6-8 weeks to maximal effect • Weight gain (fluid retention), edema, rare CHF • Increased fracture risk • Avoid in HF, liver dysfunction • May increase the risk of ischemic events	
DPP-4 inhibitor • Sitagliptin (Januvia)	• Weight neutral • ↓ hypoglycemia • Good postprandial control	• No long-term studies • Not for use in kidney or liver failure	
Incretin mimetic • Liraglutide (Victoza)	• Glucose-dependent insulin secretion • ↓ hypoglycemia • Improved postprandial control • Weight loss	• Injection • Nausea and diarrhea common, decreases with use • Minor hypoglycemia if used with sulfonylureas • Pancreatitis risk • CI: Fhx of MEN 2, medullary thyroid cancer	
Alpha-glucosidase inhibitor • Acarbose	↓ risk of hypoglycemia Weight neutral Good postprandial control	• GI side effects • Use in combination with another oral agent • Modestly effective in elderly • Hypoglycemia should be treated with glucose!	
Insulin	Greatest A1C reduction No maximum dose	• Weight gain • Risk of hypoglycemia	

Management of DM

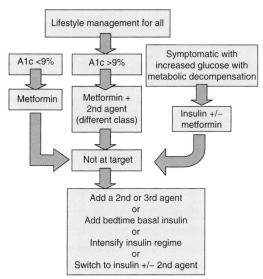

FIGURE 7-3: Management of hyperglycemia in DM type 2. Canadian Diabetes Association Clinical Practice Guidelines Expert Committee. Canadian Diabetes Association, 2008.

DM Treatment Goals (mmol/L)

	DM	Frail	No CVD and young/safe
A1C (q3-6mo):	<7%	<8%	<6%
Q 3-6 months			
FPG:	4-7		4-6
2hr PPG hours post	5-10		5-8

Frail = patients with DM and at high risk for adverse side effects from hypoglycemia

HIGH RISK OR CVD?
Also Start :
1. ACE-I/ARB
2. Statin
3. ASA/ Plavix

Complications/Chronic Disease Monitoring

1. **A1C** (glycated hemoglobin):
   (a) Test q 3 months
   (b) Target: <7.0%
   (c) Consider testing q 6 months if stable
2. **Chronic kidney disease** (screen annually):

	Normal	Micro	Macro
(a) Proteinuria	<30 mg/day	30-300 mg/day	>300 mg/day
(b) Urine ACR (albumin: creatinine ratio)	M: <2; F: <2.8	<10× normal	>10 × normal

   (c) eGFR: CKD if <60 mL/min
3. **Retinopathy** (retinal examination):
   (a) DM type 2: at diagnosis then q 1-2 years
   (b) DM type 1: 5years post diagnosis then q1 year
4. **CAD**:
   (a) ECG: q 1-2 years (age >40 years or DM >15 years)
   (b) Lipids (TC, HDL-C, LDL-C, triglycerides): q 1-3 years, if at target and no therapy. If therapy indicated, retest 6-8 weeks after any therapy change and then q 6-8 months. (DM patients are high risk for CAD.)
     □ High risk lipid targets: LDL <2.0 mmol/L and TG/HDL <4.0 mmol/L
5. **Peripheral neuropathy**: foot examination q 1 year

TABLE 7-7	Emergency/Acute Complications of DM		
	SIGNS/SYMPTOMS	LABS	TREATMENT
Hypoglycemia <3.5 mmol/L	Tachycardia Sweating Tremulous Nausea/vomit Hunger Confusion Stupor	↓ glucose	Awake—dextrose or 15 g glucose containing food q 15 minutes, until glucose > 5.0 mmol/L Unconscious— glucagon IM or 50% glucose IV

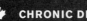
TABLE 7-7 Emergency/Acute Complications of DM (*Continued*)

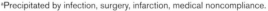

	SIGNS/SYMPTOMS	LABS	TREATMENT
Hyperglycemia	Abdominal pain Vomiting Lethargy Increased thirst Increased urination	↑ glucose	Insulin
DKA[a]	Tachycardia Vomiting Kussmaul breathing (rapid & deep) Fruity breath Lethargy Coma	↑ glucose ↑ osmolality ↑ anion-gap metabolic acidosis + Ketones ↑ K+ ([a]falsely elevated)	Insulin infusion Fluids K+
Hyperosmolar hyperglycemic syndrome[a]	Polyuria Polydipsia Polyphagia Weakness Lethargy Confusion Coma	↑↑ glucose ↑↑ osmolality ↑ anion-gap metabolic acidosis ↑ K+ ([a]falsely elevated)	Insulin infusion Fluids K+

[a]Precipitated by infection, surgery, infarction, medical noncompliance.

Acute Illness in DM—Advise for Patients
- Can lead to DKA
- If preprandial glucose >14.0 mmol/L and symptoms—test urine/serum ketones
- Increase frequency of self blood glucose testing
- Increased insulin requirements during illness/stress

Bibliography

British Columbia Medical Association. Guidelines and protocols advisory committee. *Diabetes Care.* 2010. http://www.bcguidelines.ca/guideline_diabetes.html. Accessed November 18, 2011.

Canadian Diabetes Association, Clinical Practice Guidelines Expert Committee. Prevention of diabetes. *Can J Diabetes.* 2008;32(supp.1). http://www.diabetes.ca/files/cpg2008/cpg-2008.pdf. Accessed November 20, 2011.

McCulloch DK. Overview of medical care in adults with diabetes mellitus. In: Nathan DM, Mulder JE, eds. *Uptodate.* 2012. http://www.uptodate.com/contents/overview-of-medical-care-in-adults-with-diabetes-mellitus?source=search_result&search=diabetes&selectedTitle=1~150. Accessed December 5, 2011.

O'Connor NR. Diabetes type 2. In: Slawson D, French L, Lin K, eds. *Essential Evidence Plus.* 2011. https://www.essentialevidenceplus.com/content/eee/127. Accessed December 1, 2012.

Hypertension

Priority Topic 47

Definitions

(Note: All blood pressures noted are in mm Hg.)

- Hypertensive urgency: Blood pressure ≥180/120 *without* signs of target end-organ damage
- Hypertensive emergency: Blood pressure ≥180/120 with signs of target end-organ damage
- Hypertension: Blood pressure ≥140/90
- Hypertension (DM or chronic renal failure): Blood pressure ≥130/80

Screen

- Age ≥18 years, then every 2 years
- If pre-hypertension, (120-139/80-89), recheck in 1 year

Diagnosis

- Diagnosis of hypertension depends on whether it is an ambulatory, home, or office value. Due to the variability of values and white coat syndrome, it may take several visits before diagnosis.

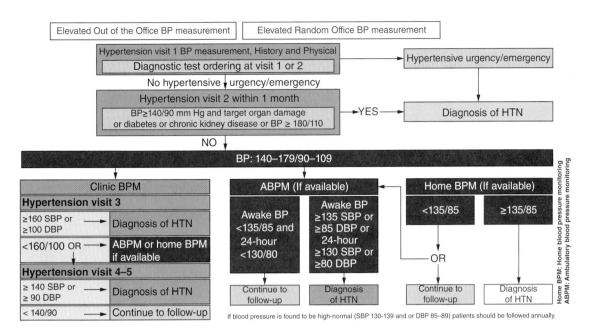

FIGURE 7-4: Steps to diagnose hypertension. Reprinted with permission from the Canadian Hypertension Education Program.

Evaluation

History

- Usually asymptomatic
- Cardiovascular risk factors for atherosclerosis (refer to Ischemic Heart Disease)

Examination

- Signs of target organ damage:
  - Cerebrovascular: TIA, ischemic or hemorrhagic stroke, vascular dementia
  - Ocular: hypertensive retinopathy
  - Cardiac: left ventricular dysfunction, angina, MI, heart failure
  - Renal: chronic kidney disease, albuminuria
  - PVD: intermittent claudication
- Suspect secondary hypertension if:
  - Sudden onset or worsening of hypertension and age >55 or <30 years
  - Hypertension resistant to three or more drugs
  - Renal/vascular symptoms: abdominal bruit, rise in creatinine >30% with use of ACE inhibitor, pulmonary edema, atherosclerosis
  - Hypokalemia (hyperaldosteronism)
  - Pheochromocytoma symptoms: headaches, palpitations, sweating, paroxysmal hypertension
  - Thyroid disease
  - Cushing syndrome: central obesity, moon face, striae, hirsutism, acne
  - Obstructive sleep apnea signs/symptoms: daytime fatigue, snoring, thick neck
  - Renal insufficiency (including polycystic kidney)
  - Drugs: NSAIDs, cold remedies (pseudoephedrine), high dose and long-term use of nasal decongestants, OCP, venlafaxine, corticosteroids, cocaine, anabolic steroids, alcohol

Labs

- Urinalysis
- Sodium, potassium, and creatinine
- Fasting glucose

- Fasting lipids (serum total cholesterol, HDL, LDL, triglycerides, total cholesterol/HDL ratio)
- ECG
- If DM or chronic kidney disease, check urine albumin
- Appropriate investigations for secondary hypertension if indicated

Management

Lifestyle

- Weight loss (target BMI 18.5-24.9 kg/m^2)
- DASH (dietary strategies against hypertension) diet
- Low sodium intake
- Physical activity: 30-60 min of moderate intensity dynamic exercise (walking, cycling, swimming) 4-7 days/week + activities of daily living
- Alcohol in moderation
- Stress management
- Smoking cessation

Medications

TABLE 7-8	Hypertension: Medications and Targets (mm Hg)	
	TARGET	TREATMENT
Uncomplicated HTN	140/90	ACE-I/ARB or thiazide or β-blocker[a] or CCB
Isolated systolic	<140	ACE-I/ARB or thiazide or CCB
Diabetes	<130/80	ACE-I/ARB ± thiazide or β-blocker/CCB (2nd line)
Diabetes with nephropathy[b]	<130/80	ACE-I/ARB ± CCB
CKD	<130/80	ACE-I/ARB ± thiazide
CAD	<140/90	ACE-I/ARB + β-blocker/CCB
Heart failure	<140/90	ACE-I/ARB + β-blocker (+ spironolactone in NYHA III or IV)

In black patients ACE-I/ARB and β-blockers are less effective. (CCB and thiazides are more effective.)
[a]Not indicated as first-line therapy if age > 60 years.
[b]Diabetes with nephropathy: albumin:creatinine ratio >2 mg/mmol in men; >2.8 mg/mmol in women.

Key Points for HTN Medication Use (See Table 7-9)

- Multiple drug therapy is required in many patients
- Useful combinations include a thiazide or CCB with either an ACE-I, ARB, or β-blocker
- Caution should be exercised in combining a nondihydropyridine CCB and a β-blocker
- The combination of an ACE-I and an ARB is not recommended
- Consider referral to specialist if blood pressure is not controlled with three anti-hypertensives

TABLE 7-9	Hypertension: Medications Adverse Effects	
DRUG	SIDE-EFFECTS	CONTRAINDICATIONS
ACE-I	Cough (10%), angioedema, hyperkalemia	Bilateral renal artery stenosis, history of angioedema, pregnancy
β-Blocker	Fatigue, insomnia, impotence, bronchospasm, mask symptom of hypoglycemia	Asthma, 2nd or 3rd degree heart block, severe PVD, uncompensated heart failure

TABLE 7-9	Hypertension: Medications Adverse Effects (*Continued*)	
DRUG	**SIDE-EFFECTS**	**CONTRAINDICATIONS**
DHP-CCB	Edema, gingival hyperplasia, dizzness, headache, flushing	Severe hypotension (SBP<90), recent MI with pulmonary edema, sick sinus syndrome, 2nd or 3rd degree heart block
Thiazide diuretics	Photosensitivity, rash; decrease sodium, potassium, magnesium, zinc; increase calcium, uric acid, glucose, cholesterol, TG	Anuria, severe sulfa allergy, gout, hyponatremia
Potassium-sparing diuretics	Hyperkalemia with impaired renal function; gynecomastia (if used in combination with ACE-I/ARB)	

Follow-up

- If lifestyle modification only: every 3-6 months
- If anti-HTN drug treatment: every 2 months until 2 consecutive readings below target; then every 3-6 months

Management of Hypertensive Urgency/Emergency

- Hypertensive urgency—treat with any of the following:
  - Nicardipine, captopril, clonidine, labetalol
- Hypertensive emergency—admit to ICU for IV medications to lower blood pressure

Hypertension in Pregnancy—Medications

- Methyldopa
- Labetelol
- Long-acting DHP-CCB (nifedipine XL)

Bibliography

Dynamed. *Hypertensive Emergency*. Ipswich, MA: EBSCO Publishing;. 2011, Oct 5. http://search.ebscohost.com.cyber.usask.ca/login.aspx?direct=true&site=DynaMed&id=113862. Accessed March, 2012.

Jensen B, Regier L, ed. RxFiles drug comparison charts. *Oral Antihypertensives Summary/Guidelines Comparison Chart*. 8th ed. Saskatoon, SK: Saskatoon Health Region: 6.

National Heart, Lung, and Blood Institute. Seventh report of the Joint National Committee on prevention, detection, evaluation and treatment of high blood pressure (JNC 7) express. *JAMA*. 2003;289,2560-2571.

Rabi DM, Daskalopoulou SS, Padwal RS, et al. The 2011 Canadian Hypertension Education Program recommendations for the management of hypertension: blood pressure measurement, diagnosis, assessment of risk, and therapy. *Can J Cardiol*. 2011;27(4):415-433.

United States Preventive Services Task Force. Screening for high blood pressure: U.S. preventive services task force reaffirmation recommendation statement. *Ann In Medicine*. 2007;147(11):783.

Hyperlipidemia

Priority Topic 46

Definition

Elevated total cholesterol, low-density lipoprotein cholesterol, or non-high-density lipoprotein cholesterol levels

Screening/Risk Factors

- Initiate screening in women ≥50 years or who are postmenopausal
- Initiate screening in men ≥40 years
- Screen every 1 to 3 years

- Screen patients with the following risk factors regardless of age:
  - Atherosclerosis
  - HIV patient on antiretroviral therapy
  - Diabetes mellitus
  - Hypertension
  - Obesity (BMI >27 kg/m^2)
  - Clinical signs of hyperlipidemia (arcus cornealis, xanthomas, xanthelasmas)
  - Erectile dysfunction
  - Inflammatory disease (SLE, rheumatoid arthritis, psoriasis)
  - Chronic kidney disease
  - Cigarette smoking
  - Family history of premature CAD (<60 years in first-degree relative)
- An additional consideration for cardiovascular disease risk: metabolic syndrome

Metabolic Syndrome (Syndrome X)

Insulin resistance syndrome

Diagnosis

Any three of the following:

1. Abdominal obesity* (males >94 cm, females >80 cm)
2. TG ≥1.6 mmol/L
3. HDL <1.0 (males), <1.3 (females)
4. BP ≥130/85
5. Fasting glucose ≥5.6 mol/L

Treatment

Lifestyle modification, prevention of DM2 and CVD

Diagnosis

- Fasting lipid profile (see management section—diagnosis values vary based on risk stratification)
- Rule out secondary causes of hyperlipidemia
  - Diabetes
  - Metabolic syndrome
  - Hypothyroid
  - Nephrotic syndrome
  - Obstructive liver disease
  - Chronic kidney disease
- Drugs (alcohol, amiodarone, β-blockers, antiepileptics, thiazides, corticosteroids, protease inhibitors)

Management and Treatment

Aim to meet the LDL targets (see Table 7-10)

In low-risk patients, may try lifestyle changes for 3 to 6 months before medications (see Tables 7-11 and 7-12) are initiated.

Lifestyle changes

- Diet modification (reduce saturated fats and refined sugar)
- Weight reduction and maintenance
- Daily exercise (30 to 60 min, moderate to vigorous)
- Stress management
- Smoking cessation

---

*People of non-Caucasian ethnicities (Aboriginal, Asian, etc) may have different waist circumference values.

TABLE 7-10	LDL Targets (2009 Canadian Cardiovascular Society Guidelines) for Primary Prevention of CAD		
FRAMINGHAM RISK[A]	GOAL LDL		INITIATE MEDICATION
High (10-year risk ≥20%)	<2 mmol/L or ≥50% decrease in LDL		>2 mmol/L
Moderate (10-year risk 10%-19%)	<2 mmol/L or ≥50% decrease in LDL		>3.5 mmol/L[b] or TC/HDL >5
Low (10 year <10%)	≥50% decrease in LDL		>5 mmol/L or TC/HDL >6

[a]www.cvdriskcheck.com/FraminghamRiskScore.aspx.
[b]If LDL is <3.5 and female >60 years or male >50 years, risk stratify with hs-CRP. If >2 mg/L → treat.

Components of the Framingham Risk Calculator: age, sex, HDL-C, total cholesterol, systolic blood pressure (treated or not treated), history of smoking, and diabetes

Other high-risk categories: CAD, PVD, atherosclerosis, DM patients (male>45, female >50, or younger with risk factors)

The Framingham Risk Score doubles if CVD is present in a first-degree relative before 60 years of age!

TABLE 7-11	Drug Choices for Hyperlipidemia
High LDL	HMG-CoA reductase inhibitors +/− resins +/− cholesterol absorption inhibitors
High LDL and high TG	HMG-CoA reductase inhibitors
High LDL and low HDL	HMG-CoA reductase inhibitors +/− fibrate/nicotinic acid
High TG	Fibrate/nicotinic acid/omega 3 fatty acid
Low HDL	Fibrate/nicotinic acid

HMG-CoA reductase inhibitor → commonly known as the statins
Resin (eg, cholestyramine)
Fibrate (eg, gemfibrozil)
Cholesterol absorption inhibitor (eg, ezetimibe)
Nicotinic acid (eg, Niacin)

TABLE 7-12	Hyperlipidemia Medications–Adverse Affects
HMG-CoA reductase inhibitors[a]	GI upset, headache, rash, sleep problems, muscle pain, increased LFTs
Fibrates	GI upset, rash, abdominal pain
Resins	Constipation, nausea, bloating
Nicotinic acid	Flushing,[b] elevated glucose, dry eyes, pruritus
Cholesterol absorption inhibitors	Headache, diarrhea, decreased intestinal cholesterol absorption

[a]Increased risk of toxicity if used concomitantly with amiodarone, clarithromycin, erythromycin, gemfibrozil, verapamil, grapefruit juice, protease inhibitor.
[b]Decrease flushing by taking ASA/ibuprofen 30 min before niacin.

Important Points on Statin Use

- When starting a statin → order LFT and CK at 0, 3, 6, and 12 months
- If muscle pain and weakness → check CK level. Concerning if CK >3 to 5 times normal levels
- Routine LFT and CK not indicated in all patients
- Annual LFT and CK for patients on high dose or at risk
  - Risk factors for statin-related myopathy: elderly, hypothyroidism, high dose, alcoholism, drug interaction

Bibliography

Dynamed. Hypercholesterolemia. Ipswich, MA: EBSCO Publishing; 2012, Feb 6. http://search.ebscohost.com.cyber.usask.ca/login.aspx?direct=true&site=DynaMed&id=113862. Accessed March, 2012.

Genest J, McPherson R, Frohlich J, Anderson T, Campbell N, Carpentier A. 2009 Canadian Cardiovascular Society/Canadian guidelines for the diagnosis and treatment of dyslipidemia and prevention of cardiovascular disease in the adult—2009 recommendations. *Canadian J Cardiol.* 2009;25(10);567-579.

Jensen B, Regier L, ed. RxFiles drug comparison charts. *Lipid Lowering Therapy: Dyslipidemia Comparison Chart.* 8th ed. Saskatoon, SK: Saskatoon Health Region; 2010: 15.

Ischemic Heart Disease
Priority Topic 54

Definition

Atherosclerosis leading to narrowing of coronary arteries. Decreased blood flow leads to ischemia of heart muscle.

Symptoms

- Typical angina
  - Provoked by exertion or emotional stress
  - Chest heaviness or tightness
  - Relieved by rest or nitroglycerin
    - If all three characteristics met → typical angina
    - May radiate to neck, jaw, arms, epigastric area, back
- Atypical (more common in women, DM, young and low risk patients)
  - If two of the three characteristics → atypical angina
  - If only one characteristic present → not likely cardiac chest pain

Cardiovascular Risk Factors for Atherosclerosis

- Modifiable
  - Diabetes
  - Dyslipidemia
  - High stress
  - Poor diet
  - Abdominal obesity
  - Sedentary lifestyle
  - Tobacco use
  - Metabolic syndrome
  - Hypertension
  - Depression
  - Chronic kidney disease (microalbuminuria, proteinuria, or eGFR<60 mL/min/1.73m^2)
  - Excess alcohol use
- Nonmodifiable
  - Age >55
  - Male
  - Family history of premature cardiovascular disease (males <55 years, females <65 years)
- Prior history of atherosclerotic disease
  - PVD
  - Previous stroke or TIA

Diagnosis

- Ischemic heart disease established if:
  - History of MI or acute coronary syndrome
  - Presence of obstructive lesions on angiographic imaging
- Ischemic heart disease presumed if:
  - Typical angina in a high-risk patient
  - Atypical angina or typical angina in an intermediate risk patient, with positive functional testing (exercise stress test, perfusion imaging, or stress echocardiography)

Management

Stable Angina

- Management of modifiable risk factors
- Pharmacotherapy:

  Antianginal medications:
  - β-Blocker (first-line therapy and mortality benefit)
  - Calcium channel blocker
  - Nitroglycerin (for symptom control)

  Risk-modifying medications:
  - ASA
  - ACE-I
  - Statin
  - Clopidogrel if recent acute coronary syndrome (NSTEMI—combination with ASA for 12 month; STEMI – ASA+ clopidogrel for 4 weeks if started in the first 24 hours of MI)
- Patient education and self-management
  - If angina, use sublingual nitro × 1. If no relief after 5 minutes, call emergency services immediately
  - If increased frequency of angina, call physician
  - If there is a change in symptoms, call physician
- Follow-up care
  - Symptom control
  - Medication adherence
  - Lifestyle modification
  - Impact on daily activity

Acute Coronary Syndrome

- ASA chewed
- Nitroglycerin (0.4 mg sublingually every 5 minutes for up to three doses)
- Oxygen if arterial saturation is <90%
- β-Blocker and ACE-I within the first 24 hours
- If persistent symptoms after β-blocker and nitroglycerin, then long-acting CCB +/− morphine

Post-MI Management: Secondary Prevention

- ACE-I (or ARB) indefinitely
  - Start low dose and titrate up to target dose
  - Mortality benefit
  - Prevents ventricular remodeling and decreases proteinuria
- β-Blocker indefinitely
  - Start low dose and titrate up to target dose
  - Mortality benefit
  - Decreases reinfarction, arrhythmia, and sudden death

DRUGS WITH MORTALITY BENEFITS

MI: β-blocker, ASA, ACE-I, statin

CHF: β-blocker, ACE-I, spironolactone

COPD: home O_2, smoking cessation

MODIFIABLE CARDIOVASCULAR RISKS

Risk Factor	Target
Blood Pressure	<140/90
	<130/80 (DM)
Lipids	LDL <2
	Tot Chol/HDL <4
Glucose	A1C <7%;
	FBG 4-7 mmol/L
2hr PPG	5-10 mmol/L
Smoking Cessation	–

- Statin in all patients (even when baseline LDL <2.5 mmol/L)
  - Start at target dose, unless high risk for side effects
- ASA (75-162 mg) indefinitely
- Manage modifiable cardiovascular risk factors
  - Blood pressure: <140/90 (<130/80 with diabetes)
  - Lipids: LDL <2, Total cholesterol/HDL <4
  - Glucose: A1C <7%, FBG 4 to 7 mmol/L, PPBG (2 hours) 5 to 10 mmol/L
  - Smoking cessation counseling
- Patient education to avoid NSAID/COX-2 Inhibitors in post MI
- Referral to cardiac rehabilitation program

Bibliography

Dynamed. *Chest Pain.* Ipswich, MA: EBSCO Publishing; 2012, March 15. http://search.ebscohost.com.cyber.usask.ca/login.aspx?direct=true&site=DynaMed&id=113862. Accessed March, 2012.

Dynamed. *Coronary Artery Disease (CAD).* Ipswich, MA: EBSCO Publishing; 2012, March 2. http://search.ebscohost.com.cyber.usask.ca/login.aspx?direct=true&site=DynaMed&id=113862. Accessed March, 2012.

Finnish Medical Society Duodecim. Coronary heart disease. 2010. http://www.guideline.gov/content.aspx?id=24713. Accessed March, 2012.

Jensen B, Regier L, ed. RxFiles drug comparison charts. *Post-MI—Drug & Dosage Considerations.* 8th ed. Saskatoon, SK: Saskatoon Health Region; 2010:12.

National Institute for Health and Clinical Excellence. Secondary prevention in primary and secondary care for patients following myocardial infarction. NICE Clinical Guideline 48. 2007. Accessed March 2012.

Safer Health Care Now. Improved care for acute myocardial infarction: Getting started kit. 2007. http://www.saferhealthcarenow.ca. Accessed March, 2012.

Congestive Heart Failure

Supplementary Priority Topic

Definition and Types

A clinical syndrome defined by symptoms suggestive of impaired cardiac output and/or volume overload with concurrent cardiac dysfunction.

- **Systolic heart failure (SHF)**
  - Left ventricular ejection fraction <40%
  - Worse prognosis
- **Heart failure with preserved systolic function (HFPSF; previously called diastolic heart failure)**
  - Left ventricular ejection fraction ≥40% (abnormal filling)
  - Half of all cases of HF

Etiology

The most common cause of right ventricular failure is left ventricular failure.

TABLE 7-13 Heart Failure Causes

CARDIAC		NONCARDIAC
SHF	HFPSF	
• Coronary artery disease • Hypertension • Valvular lesions (AS, AR, and MR) • Atrial fibrillation • Dilated cardiomyopathy	• Pericarditis • Hypertrophy • Fibrosis • Tamponade • Scarring	• Infiltrative disorders • HIV • Muscular dystrophy • Anemia • Thyrotoxicosis • Nonadherence with medications • Excess dietary sodium • Drugs (eg, alcohol, NSAIDs, cocaine, estrogens, corticosteroids)

Evaluation

Assess volume status, risk factors, comorbid conditions, assign NYHA class.

Signs/Symptoms

- Fatigue (decreased exercise tolerance)
- Dyspnea, orthopnea, paroxysmal nocturnal dyspnea
- Fluid retention/weight gain/peripheral edema
- Cough
- Nocturia
- Rales
- Hepatomegaly
- Increased JVD
- S_3 gallop (systolic failure)
- S_4 (diastolic failure)

Investigations

- ECG
- Chest x-ray
- Transthoracic echocardiogram—diagnostic in combination with clinical picture
- Labs: CBC, renal function, lytes, lipids, TSH, microalbuninuria (a marker of underlying endothelial dysfunction)
- BNP (if diagnosis is unclear)

Screening

- Not routine if asymptomatic
- Consider echocardiogram if multiple risk factors

Management

Chronic Heart Failure

- All patients:
  - Education
  - Daily weights (report a weight gain of 2.5 kg/week)
  - Limit sodium intake (2-3 g/day; 6 g salt = 1 tsp salt = 2.4 g sodium)
  - Fluid restriction (1.5-2 L/day) for patients with fluid retention, significant renal impairment, or hyponatremia
  - Decrease alcohol consumption (1 drink/day maximum)
  - Physical activity if stable HF
  - Immunizations (one time pneumococcal and annual influenza)
  - **Treat all cardiac risk factors and underlying causes**
- Pharmacotherapy:
  - NYHA I — ACE-I (or ARB if intolerant)
  - NYHA II — ACE-I, β-blocker
  - NYHA III-IV — ACE-I, β-blocker, spironolactone, digoxin +/− nitrates
  - Loop diuretics if evidence of fluid retention/symptomatic
  - Add low dose ASA if atherosclerosis

Acute Heart Failure

- Treat the precipitating causes
- Supplemental oxygen
- Assess perfusion and volume status
  - Warm and wet (well perfused and volume overloaded):
    - IV diuretic (double usual PO dose and give it IV, reassess after 60-90 min and titrate dose prn)

HF SYMPTOM TRIAD

Fatigue, dyspnea, fluid retention

EXTRA HEART SOUNDS

S_3–dilated LV with rapid filling

S_4–atrial contraction against a stiff ventricle

NEW YORK HEART ASSOCIATION CLASSIFICATION

Class 1–asymptomatic

Class 2–symptomatic with ordinary activity

Class 3–symptomatic with less than ordinary activity

Class 4–symptomatic at rest

CHF RISK FACTORS

- Hypertension
- Ischemic heart disease
- Diabetes mellitus
- Dyslipidemia
- Smoking

CHF DRUGS WITH MORTALITY BENEFITS

ACE-I/ARB

β-Blocker

Spironolactone

ACE-I/ARB–monitor creatinine and potassium upon initiation and within 3 to 7 days of starting or adjusting dose.

- Vasodilator (nitroglycerin or nitroprusside)
- Morphine
- Cold and wet (cardiogenic shock):
  - Inotropes to stabilize (dopamine or dobutamine)
  - When stable, add diuretics and vasodilators (ACE-I, hydralazine, nitrates)

Prognosis

Poor prognostic factors include:

- Age >75
- Female
- Ventricular arrhythmias
- Atrial fibrillation
- NYHA Classes III and IV
- Left ventricular ejection fraction <35%
- Recurrent hospitalizations for acute HF
- High BNP
- Sodium <132 mmol/L
- Hypocholesterolemia
- Marked left ventricular dilation

Bibliography

Dynamed. *Heart Failure*. Ipswich, MA: EBSCO Publishing; 2012, Mar 13. http://search.ebscohost.com. cyber.usask.ca/login.aspx?direct=true&site=DynaMed&id=113862. Accessed March, 2012.

Guidelines and Protocols Advisory Committee (BC). Heart Failure Care. 2008. http://www.bcguidelines. ca/guideline_heart_failure_care.html#recommendation1.

Jensen B, Regier L, ed. (2010). RxFiles drug comparison charts. *Heart Failure—Treatment Overview*. 8th ed. Saskatoon, SK: Saskatoon Health Region; 12.

Fatigue

Priority Topic 38

Definition

Reduced ability to start and maintain activity, as well as difficulty with short-term memory and concentration

- 50% psychogenic
- 30% medical causes
- 20% idiopathic

Differential Diagnosis

Medical causes of fatigue: Patients often associate fatigue with activities they are no longer able to finish (decreased exertional capacity).

Psychogenic fatigue: Patients report being tired all of the time. Fatigue is not necessarily related to exertion, and does not improve after rest.

Ask open ended questions: "What do you mean by fatigue?"

	TABLE 7-14	Causes of Fatigue - PS VINDICATE
P	**Psychogenic**	depression, dysthymia, anxiety, sleep disorder, CFS, life stress, fibromyalgia
S	Sedentary	unhealthy/sedentary lifestyle
V	Vascular	stroke
I	**Infectious**	mononucleosis, TB, hepatitis, HIV
N	Neurogenic	myasthenia gravis
	Neoplastic	malignancy
	Nutrition	anemia (iron deficiency, B_{12} deficiency)
D	**Drugs**	β-blockers, benzodiazepines, antihistamines, anticholinergics, etc

TABLE 7-14		Causes of Fatigue - PS VINDICATE (*Continued*)
I	Idiopathic	
C	Chronic illness	CHF, COPD, renal failure, chronic liver disease
A	Autoimmune	SLE, RA, polymyalgia rheumatica, mixed connective tissue disease
T	Toxin	substance abuse (ie, ETOH, illicit drugs), heavy metal
E	Endocrine	hypothyroidism, DM, pregnancy, adrenal insufficiency, Cushing syndrome

Adapted with permission from *Toronto Notes*.

Approach to Patient With Fatigue

First Visit

- Assess fatigue: onset, duration, severity, exacerbation and palliative factors, impact on function, PHQ-9, drug/ETOH screen, celiac screen, malignancy screen: **RED FLAGS!**
- Review current medications
- Complete a physical examination
- Initial testing can include CBC, TSH, ESR, glucose, renal panel, liver panel, U/A
- Clinically indicated testing: CXR, BHCG, HIV, hepatitis, Lyme disease, tuberculin skin test, mononucleosis, ANA, RF, CK, cortisol, IgA tissue transglutaminase

Second Visit

- Review labs: any abnormal?
- Schedule frequent, brief follow-ups
- Patient education, support, and reassurance

Prognosis

Factors at presentation that predict persistent symptoms:

- Age >38 years old
- More than 1.5 years of chronic fatigue
- History of dysthymia
- Less than 16 years of formal education
- Less than 8 years of medically unexplained physical symptoms

Management

- Schedule frequent, brief follow-ups
- Patient education, support, and reassurance
- Treat medical causes: anemia, hypothyroid, depression
- Consider trial of antidepressants for 6 to 8 weeks
- Recommend: CBT, daily exercise, sleep hygiene, counseling, group therapy, nutritious diet

Fatigue - RED FLAGS!
- Weight loss
- Fever
- Night sweats
- Neurological defects
- Ill appearing

Fatigue is more common in women than in men.
Patients who are experiencing domestic violence may initially present with fatigue.

FIBROMYALGIA

Definition/ Diagnosis

Chronic widespread pain with:

- Characteristic tender points
- Pain for >3 months in four quadrants of the body
- Diagnosis of exclusion: absence of identifiable disease
- Labs:
  - Normal CBC, ESR, TSH, CK, renal and liver function tests

- Multifactorial Signs/Symptoms:
  - Fatigue, impaired social and occupational function, sleep disturbance, depression/anxiety, hyperalgia, paresthesia, IBS, migraine

Treatment Combination therapy to reduce key symptoms

- Pharmacological (intended for relief of certain symptoms):
  - **Amitriptyline (TCA)**
  - Cyclobenzaprine (muscle relaxant)
  - SSRI for treatment of depression, anxiety
  - Zopiclone (non-benzodiazepine sedative hypnotic) for sleep disturbance **short term**
  - NSAIDs (anti-inflammatory)
  - Tramadol (opioid analgesic)
  - Acetaminophen (analgesic)
  - Gabapentin (antiepileptic)
- Non-pharmacological:
  - **Daily exercise**
  - Patient education
  - **Sleep hygiene**
  - CBT
  - Stress reduction
  - Acupuncture
  - Biofeedback
  - Scheduled visits

Complications

- Negative impact of social and occupational life
- Chronic pain

CHRONIC FATIGUE
- Primarily affects young to middle aged adults
- More common in women

CHRONIC FATIGUE SYNDROME

Definition/Diagnosis

- Diagnosis of exclusion
- Diagnosis requires the following:
  - Unexplained, persistent relapsing fatigue of new onset:
    - Not related to exertion
    - Not alleviated with rest
    - Results in dysfunction
- **And** four or more of following for >6 months:
  - Change in short-term memory or concentration
  - Sore throat
  - Tender cervical or axillary nodes
  - Headaches (new pattern/severity)
  - Non-rejuvenating sleep
  - Post-exertional malaise ≥24 hours

Bibliography

Bono NA, Shflin DO. Fatigue. In: Ebell MH, Brown SR, Lindbloom E. eds. *Essential Evidence Plus.* 2011. https://www.essentialevidenceplus.com/content/eee/433. Accessed March 15, 2012.

Centers for Disease Control and Prevention. Chronic Fatigue Syndrome: A toolkit for providers. 2011. http://www.cdc.gov/cfs/toolkit/index.html. Accessed March 15, 2012.

Chen YA, Tran C. *Toronto Notes—Comprehensive Medical Reference & Review for MCCQE I and USMLE II.* Toronto, Canada: Toronto Notes for Medical Students Inc; 2011.

Craig T, Kakumanu S. Chronic fatigue syndrome: Evaluation and treatment. *Am Fam Phy.* 2002;15;65(6):1083-1091. http://www.aafp.org/afp/2002/0315/p1083.html. Accessed March 15, 2012.

Ebell MH. What is a reasonable initial approach to the patient with fatigue? In: Belden JL, ed. *Pepid. Primary Care Plus Platinum v. (12.1)*, 2001.

Fosnocht KM. and Ende J. Approach to the adult with fatigue. In: Fletcher RH, Sokol HN, eds. *Uptodate*. 2011. http://www.uptodateonline.com; http://www.uptodate.com/contents/approach-to-the-adult-patient-with-fatigue?source=search_result&search=fatigue&selectedTitle=1~150. Accessed March 15, 2012.

Gluckman SJ. Treatment of chronic fatigue syndrome. In: Weller PF, Thorner AR, eds. *Uptodate*. 2011. http://www.uptodateonline.com; http://www.uptodate.com/contents/treatment-of-chronic-fatigue-syndrome?source=search_result&search=fatigue&selectedTitle=3~150. Accessed March 15, 2012.

Goldberg DL. Treatment of fibromyalgia in adults. In: Schur PH, Roman PL, eds. *Uptodate*. 2011. http://www.uptodateonline.com; http://www.uptodate.com/contents/treatment-of-fibromyalgia-inadults?source=search_result&search=fibromyalgia&selectedTitle=1~134. Accessed March 15, 2012.

Sandore R. Approach to chronic fatigue syndrome. In: Rosenbloom M. ed. *Pepid. Primary Care Plus Platinum v. (12.1)*, 2005.

8

Preventative Medicine

Periodic Health Assessment
Priority Topic 72

DEFINITION

A dedicated appointment that incorporates evidence-based recommendations for adults from various professional bodies in several domains:

- Education/counseling
- Functional inquiry
- Physical examination
- Laboratory investigations
- Immunizations

PURPOSE

- Primary prevention—identifies risk factors and implements strategies to prevent disease onset
- Secondary prevention—pre-symptomatic detection of disease so as to prevent disease progression and complications
- Health promotion—enables patients to increase control over and improve their health
- Create and maintain an up-to-date patient profile—optimizes both acute and chronic care (ie, current medications, allergies, hospitalizations)
- Enhance therapeutic relationship

PROBLEMS AND CONTROVERSIES

- Low SES and minority group access
- High cost and demand on time (21.4 million half hour visits, $2 billion in costs)
- Debated impact (effect on mortality and morbidity) of dedicated periodic health examination (PHE) versus appropriate case-finding maneuvers during other visits (chronic disease management visits or symptom-based visits)

GUIDES AND CHECKLISTS

Checklists highlight best practices for average risk populations, which include recommendations (those with good and fair evidence) from the CTFPH as well as other screening guidelines from various Canadian agencies.

FUNCTIONAL INQUIRY

"Screening" for depression is the only evidence-based maneuver (grade B evidence)

Over the past 2 weeks:

- Have you felt little pleasure in doing things?
- Have you felt down, depressed, or hopeless?

Other inquiry identifies and targets symptom-based problems for investigation, management, and discussion.

PHYSICAL EXAMINATION

Evidence is either **level A** or level B (Table 8-1)

Table 8-1	Preventative Health: Physical Exam Components	
MANEUVER	**INDICATION**	**COMMENT**
BP	**Treating to prevent stroke, CAD, and death** Screening for hypertension	General population <140/90; CKD or DM 2 <130/80
BMI	Prevention of obesity-related disease	For obese adults
Waist to hip ratio	Screening for abdominal obesity	High risk for more intensive screening
Waist circumference	Increased risk of DM 2, hypertension, and CAD	Men <102 cm Women <88 cm
Sensorium testing	In the elderly	Whispered test vs audiometry vs inquiry are all equivalent Snellen for visual acuity
Pap smear	Reduce the risk of invasive cervical cancer	Sexually active women based on provincial guidelines

CFPC Explanations, 2012.

LABS AND INVESTIGATIONS

Sexually Transmitted Infections

In high-risk populations (<30 years with two partners in last year, >16 at coitarche, prostitutes, sexual contact of known case)

- Syphilis serology
- Gonorrhea and Chlamydia → urethral/cervical swab or urine
- HIV serology
- HBV serology (HBsAg)

Cancer Screening Maneuvers

Cervical Cancer

- Provincial guidelines and screening programs vary
- Most are moving toward screening women >21 years of age or women who are >3 years from coitarche, whichever comes later
- Pap smears should be done every 2 to 3 years, with changes in frequency depending on previous results

See Figure 8-1 for management of abnormal PAP cytology.

MANAGEMENT OF ABNORMAL CYTOLOGY

Pap Result	Recommended Management
Unsatisfactory	Repeat Pap test in 3 months
Atypical squamous cells of undetermined significance (ASC-US) and Low-grade squamous intraepithelial lesion (LSIL)	Women 21 years and older: Repeat Pap test every 6 months for 1 year (two tests) (*tests must be at least 6 months apart*) • If all negative return to routine screening • If either result is ASC-US or greater refer for colposcopy
	Women <21 years: (*although routine cervical screening is not recommended*) Repeat Pap test every 12 months for 2 years (two tests): • At 12 months: Only high-grade lesions should be referred to colposcopy • At 24 months: Negative results return to routine screening ASC-US or greater refer to colposcopy
Atypical squamous cells—cannot exclude HSIL (ASC-H)	Refer for colposcopy
High-grade squamous intraepithelial lesion (HSIL)	Refer for colposcopy
Atypical glandular cells (AGC), Adenocarcinoma in situ (AIS)	Refer for colposcopy
Squamous carcinoma, adenocarcinoma, other malignancy	Refer to specialist care
Endometrial cells	After the age of 40 should be managed or referred as appropriate

The Saskatchewan Cancer Agency's Prevention Program for Cervical Cancer (PPCC) tracks compliance with recommended follow-up of abnormal and unsatisfactory results to ensure women receive appropriate and timely follow-up. If follow-up cytology, histology, and/or colposcopy information is not received by the PPCC within the recommended follow-up time the care provider office will receive a letter from the PPCC requesting follow-up information. If no response to the letter or follow-up information is received by the PPCC, a fax reminder will be sent followed by telephone calls.

FIGURE 8-1: Management of abnormal PAP cytology. *Source*: Saskatchewan Cancer Agency.

- Repeated normal results warrant less frequent screening
- Abnormal results warrant more frequent surveillance or screening, particularly among older women
- Health status (ie, immunocompromised) intensifies screening frequency

Breast Cancer (Canadian Task Force on Preventative Health, 2011)

- Provincial guidelines and screening programs vary
- Discuss the risks and benefits of screening with all women, and ascertain individual preferences
  - Number needed to screen to prevent one breast cancer death is 720 every 2 to 3 years for 11 years
  - In that time, 204 will have false positive results on mammography, and 26 will have unnecessary biopsies
- Screen average risk women between the ages of 50 to 74 with mammography every 2 to 3 years
- Clinical breast examination is no longer recommended (weak recommendation; same strength of evidence as the above recommendation to screen with mammography)
- Advising women to perform self-breast examination is also not recommended

Colorectal Cancer (Canadian Association of Gastroenterology Position Statement, 2010)

- Screen average risk adults >50 years with
  - Guaiac-based fecal occult blood test (FOBT) or more sensitive fecal immunochemical test (FIT) every 2 years

- Flexible sigmoidoscopy +/− FOBT every 5 years
- Double contrast barium enema every 5 years
- Colonoscopy every 10 years
- Higher risk patients have unique screening/surveillance schedules
  - First-degree with diagnosis in relative <60 years → every 5 years starting at age 40 or 10 years before relative's diagnosis
  - Genetic syndromes
    - Familial adenomatous polyposis → annual colonoscopy starting at age 10 to 12
    - Hereditary non-polyposis colorectal cancer → colonoscopy every 1 to 2 years starting at age 20 or 10 years before earliest relative's diagnosis
  - Inflammatory bowel disease → colonoscopy 8 years after diagnosis
  - Polyps on previous colonoscopy
    - One to two adenomas <1 cm → repeat colonoscopy in 5 years
    - More than two adenomas → repeat colonoscopy in 3 years

Prostate Cancer (Canadian Urological Association, 2011)

See section on Men's GU Health

- Discuss the risks and benefits of screening with all men, and ascertain individual preferences
  - Number needed to screen to prevent one prostate cancer death is 503
  - Important health and psychological risks of over-diagnosis, biopsy, and treatment for cancers that may not have been clinically significant
- Offer yearly digital rectal examination and prostate-specific antigen testing between 50 and 75
- Start at age 40 with risk factors (or 10 years before relative's diagnosis)
- Do not screen men whose life expectancy is <10 years

Chronic Diseases

Diabetes Mellitus Type 2

See section on diabetes mellitus type 2

- Fasting blood glucose every 3 years starting at age 40
- Earlier and more frequently in patients with the following comorbidities:
  - First-degree relative
  - Presence of complications associated with DM 2
  - Hypertension or other vascular disease
  - Dyslipidemia
  - Overweight or abdominal obesity
  - High-risk population (Aboriginal, Hispanic, Asian, South Asian, African descent)
  - History of impaired glucose tolerance, impaired fasting glucose, gestational diabetes mellitus, or macrosomic infant
  - Other comorbidities: PCOS, schizophrenia

Osteoporosis

See section on osteoporosis

BMD testing is indicated in the following groups:

- Everyone >65
- 50 to 64 years with risk factors:
  - Fragility fracture
  - High-risk medication: prolonged glucocorticoid use (>3 months of >7.5 mg prednisone-equivalent/day, aromatase inhibitors, androgen deprivation therapy)
  - Parental hip fracture
  - Vertebral fracture or osteopenia on x-ray

- Lifestyle: current smoking, high alcohol intake
- Low body weight (<60 kg) or major weight loss (>10% of weight at age 25 years)
- Comorbidities: rheumatoid arthritis, others (see Osteoporosis section for full list)

■ <50 with risk factors:
  - Fragility fracture
  - High-risk medications (same as above)
  - Hypogonadism or premature menopause
  - Malabsorption syndrome
  - Primary hyperparathyroidism
  - Other disorders strongly associated with rapid bone loss and/or fracture

Coronary Artery Disease

See hyperlipidemia section

■ Fasting lipid profile on all men >40 and all women >50 or postmenopausal
■ All patients, regardless of age, with:
  - Chronic diseases: diabetes, hypertension, inflammatory diseases (SLE, RA, psoriasis), CKD (eGFR <60), HIV on HAART
  - Risk factors: current cigarette smoking, obesity
  - Family history of premature CAD (<60 years)
  - Evidence of atherosclerosis
  - Clinical manifestation of hyperlipidemia
  - Children with family history of hypercholesterolemia or chylomicronemia
■ Stratify patients into low, medium, or high risk (based on Framingham criteria or other risk calculator) then treat to target (see Table 8-2)

TABLE 8-2	Cardiovascular Risk Stratification	
RISK	TREAT IF	TARGET
Low (<10% over 10 years)	LDL >5.0 (or total/HDL >6)	LDL drop by >50%
Medium (10%-19% over 10 years)	LDL >3.5 (or total/HDL >5, hsCRP >2.0 or Apo B >1.0)	LDL drop by >50% or <2.0 Apo B <0.80
High (>20% over 10 years)	Everyone	LDL <2.0 or Apo B <0.80

Summarized from Genest J, et al. 2009.

IMMUNIZATIONS

Evidence: **Level A,** level B

Tetanus and Diphtheria (Td) +/− Pertussis (Tdap)

■ Td booster every 10 years with one Tdap booster if not previously immunized
■ Primary series: three doses at 0, 1 to 2, and 6 to 12 months (two doses Td, one dose Tdap)

Pneumococcal

■ Everyone >65 years
■ All persons >5 years at high risk:
  - Common high-risk groups:
    ○ Immunosuppressed: asplenia, HIV infection, sickle cell disease, lymphoma, Hodgkin disease, organ transplant recipients
    ○ Chronic diseases: diabetes, cardiopulmonary disease (except asthma), kidney disease, cirrhosis, smokers
    ○ Marginalized populations (IVDUs, homeless)

Influenza A: Immunize Annually in The Autumn

- Those at high risk for influenza complications or those more likely to require hospitalization:
  - Cardiopulmonary diseases, metabolic diseases (including diabetes), kidney disease, anemia or hemoglobinopathies, nursing home residents
- Those >65 years and <23 months, healthy pregnant women
- Those capable of transmitting to those at high risk
  - Health care workers (HCWs), childcare workers, household contacts of those above

Rubella

- One dose to nonpregnant women of child-bearing age unless evidence of immunity (records, serology)

  Varicella:

- Determine status by history or serology
- Two doses at least 4 weeks apart to high-risk groups: HCWs, women of reproductive age who are not pregnant, teachers and daycare workers, newly arrived immigrants, household contact of immunocompromised

No A or B level evidence for the following

HPV

- Recommended for females 9 to 13, indicated for women up to age 26
- Indicated for boys age 9 to 26 years, but not covered by any provincial vaccination program currently

Pertussis

- Single dose to nonimmunized adults

Meningococcal

- To all high-risk groups:
  - Recent contacts of known cases
  - Occupational: military recruits, lab workers exposed to meningitis
  - Travelers to endemic areas
  - Medical: asplenia, deficiencies (factor D, complement, properdin)

Herpes Zoster

- Indicated for prevention of herpes zoster and its complications in >60 years but NNT = 91

Travel immunizations vary

EDUCATION AND COUNSELING

Evidence is either **level A** or level B for interventions listed below (see Table 8-3)

TABLE 8-3	Preventative Health: Dietary Supplements	
INTERVENTION	INDICATION	COMMENT
Folic acid	Prevent neural tube defects in women of reproductive age	**Low risk: 0.4-0.8 mg/d for 1 month pre- and 3 months post-conception** **High risk: 4 mg/d for 3 months pre- and post-conception**
Calcium (B)	Prevent osteoporosis	OSC: 1000-1500 mg/d; >1200 mg/d for women >50 SOGC: 1500 mg/d if postmenopausal
Vitamin D	Prevent osteoporosis (B) and hip fractures	OSC: 400-1000 IU/d; 800-1000 IU if >50 or moderate risk of vitamin D deficiency SOGC: 800 IU/d if postmenopausal
Diet (B)	Prevent CAD, colon cancer	Lower use of saturated and total fat; lower cholesterol; increase fiber intake Consider referral to nutritionist if at high risk

TABLE 8-3	Preventative Health: Dietary Supplements (*Continued*)	
INTERVENTION	**INDICATION**	**COMMENT**
Physical activity (B)	Prevent hypertension and CAD Contribute to preventing DM 2 and osteoporosis	Moderate physical activity for 30 min/day on most days of the week
Sun exposure	Prevent skin cancer	Avoid excessive midday sun exposure with protective clothing
Safe sex	Prevent STI transmission	Abstinence Condoms
Obesity (BMI >30)		Multimodal strategy to achieve weight loss of 5%-10% at rate of 5-10 kg/week for 6 months
Smoking cessation	Prevent tobacco-caused diseases	**Counseling for smoking cessation** and use of nicotine replacement +/− bupropion Refer to cessation program
Oral hygiene	Prevent oral cancer and periodontal disease	Brushing and flossing with fluoride-containing toothpaste in areas where water is not fluoridated Smoking cessation to prevent oral cancer and periodontal disease
Alcohol	Prevent alcohol-related morbidities	Standardized inquiry (CAGE) Counsel for problem drinking (CAGE 2/4 is sensitive and specific for problem drinking) **At risk drinking: Women (>7 units/week or >3/occasion), Men (>14 units/week or >4/occasion)**
Elderly	**Cognitive decline** **Fall assessment**	When caregiver expresses concern with either
Personal safety	Various	Noise control protection or protection to prevent injures Seatbelts to prevent MVA-related injuries

Bibliography

Canadian Task Force on Preventive Health. Recommendations on screening for breast cancer in average risk women aged 40-74 years. *Can Med Asson J.* 2010;183(17):1991-2001.

CFPC. Explanations for the Preventive Care Checklist Form. http://www.cfpc.ca/ProjectAssets/Templates/Resource.aspx?id=1184&langType=4105. Accessed November 11, 2012.

Genest J, et al. Canadian Cardiovascular Society guidelines for the diagnosis and treatment of dyslipidemia and prevention of cardiovascular disease in the adult—2009 recommendations. *Can J Cardiol.* 2009;25(10):567-579.

Howard-Tripp M. Should we abandon the periodic health examination? Yes. *Can Fam Phy.* 2011;57:159-160.

Leddin DJ, Enns R, Hilsden R, et al. Canadian Association of Gastroenterology position statement on screening individuals at average risk for developing colorectal cancer. *Can J Gastroenterol.* 2010;24(12):705-714.

Mavriplis C. Should we abandon the periodic health examination? No. *Can Fam Phy.* 2011;57:159-161.

National Advisory Committee on Immunization. Canadian Immunization Guide. 7th ed. 2006. http://www.phac-aspc.gc.ca/im/is-cv/index-eng.php#b. Accessed November 11, 2012.

Men's Genitourinary Health
Priority Topic 77

LOWER URINARY TRACT SYMPTOMS

Lower urinary tract symptoms (LUTS): categorized as irritative or obstructive

- Irritative: frequency, urgency, nocturia, urge incontinence
- Obstructive: hesitancy, poor flow, dribbling, incomplete voiding, retention

Benign Prostatic Hyperplasia
Definition

- Benign, often progressive disorder due to prostate enlargement

Symptoms and Characteristics

- Most common, but not exclusive, cause of LUTS in men

Risk Factors

- Advancing age
- BPH puts men at higher risk for sexual dysfunction
- BPH is not a risk factor for prostate cancer

Diagnosis

- Diagnosis is clinical, based on history, physical, and basic investigations

Physical Examination

- May be normal
- Digital rectal examination (DRE) may reveal symmetric, smooth, non-painful, enlarged prostate
- Abdominal examination may reveal distended bladder

Investigations

- Urinalysis and urine culture and sensitivity (C&S) to rule out infection
- Prostate-specific antigen (PSA) if life expectancy >10 years and knowledge of prostate cancer would change management; if starting on 5-alpha reductase inhibitors (5-ARIs)
- Other investigations as indicated by presentation (post-void residual, urine cytology, urodynamics, serum creatinine)

Management

- Use of a symptom inventory (International Prostate Scoring System) is helpful to assess "bother" (impact on patient), deciding on treatment, and in monitoring
- Consider screening for sexual dysfunction
- New focus on early treatment over watchful waiting
  - Delay symptom progression
  - Prevent complications (surgery, acute urinary retention)
- Lifestyle:
  - Fluid restriction
  - Avoiding irritants
  - Timed voiding
  - Pelvic floor exercises
  - Medication review
- Pharmacotherapy:
  Based on symptoms severity, bother, and patient preference
  - Alpha-blockers:
    - Non-selective (doxazosin, terazosin) → more side-effects
    - Selective (tamsulosin) → expensive
    - Choice based on patient comorbidities and tolerability

- 5-alpha reductase inhibitors (finasteride, dutasteride)
  - With documented large prostate (larger than 40 g)
  - Benefits: limits prostate growth and prevents cancer, urinary retention, need for surgery
  - Side-effects: sexual dysfunction, gynecomastia, decreased libido
  - Monitor with PSA 6 months post-initiation → PSA must decrease by 50% or warrants urological referral
- Either class alone or in combination is acceptable

Consider alternative diagnosis, especially if no response to treatment:
- Prostatitis
- UTI
- Overactive bladder

Key Points
- BPH is progressive—early treatment may reduce complications
- Referral to urology if abnormal DRE
- PSA must be followed with 5-alpha reductase inhibitor use

Prostate Cancer
Definitions
- Informed screening:
  - Early detection and treatment of asymptomatic cancer to extend life
  - Requires accurate, reliable, easy-to-administer test that detects disease of clinical importance at a pre-clinical stage

Screening (See Table 8-4)

Both patient and clinician must understand that screening for prostate cancer with PSA or DRE does not fulfill many of these criteria.

TABLE 8-4	Prostate Cancer Screening Recommendations		
RECOMMENDATION FOR SCREENING	CANADIAN UROLOGICAL ASSOCIATION	AMERICAN UROLOGICAL ASSOCIATION	US PREVENTIVE SERVICES TASK FORCE
Age to offer	40 for high risk, otherwise age 50-75	40 for everyone	No one
Maneuver	DRE and PSA	DRE and PSA	None
Frequency	Yearly (do not screen if life expectancy <10 years)	Yearly	N/A

- Screening: controversial
- Extremely large numbers needed to screen (to prevent 1 death = 503) (503 in ERSPC pooled and extrapolated data—*NEJM* article)
- Questionable impact on mortality versus financial cost to system and potential negative impacts on patient QOL
- Risks of screening:
  - Worry → cancer can exist with normal PSA and DRE
  - Risks of invasive investigations → bleeding, pain, infection
- Risks of diagnosis:
  - Risks of therapies → sexual, urinary, and bowel dysfunction
  - At least one-fourth of diagnoses are over-diagnosis → cancer would not have become clinically significant
- Benefits of screening:
  - Small mortality benefit, unproven in RCTs
  - Relief and reassurance

Symptoms
- Frequently asymptomatic
- LUTS
- Hip or vertebral pain

Risk Factors

- Age >50 → 30% of those above 50 will have autopsy-proven cancer; 70% of more than 70
- Black → higher incidence and more advanced stage at diagnosis
- Positive family history (first-degree relative <65) → doubles risk

Physical Examination

- Frequently normal
- Abnormal DRE → nodular, firm, irregular, often peripheral zone affected

DRE does not cause elevated PSA.

Differential Diagnosis of Elevated PSA

Inflammation, urinary retention, instrumentation, cancer, frequent/recent ejaculation, **not DRE!**

- PSA half-life is 2 to 3 days → stays elevated for roughly 2 weeks (5½ lives)
- PSA variability is 20% (*CMAJ* article)

Workup

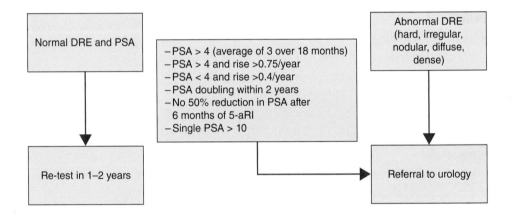

Normal DRE and PSA

- PSA > 4 (average of 3 over 18 months)
- PSA > 4 and rise >0.75/year
- PSA < 4 and rise >0.4/year
- PSA doubling within 2 years
- No 50% reduction in PSA after 6 months of 5-aRI
- Single PSA > 10

Abnormal DRE (hard, irregular, nodular, diffuse, dense)

Re-test in 1–2 years

Referral to urology

Diagnosis

- Requires transrectal ultrasound guided biopsy

Treatment

TABLE 8-5	Risks and Benefits of Various Treatments Options	
TREATMENT	**RISKS**	**COMMENTS**
Surgery	Incontinence, impotence	Relative hazard reduction of 50%
Radiation	Incontinence, impotence, GI dysfunction	Improved mortality benefit with hormonal therapy
Chemotherapy	Systemic side effects	No role alone
Hormonal	Low libido, increased weight, impotence, bone loss, no surgery after	Improved mortality benefit with radiation
No treatment		Most low grade cancers will be subclinical

Treatment is based on staging, which is grouped from I to IV, and arrived by combination of T (clinical and pathological) N, M, serum PSA level, and Gleason score.

Localized disease:

- Active surveillance for Gleason <6, locally confined
  - Trials underway

- Radical prostatectomy
  - Group I and II (all tumor confined to prostate)
  - Men >70 unlikely to be offered surgery as greatest benefit is in those <70 years
- Radiation: either external-beam radiation therapy (EBRT) or brachytherapy
  - EBRT → GI and GU side-effects; comparable to radical prostatectomy
  - Brachytherapy is comparable to EBRT with Gleason <6, PSA <10
  - Group 3 (includes some extra-prostatic tumor): either radical prostatectomy or radiation

Metastatic disease or local extension:
- Group 3: either radical prostatectomy or radiation
- Group 4 (metastatic): androgen deprivation therapy
- Chemotherapy for hormone-refractory tumors
  - Hormonal resistance occurs within 5 years, sometimes earlier

Follow-Up
- Local spread: low back pain, hip pain, LUTS, well-being, appetite, lymphadenopathy
- Distant metastases: bone, lung, liver, adrenals
- Labs: CBC, liver enzymes and function, renal function, PSA

Issues
- Fear of mortality and morbidity versus apprehension surrounding investigations and treatments
- A few comforting thoughts:
  - Roughly 20% of men will be diagnosed with prostate cancer
  - Most die with it, few die from it

Key Points
- Assessing patient values
- Shared decision-making
- Use of a decision aid for patients are all keys

Guideline Summary
Canadian Urological Association
- Offer yearly DRE and PSA between 50 and 75
- Start at age 40 with risk factors (or 10 years before relative's diagnosis)
- Do not screen men whose life expectancy is <10 years

Prostatitis
There are three forms of clinically relevant prostatitis
- Acute prostatitis
- Chronic bacterial prostatitis
- Chronic prostatitis/pelvic pain syndrome

Acute Prostatitis

Definition
- Acute bacterial infection of the prostate gland

Symptoms
- Pain (rectal, perianal, low back, with ejaculation), LUTS, systemic (fever, chills)

Physical Examination
- Generally unwell and uncomfortable
- DRE → boggy, very tender prostate

Investigations
- Urinalysis → bacteria, hematuria, pyuria
- Urine C+S → positive for *Escherichia coli, Staphylococcus aureus,* Gram-negative bacilli
- Urine PCR for Chlamydia and Gonorrhea
- CBC → increased WBCs
- No role for PSA
- Bladder ultrasound with severe obstructive symptoms

Treatment
- Severe illness may require admission
- Antibiotics for 2 to 4 weeks post resolution of symptoms
  - Severe: IV aminoglycoside + ampicillin *or* broad-spectrum penicillin +beta-lactamase inhibitor *or* third-generation cephalosporin
  - Mild-moderate: oral fluoroquinolone

Chronic Bacterial Prostatitis

Definition
- Chronic bacterial infection, +/− symptoms, often the cause of recurrent urinary tract infections (UTI) with consistent pathogen

Symptoms
- Presentation may be subtle or nonspecific (pain may or may not be present)
- Symptom scoring system is helpful (NIH—Chronic Prostatitis Symptom Index) in symptom evaluation and monitoring treatment

Physical Examination
- May be normal

Diagnosis
- Diagnosis is usually made through careful history
- Guidelines recommend the 4 glass or 2 glass test to establish existence of bacterial pathogen
- Sequential urine cultures before and after prostatic massage

Treatment

Check susceptibility and treat for 6 to 12 weeks
- First-line: ciprofloxacin 1 g daily or levofloxacin 500 mg daily
- Second-line: TMP-SMX 1 double-strength tab twice daily
- Consider urological referral if refractory to treatment

Chronic Prostatitis/Pelvic Pain Syndrome

Definition
- Chronic pelvic pain +/− voiding symptoms in the absence of UTI

Physical Examination
- Extraprostatic pain is suggestive

Workup
- 4 glass or 2 glass test to rule out bacterial pathogen
- Urine cytology
- Post-void residual volume
- Flow rate

Treatment
- No single modality has been shown to be effective on its own.
- Multimodal treatment plan targeted to improve symptoms:
  - Antibiotics for newly diagnosed or anti-microbial naïve
  - Alpha-blockers for obstructive symptoms
  - Anti-inflammatories for short-term analgesia
  - Neuromodulating drugs (+/− muscle relaxants) and techniques (acupuncture, pudendal nerve modulation) for long-term analgesia
  - Phytotherapies (quercetin, pollen) for local tenderness
  - Other modalities: physiotherapy, 5-alpha reductase inhibitors, electromagnetic stimulation, psychotherapy

Key Points
- Chronic prostatitis/pelvic pain syndrome—recurrent use of antibiotics for isolated pathogens only
- Individualize treatment—target to symptoms and response

ACUTE SCROTAL PROBLEMS–SWELLING PREDOMINANT

TABLE 8-6 Differential Diagnosis and Physical Examination Findings of Scrotal Swelling

MASS	PALPATION	TRANSILLUMINATION	EFFECT OF VALSALVA
Tumor	*Firm*	No	Unchanged
Varicocele	Fluid filled	No	*Increase*
Hydrocele	Fluid filled	Yes	Unchanged
Spermatocele	Fluid filled	Yes	Unchanged

Spermatocele is superior to testicle, and should be isolatable, unlike a hydrocele.
Brenner and Aderonke, 2012.

Hydrocele
Definition
Filling of the tunica vaginalis' potential space (between parietal and visceral layers) with peritoneal fluid
- Communicating → fluid flows through patent processus vaginalis from peritoneal cavity (with potential for other abdominal contents)
- Non-communicating → imbalance between absorption and resorption

Symptoms
- Swelling, dull pain may be present with large volume.

Physical Examination
- See Table 8-6. Increase in swelling at end of day or with Valsalva suggests communicating hydrocele.

Investigation
- Ultrasound may be necessary to rule out secondary or reactive hydrocele
  - May be secondary to neoplasm or torsion

Management
- Referral to urology if symptomatic, otherwise conservative
- Communicating hydrocele carries with it high risk of herniation and strangulation of bowel/mesentery → must be surgically corrected

Varicocele

Definition

- Dilation of pampiniform plexus or spermatic vein

Symptoms and Characteristics

- Typically left hemiscrotal swelling (due to increased pressure in left gonadal vein from the 90 degree angle made when draining to left renal vein)
- Dull pain may be present, worsens with straining
- Testicular atrophy secondary to increased temperature
- Ten to fifteen percent present in the context of male infertility or subfertility

Physical Examination

- See Table 8-6
- Standing and supine examination
- Persistence in supine position is a red flag for possible inferior vena cava (IVC) obstruction

Investigations

- Semen analysis
- Doppler ultrasound if concerned about IVC obstruction

Management

- Patients with completed families → NSAIDs, scrotal supports
- Patients without completed families or fertility concerns → semen analysis
  - If normal, management may be supportive
  - If abnormal → refer for either surgical ligation or embolization
- Other criteria favoring intervention:
  - Reduced volume by 2 mL or 10%
  - Reduction with reduced sperm count
  - Symptomatic

Cystic Scrotal Swelling (Spermatocele, Epididymal Cyst)

Definition

- Fluid-filled (nonviable sperm) collection of the head of the epididymis >2 cm → spermatocele; <2 cm → epididymal cyst

Symptoms

- Painless swelling

Physical Examination

- See Table 8-6
- Cystic mass superior to and separate from body of testis

Testicular Cancer

Characteristics

- Most common solid tumor in men ages 18 to 40

Symptoms

- Typically painless mass or swelling

Risk Factors

- Cryptorchidism, personal or family history of testicular cancer, HIV, testicular carcinoma in situ

Physical Examination

- See Table 8-6
- Typically nontender

Investigations

- Imaging: ultrasound, or MRI if ultrasound is equivocal
- Serum: alpha fetoprotein, beta-hCG (establishes risk)

Management

- Depends on specific diagnosis and risk profile

ACUTE SCROTAL PROBLEMS—PAIN PREDOMINANT

Pain-Predominant Scrotal Problems

Differential Diagnosis

Children and adolescents

- Torsion
- Torsion of appendage
- Strangulated inguinal hernia (testicle not tender)
- Trauma
- Orchitis (very rare)
- Henoch-Schonlein Purpura

In adults, consider:

- Testicular cancer (pain an uncommon symptom)
- Fournier's gangrene
- Post-vasectomy

TABLE 8-7	Differentiating Acute Scrotal Pain			
ETIOLOGY	DOPPLER U/S	CREMASTERIC REFLEX	AGE	FEATURE
Torsion	Decreased	Absent	12-18 years	Negative Prehn sign
Torsion of appendage		Present	Prepubertal	Blue dot sign
Epididymitis	Increased	Present	Sexually active	Positive Prehn sign

Epididymitis

Definition

- Infection (usually bacterial) of the epididymis

Symptoms

- Acute onset of unilateral testicular pain
- May have urethral discharge, dysuria, and fever

Risk Factors

- Sexually active males

Physical Examination

- See Table 8-7
- Relief of pain with elevation of the testicle (Prehn sign) → not reliable
- Unilateral swelling becoming generalized
- Exquisite tenderness
- Preserved cremasteric reflex

Investigations

- See Table 8-7
- Urinalysis and urine C + S → often pyuria
- Urine PCR for Chlamydia and Gonorrhea

Prevention

- Safe sex

Treatment

For 10 to 14 days

- Age <35, likely organism Chlamydia or Gonorrhea → cefixime and doxycycline
  - Treat sexual partner also
- Age >35, likely organism *E. coli*
- Oral fluroquinolone to >35 years

Key Points

- Pubertal males, usually sexually transmitted
- Rule out other causes with history and physical
- Emergency referral to urology if any suspicion of torsion

Testicular Torsion

Definition

- Greater than 180 degree rotation of testis causing strangulation of blood supply.

Symptoms

- Severe scrotal pain
- Testicle may be swollen, erythematous, +/− induration, elevation
- Associated nausea and vomiting

Physical Examination

- See Table 8-7
- Testicle may be swollen, erythematous, +/− indurated, elevated

Investigations

- See Table 8-7

Treatment

- Emergency urological referral, ideally within 6 hours of onset

Key Points

- Ruling out torsion can be difficult as reliability of signs is examiner dependent → referral to urology within 6 to 8 hours of onset if suspicious

Torsion of the Appendage of the Testicle

Definition

- Twisting of testicular/epididymal vestigial appendix

Symptoms

- Severe scrotal pain and swelling

Physical Examination

- See Table 8-7
- Less pain than torsion
- May have point tenderness over superior-posterior testicle

Treatment

- Analgesia as is self-limited within 1 week

Key Points

- Difficult to confidently exclude testicular torsion with acute presentation

Bibliography

Brenner JS, Aderonke O. Causes of scrotal swelling in children and adolescents. In: Basow DS, ed. *UptoDate*. Waltham, MA: UptoDate; 2011.

Canadian Urological Association. Prostatitis guidelines (draft). 2011. http://www.cua.org/guidelines_e.asp.

Canadian Urological Association. Prostate cancer screening: Canadian guidelines 2011. 2011. http://www.cua.org/guidelines_e.asp.

Canadian Urological Association. 2010 Update: Guidelines for the management of benign prostatic hyperplasia. 2010. http://www.cua.org/guidelines_e.asp.

Eyre RC. Evaluation of the acute scrotum in adults. In: Basow DS, ed. *UptoDate*. Waltham, MA: UptoDate;2012.

Hoffman RM. Screening for prostate cancer. *NEJM*. 2011;365:2013-2019. http://www.nejm.org/doi/full/10.1056/NEJMcp1103642.

Kantoff PW, Taplin M. Clinical presentation, diagnosis, and staging of prostate cancer. In: Basow DS, ed. *UptoDate*. Waltham, MA: UptoDate; 2012.

Osteoporosis

Priority Topic 69

Definitions

World Health Organization definition of postmenopausal osteoporosis in women without fragility fractures:

- T-score is bone density expressed as number of standard deviations (SD) above or below mean bone mineral density (BMD) value for a normal young adult, based on BMD measurement at spine, hip, or forearm by dual-energy x-ray absorptiometry (DEXA)
  - Normal is BMD within 1 SD of young adult mean (T-score at −1 and above)
  - Osteopenia is BMD within −1 SD and −2.5 SD below young adult mean (T-score between −1 and −2.5)
  - Osteoporosis is BMD ≤−2.5 SD below young adult mean (T-score at or below −2.5)
  - Clinical diagnosis of osteoporosis is fragility fracture regardless of T-score

> Fragility fracture is hip, vertebral, or extremity fracture sustained from fall from standing height.

Symptoms

Essentially asymptomatic until fragility fracture occurs, "the silent thief"

Characteristics

- Common: 40% lifetime risk (equivalent to cardiovascular disease), 80% will get a second fragility fracture
- Costly:
  - Financial: $1.9 billion are spent each year in Canada for treating osteoporosis and associated fractures
  - Human: High mortality (23% with hip fractures at 1 year), high morbidity (60% will require help with activities of daily living and 40% will require mobility aids after hip fracture)
  - Gap in care: <20% of women and 10% of men with fragility fracture receive appropriate care

Risk Factors

Focus since 2010 is on constellation of risk factors versus BMD score alone, with BMD being one among several independent risk factors

All patients should get BMD testing if:

- Advancing age—men and women at or over age 65
- Men and women at or over age 50 with risk factors:
  - Fragility fracture after age 40
  - High-risk medications
    - Corticosteroids (prednisone 7.5 mg daily for 3 months or equivalent)
    - Others (aromatase inhibitors, androgen deprivation therapy)
  - Parental hip fracture
  - Radiographic (vertebral fracture)
  - Current smoking
  - Alcohol (>3 drinks/day)
  - Low or loss of weight (<60 kg or loss of 10% of body weight from age 25)
  - Medical illnesses (rheumatoid arthritis, premature menopause, malabsorption, hypogonadism, chronic liver disease, inflammatory bowel disease)

Physical Examination

Findings on periodic health examination that may suggest osteoporosis:

- Loss of height of 2 cm/year or historical loss of 6 cm → consider lateral spine x-ray to identify possible fracture
- Loss of ilio-costal distance greater than two finger breadths
- Kyphosis >5 cm

Fall Assessment

- "Get up and go" screening test
- Assess and modify medications (polypharmacy, benzodiazepines, opioids, anti-hypertensives, TCAs, SSRIs)
- Home assessment
- Optimize vision, cardiovascular, neurological, musculoskeletal conditions

Diagnosis

Made by fragility fracture, vertebral fracture (>25% loss of vertebral body height on lateral spine x-ray), or BMD of −2.5 or lower

Investigations

- To rule out secondary causes of osteoporosis once diagnosis has been made
- Corrected calcium, CBC, creatinine, ALP, TSH, S-PEP, 25-OH vitamin D (initially and once after 3-4 months of supplementation)
- Frequent, repetitive BMD testing is an area of controversy:
  - Baseline BMD better than repeat BMD for predicting fracture risk over 8-year period
  - Repeat BMD in 1 to 3 years for high-risk patients to identify "early losers"; benefit from referral to rheumatology

Prevention

Optimize bone health with adequate calcium, vitamin D, smoking cessation, alcohol moderation, weight-bearing exercise as a young adult (bone density peaks at age 16 for women, 20 for men), and beyond

Treatment

Risk stratify with either tool

- CAROC → requires BMD
- FRAX → does not require BMD, but score improves with its addition

1. Low-risk/all groups:
   - 1200 mg of elemental calcium (supplement as needed, typically 500 mg daily)
   - 800 to 2000 IU of vitamin D_3 daily
   - Fall prevention strategies
   - Hip protectors for institutionalized patients
   - Regular active weight-bearing exercise
2. Medium risk:
   - Consider pharmacotherapy. Patients with risk factors (steroid use, more than two falls in last 12 months, previous wrist fracture, or lumbar spine T-score significantly lower than femoral neck T-score) are more likely to benefit from pharmacotherapy
3. High risk:
   - Initiate pharmacotherapy

Pharmacotherapy

First line:

■ Prevention of all fractures: bisphosphonates

■ Prevention of vertebral fractures: SERM (raloxifene) if breast cancer indication, HRT if indicated for vasomotor symptoms

■ Bisphosphonates: decrease bone resorption and turnover which increases BMD
   - Essentially all equivalent
   - Benefits
     ◦ Vertebral fracture > non-vertebral (NNTs 13-50 vs NNTs of 91)
     ◦ Alendronate
     ◦ Risedronate: monthly dosing available
     ◦ Zoledronic acid: yearly IV infusion possible (if covered)
     ◦ Risks: osteonecrosis of jaw (ONJ), atypical sub-trochanteric hip fractures, esophagitis.
     ◦ Treat for 5 years, then consider drug holiday.

Second line (if bisphosphonate-resistant or intolerant): calcitonin or parathyroid hormone (teriparatide)

Guideline Summary

See Quick Reference Guide from Osteoporosis Canada (Figure 8-2)

Key Points

■ Risk factor assessment is more important than BMD

■ Ensure adequate calcium (1200 mg daily) and vitamin D (800-2000 IU daily) intake

■ Treat high-risk patients with bisphosphonates

■ ONJ, atypical sub-trochanteric hip fractures are important side effects of bisphosphonates

Bibliography

Journal Watch. Baseline BMD better than repeat BMD for predicting fracture risk over 8 year period. *Arch Intern Med.* 2007 Jan 22;167:155-160.

Osteoporosis Canada. Facts and statistics. 2011. http://www.osteoporosis.ca/index.php/ci_id/8867/la_id/1.htm. [Information page].

Rx Files. Potpourri of Q & As: osteoporosis, vitamin D, SMBG, & anti-infectives. 2010. http://www.rxfiles.ca/rxfiles/uploads/documents/QA-Remake.htm.

Rx Files. Osteoporosis treatment comparison chart. *Drug Comparison Charts.* 8th ed. 2010:72-73.

Scientific Advisory Council of Osteoporosis Canada. 2010 clinical practice guidelines for the diagnosis and management of osteoporosis in Canada: summary. *Can Med Assn J.* 2010. DOI:10.1503/cmaj.100771.

SOGC. Menopause and osteoporosis update. *J Obst Gynecol Can.* 2009;31(1).

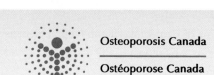

Quick Reference Guide

2010 Clinical Practice Guidelines for the Diagnosis and Management of Osteoporosis in Canada

This guide has been developed to provide healthcare professionals with a quick-reference summary of the most important recommendations from the **2010 Clinical Practice Guidelines for the Diagnosis and Management of Osteoporosis in Canada**. For more detailed information, consult the full guideline document at www.osteoporosis.ca.

Recommendations for Clinical Assessment

Assessment	Recommended Elements of Clinical Assessment
History	☐ Identify risk factors for low BMD, fractures and falls: ☐ Prior fragility fractures ☐ High alcohol intake (≥3 units/day) ☐ Parental hip fracture ☐ Rheumatoid arthritis ☐ Glucocorticoid use ☐ Inquire about falls in the previous 12 months ☐ Current smoking ☐ Inquire about gait and balance
Physical Examination	☐ Measure weight (weight loss of >10% since age 25 is significant) ☐ Measure height annually (prospective loss >2 cm) (historical height loss >6 cm) ⎤ ☐ Measure rib to pelvis distance ≤2 fingers' breadth } Screening for vertebral fractures ☐ Measure occiput-to-wall distance (for kyphosis) >5 cm ⎦ ☐ Assess fall risk by using Get-Up-and-Go Test (ability to get out of chair without using arms, walk several steps and return)

Recommended Biochemical Tests for Patients Being Assessed for Osteoporosis

☐ Calcium, corrected for albumin   ☐ Thyroid stimulating hormone (TSH)
☐ Complete blood count   ☐ Serum protein electrophoresis for patients with vertebral fractures
☐ Creatinine   ☐ 25-hydroxy vitamin D (25-OH-D)*
☐ Alkaline phosphatase

Should be measured after 3-4 months of adequate supplementation and should not be repeated if an optimal level ≥75 nmol/L is achieved.

Indications for BMD Testing

Older Adults (age ≥50 years)	Younger Adults (age <50 years)
• All women and men age ≥65 years • Menopausal women, and men aged 50-64 years with clinical risk factors for fracture: – Fragility fracture after age 40 – Prolonged glucocorticoid use[†] – Other high-risk medication use* – Parental hip fracture – Vertebral fracture or osteopenia identified on x-ray – Current smoking – High alcohol intake – Low body weight (<60 kg) or major weight loss (>10% of weight at age 25 years) – Rheumatoid arthritis – Other disorders strongly associated with osteoporosis such as primary hyperparathyroidism, type 1 diabetes, osteogenesis imperfecta, uncontrolled hyperthyroidism, hypogonadism or premature menopause (<45 years), Cushing's disease, chronic malnutrition or malabsorption, chronic liver disease, COPD and chronic inflammatory conditions (eg, inflammatory bowel disease)	• Fragility fracture • Prolonged use of glucocorticoids* • Use of other high-risk medications[†] • Hypogonadism or premature menopause • Malabsorption syndrome • Primary hyperparathyroidism • Other disorders strongly associated with rapid bone loss and/or fracture

[†] ≥ 3 months in the prior year at a prednisone equivalent dose ≥7.5 mg daily; *eg, aromatase inhibitors, androgen deprivation therapy.*

Assessment of Basal 10-year Fracture Risk: 2010 CAROC System

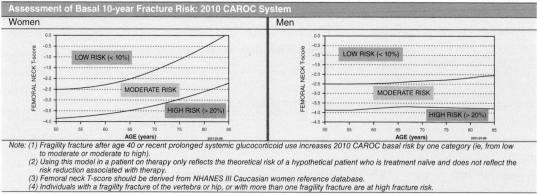

Note: (1) Fragility fracture after age 40 or recent prolonged systemic glucocorticoid use increases 2010 CAROC basal risk by one category (ie, from low to moderate or moderate to high).
(2) Using this model in a patient on therapy only reflects the theoretical risk of a hypothetical patient who is treatment naïve and does not reflect the risk reduction associated with therapy.
(3) Femoral neck T-score should be derived from NHANES III Caucasian women reference database.
(4) Individuals with a fragility fracture of the vertebra or hip, or with more than one fragility fracture are at high fracture risk.

Adapted from Papaioannou A et al. Clinical practice guidelines for the diagnosis and management of osteoporosis in Canada. CMAJ 2010 http://www.cmaj.ca/cgi/doi/10.1503/cmaj.100771. With permission from the publisher. © Osteoporosis Canada, October 2010. v-09-03-11.

FIGURE 8-2A: Quick reference guide from Osteoporosis Canada.

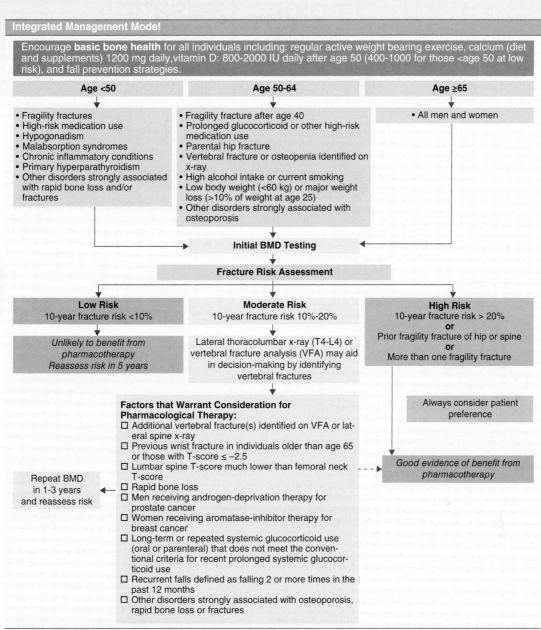

Integrated Management Model

Encourage **basic bone health** for all individuals including: regular active weight bearing exercise, calcium (diet and supplements) 1200 mg daily, vitamin D: 800-2000 IU daily after age 50 (400-1000 for those <age 50 at low risk), and fall prevention strategies.

Age <50	Age 50-64	Age ≥65
• Fragility fractures • High-risk medication use • Hypogonadism • Malabsorption syndromes • Chronic inflammatory conditions • Primary hyperparathyroidism • Other disorders strongly associated with rapid bone loss and/or fractures	• Fragility fracture after age 40 • Prolonged glucocorticoid or other high-risk medication use • Parental hip fracture • Vertebral fracture or osteopenia identified on x-ray • High alcohol intake or current smoking • Low body weight (<60 kg) or major weight loss (>10% of weight at age 25) • Other disorders strongly associated with osteoporosis	• All men and women

Initial BMD Testing

Fracture Risk Assessment

Low Risk 10-year fracture risk <10%	Moderate Risk 10-year fracture risk 10%-20%	High Risk 10-year fracture risk > 20% or Prior fragility fracture of hip or spine or More than one fragility fracture

Unlikely to benefit from pharmacotherapy Reassess risk in 5 years

Lateral thoracolumbar x-ray (T4-L4) or vertebral fracture analysis (VFA) may aid in decision-making by identifying vertebral fractures

Always consider patient preference

Factors that Warrant Consideration for Pharmacological Therapy:
- ☐ Additional vertebral fracture(s) identified on VFA or lateral spine x-ray
- ☐ Previous wrist fracture in individuals older than age 65 or those with T-score ≤ –2.5
- ☐ Lumbar spine T-score much lower than femoral neck T-score
- ☐ Rapid bone loss
- ☐ Men receiving androgen-deprivation therapy for prostate cancer
- ☐ Women receiving aromatase-inhibitor therapy for breast cancer
- ☐ Long-term or repeated systemic glucocorticoid use (oral or parenteral) that does not meet the conventional criteria for recent prolonged systemic glucocorticoid use
- ☐ Recurrent falls defined as falling 2 or more times in the past 12 months
- ☐ Other disorders strongly associated with osteoporosis, rapid bone loss or fractures

Repeat BMD in 1-3 years and reassess risk

Good evidence of benefit from pharmacotherapy

First Line Therapies with Evidence for Fracture Prevention in Postmenopausal Women*

Type of Fracture	Antiresorptive Therapy						Bone Formation Therapy
	Bisphosphonates			Denosumab	Raloxifene	Estrogen** (Hormone Therapy)	Teriparatide
	Alendronate	Risedronate	Zoledronic Acid				
Vertebral	✓	✓	✓	✓	✓	✓	✓
Hip	✓	✓	✓	✓	–	✓	–
Non-vertebral†	✓	✓	✓	✓	–	✓	✓

†In Clinical trials, non-vertebral fractures are a composite endpoint including hip, femur, pelvis, tibia, humerus, radius, and clavicle.
*For postmenopausal women, ✓ indicates first line therapies and Grade A recommendation. For men requiring treatment, alendronate, risedronate, and zoledronic acid can be used as first-line therapies for prevention of fractures (Grade D).
**Hormone therapy (estrogen) can be used as first-line therapy in women with menopausal symptoms.

www.osteoporosis.ca

Adapted from Papaioannou A et al. Clinical practice guidelines for the diagnosis and management of osteoporosis in Canada. CMAJ 2010 http://www.cmaj.ca/cgi/doi/10.1503/cmaj.100771. With permission from the publisher. © Osteoporosis Canada, October 2010. v-09-03-11.

FIGURE 8-2B: Quick reference guide from Osteoporosis Canada.

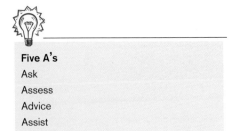

Five A's
Ask
Assess
Advice
Assist
Arrange

Smoking Cessation

Priority Topic 85

The five As: a brief intervention for smoking cessation

ASK AND ASSESS WILLINGNESS TO QUIT

Frequent starts and stops are common

Review amount, habits, and previous quit attempts

Assess willingness to quit using stages of change model (Table 8-8)

TABLE 8–8	Stages of Change
STAGE	ACTION
Precontemplation	Increase patient's awareness of risks in nonjudgmental manner, avoid resistance
Contemplation	Discuss pros and cons of quitting, understand ambivalence
Preparation	Offer practical advice and anticipate difficulties
Action	Support, reward, prevent relapse, review action plan
Maintenance	Address stressors and anticipate temptations

Patients unwilling to quit may benefit from multiple, short sessions using principles of motivational interviewing (the five Rs may be a helpful mnemonic):

Relevance to patient

Risks of smoking

Rewards of quitting

Roadblocks to quitting

Repetition at each visit

ADVISE TO QUIT

Brief advice from a physician increases cessation rate

Health benefits:

- Leading cause of preventable death
- Death an average of 6.5 to 9 years prematurely
- Reduced risk of mortality from myocardial infarction
- Reduced stroke risk
- Improvement in chronic lung disease
- Reduced number and severity of pulmonary infections
- Reduced cancer risk (bladder, cervical, stomach, oropharyngeal)
- Reduced risk of osteoporosis and fractures
- Reduced risk of peptic ulcer disease
- Improved healing
- Improved health of family/cohabitants

Improved quality of life:

- Less sexual dysfunction
- Financial gains (on average $3600/year)

ASSIST IN IMPLEMENTING A PLAN

Multi-strategy approach may include some or all of the following:

- Establishing a quit day

- Pre-quit exercise program
- Alternative oral behaviours—gum, lozenges
- Anticipate obstacles such as withdrawal, weight gain, triggers
- Support groups
- Counseling and cognitive behavioural therapy
- Hypnosis/acupuncture
- Repetition
- Pharmacotherapy (see Table 8-9)
  - Nicotine replacement
    - Gum, patch, inhaler, nasal spray
  - Bupropion
  - Varenicline

TABLE 8-9	Pharmacotherapy	
DRUG (VS PLACEBO)	BUPROPION	VARENICLINE
NNT	8 vs placebo	8 vs placebo
SEs	Insomnia, headache, dizziness, tachycardia, xerostomia, weight loss, pharyngitis, nausea	Insomnia, h/a, abnormal dreams, GI upset
Tolerability	29% discontinued due to SEs	Better
Caution	ESRD, cirrhosis → adjust dose. Depression with suicide potential → monitor mood	ESRD → adjust dose. Depression with suicide potential → monitor mood. Stable CAD → currently under Health Canada and FDA review
Contraindication	Seizure disorder, eating disorder, MAO-I use, sedative withdrawal	None

ARRANGE FOLLOW-UP

- Peak withdrawal at 2 to 3 days
- Improvement in withdrawal at 2 to 3 weeks
- Highest relapse at 2 to 3 months

Bibliography

Lai DTC, Cahill K, Qin Y, Yang JL. Motivational interviewing for smoking cessation. *Cochrane Database Syst Rev.* 2010, Issue 1. DOI: 10.1002/14651858.CD006936.pub2.

Mahoney MC, Cummings K. Chapter 57. Tobacco cessation. In: South-Paul JE, Matheny SC, Lewis EL, eds. *Current Diagnosis & Treatment in Family Medicine.* 3rd ed. 2011. http://www.accessmedicine.com/content.aspx?aID=8158522. Accessed November 12, 2012.

Rx Files. Tobacco/smoking cessation pharmacotherapy. *Drug Comparison Charts.* 8th ed. 2010:115.

Statistics Canada. Canadian Tobacco Use Monitoring Survey. 2003. http://www.hc-sc.gc.ca/hc-ps/tobac-tabac/research-recherche/stat/_ctums-esutc_fs-if/2003-smok-fum-eng.php. Accessed November 12, 2012.

Stead LF, Bergson G, Lancaster T. Physician advice for smoking cessation. *Cochrane Database Syst Rev.* 2008; Issue 2. DOI: 10.1002/14651858.CD000165.pub3.

Toronto Notes. Smoking cessation. *Family Medicine.* 24th ed. 2008:FM8-9.

9

Sexual Health

Gender-Specific Issues
Priority Topic 42

- Appreciate and anticipate that males and females may have different presentations of the same condition or disease.
- Be aware and consider the possibility of domestic violence in women with health concerns.
- Assess the possibility of role-balancing issues when presented with men or women experiencing stress-related health concerns.
- Ensure your office and practice provides comfort and choice, especially around sensitive examinations such as rectal or pelvic examinations.
- Be sure to interpret and use evidence-based medicine while being cognitive of the gender bias in clinical studies.

Bibliography
The College of Family Physicians of Canada. http://www.cfpc.ca/uploadedFiles/Education/Priority%20 Topics%20and%20Key%20Features.pdf.

Infertility
Priority Topic 52

Definition
Failure to conceive after 1 year of regular, unprotected sex for women under 35 years
- Primary infertility
  - No prior pregnancies
- Secondary infertility
  - Previous conception

Investigations
- When?
  - Women <35 years: after 1 year of trying to conceive
  - Women 35 to 40 years: after 6 months of trying to conceive
  - Women >40 years: immediately

- Sooner if history of:
  - PID
  - History of infertility
  - Prior pelvic surgery
  - Chemotherapy or radiation in either partner
  - Recurrent pregnancy loss
  - Moderate-severe endometriosis
- Who?
  - Both partners
    - Female factor approximately 30%
    - Male factor approximately 30%
    - Both male and female factors approximately 30%

Etiology
Female
- Ovulatory dysfunction
  - Polycystic ovarian syndrome (PCOS)
  - Premature ovarian failure
- Tubular disease
  - Pelvic inflammatory disease
  - Adhesions
- Uterine abnormalities
  - Fibroids
  - Asherman syndrome
- Cervical abnormalities
  - Cervical stenosis

Sperm lives longer than eggs. Therefore, it is better to advise patients to have sex a few days prior to ovulation, rather than wait until the day they think they are ovulating. Some recommend sex three times per week.

Male
- Idiopathic
- Primary hypogonadism
  - History of cryptorchidism
  - Androgen insensitivity
  - Medication/radiation
  - Varicocele
- Altered sperm transport
  - Obstructed or absent vas deferens
  - Retrograde ejaculation
- Secondary hypogonadism

Diagnosis
- History
  - Female
    - Menstrual cycle
      - Frequency and duration
      - Regular or irregular
      - Changing
      - Intermenstrual bleeding
    - Coitus
      - Frequency
      - Timing

Always rule out pregnancy in "infertility".

- PMHx
  - PID
  - Surgery
  - Systemic symptoms
  - Symptoms of PCOS
  - Nipple discharge/lactation
- Male
  - Fevers
  - Trauma
  - Previous successful pregnancies
  - Systemic symptoms
  - Erections

Investigations

- Female
  - Day 3 FSH (test of ovarian reserve)
  - LH
  - TSH
  - DHEA
  - Testosterone
  - Prolactin
  - Day 21 to 23 serum progesterone (test of ovulation)
  - Histosalpingogram
  - Laparoscopy
  - Karyotype
- Male
  - Semen analysis
  - Free testosterone
  - Karyotyping

Treatment

- Ovulation induction (clomiphene citrate)
- Tuboplasty
- Lysis of adhesions
- Artificial insemination
- IVF
- ICSI (intracytoplasmic sperm injection)
- IUI (intrauterine insemination)
- Sperm or ova donation
- Consider discussing adoption

POLYCYSTIC OVARIAN SYNDROME

Etiology

- Steady state gonadotropin production such that there is no LH surge to induce ovulation
- Most common in 15 to 35 years

Symptoms

- Hirsutism
- Hyperandrogenism
- Infertility

- Insulin resistance
- Acanthosis nigricans
- Anovulation
- Menorrhagia

Investigations
- Transvaginal ultrasound
  - String of pearls—polycystic ovaries
- LH:FSH > 2:1
- Fasting glucose
- Increased DHEAS
- Increased free testosterone

Treatment
- Cycle control
  - Weight loss
  - Increased exercise
  - OCP
  - Oral hypoglycemic (metformin)
  - Tranexamic acid for menorrhagia
- Infertility
  - Weight loss
  - Medical induction of ovulation—clomifene +/− metformin
  - Bromocriptine if increased prolactin levels
- Hirsuitism
  - OCP +/− spironolactone for antiandrogen effect

Bibliography

Chen AY, Tran C. *Toronto Notes*. Toronto, ON: Type & Graphics Inc; 2011.

Simon C, Everitt H, van Dorp F. *Oxford Handbook of General Practice*. Oxford, UK: Oxford University Press; 2010.

Sex

Priority Topic 82

Definitions
- Paraphilias: sexual arousal as a result of nonhuman objects
- Gender identity disorder: cross gender identifications
- Sexual response
  1. Desire
  2. Arousal
  3. Orgasm
  4. Resolution

FEMALE SEXUAL DYSFUNCTION

Etiology
- Intrapsychic
- Relationship issues
- Physical/organic

Top Three Classifications of Female Sexual Dysfunction

1. Lack of desire (60%–70%)
2. Lack of arousal
3. Dyspareunia (vaginismus, vulvodynia, vulvar vestibulitis)

Treatment Options for Women

- Rule out organic causes!
- Relationship therapy
- Self-exploration
- Kegel exercises
- Dilators
- Psychotherapy
- Lubricants
- Sexual position—female on top (more control for female)
- Hormone replacement therapy if indicated

MALE SEXUAL DYSFUNCTION

Erectile dysfunction: inability to obtain or maintain an adequate erection for sexual performance

Etiology

- Psychogenic (10%)
  - Morning erections are present
  - Younger men
  - Performance anxiety
- Organic (90%)
  - Circulation—cardiovascular disease, diabetes
  - Neurologic—post prostate surgery, trauma
  - Respiratory—COPD
  - Hormonal—hypogonadism
  - Drug side effects—β-blockers, SSRIs, diuretics
  - Smoking
  - Alcohol
  - Cocaine

Diagnosis

- Generally self-reported, but may require physician-directed inquiry to illicit symptoms
- ED Intensity Scale or ED Impact Scale can be used to assess patient

Treatment

- Psychogenic—non-drug treatments
- Organic—lifestyle changes (quit smoking, decrease alcohol) and medication
  - Phosphodiesterase-5 (PDE-5) inhibitors are first-line medication.
    - Sildenafil (Viagra)
    - Tadalafil (Cialis)
    - Vardenafil (Levitra)
  - Other options include prostaglandins, vasodilators, implants, and vascular surgery
- PDE-5 inhibitors
  - Contraindications
    - Patient taking nitrates or alpha-1 blockers

- Side effects
  - Common: flushing, headache, dyspepsia
  - Rare: MI, priapism (>4 h)

Bibliography

Chen YA, Tran C. *Toronto Notes—Comprehensive Medical Reference & Review for MCCQE I and USMLE II.* Toronto, Canada: Toronto Notes for Medical Students Inc; 2011.

Rx Files. Erectile dysfunction comparison chart. *Drug Comparison Charts.* 8th ed. 2010;46.

Sexually Transmitted Infections
Priority Topic 83

CHLAMYDIA

Most common STI in Canada.

Etiology

- *Chlamydia trachomatis*

Symptoms

- May be asymptomatic (80% of women)
- Vaginal or urethral discharge
- UTI symptoms (frequency, urgency, dysuria)
- Pelvic pain
- Postcoital bleeding

Diagnosis

- Nucleic acid amplification test (NAAT) on "dirty" urine sample (no cleaning of genitalia prior, first catch)

Prevention

- Condom use with every sexual contact

Complications

- Pelvic inflammatory disease
- Reactive arthritis (sterile arthritis, urethritis, conjunctivitis)
- Infertility
- Chronic pelvic pain
- Increased rate of ectopic pregnancy

Treatment

- Azithromycin 1 g po × 1 *or*
- Doxycycline 100 mg po bid × 7 days
- Always treat for gonorrhea as well, as often coinfected

Key Points

- Reportable disease in most jurisdictions and must treat partners
- In pregnant women, use azithromycin to avoid fetal bone and teeth effects
- If treating during pregnancy, must retest patients 3 to 4 weeks after treatment to ensure cure
- Abstain from sex until 7 days after completed treatment

GONORRHEA

Symptoms
- May be asymptomatic (80% of women)
- Vaginal or urethral discharge
- UTI symptoms (frequency, urgency, dysuria)
- Pelvic pain
- Postcoital bleeding
- May also have pharyngeal infection

Diagnosis
- Urine PCR for screening. In symptomatic MSM, nongenital infections, or exposure to known resistant gonorrhea, swab, and culture is recommended

Prevention
- Condom use with every sexual contact

Complications
- Same as for chlamydia

Treatment
- Cefixime 800 mg po × 1 *or*
- Ceftriaxone 250 mg IM × 1
- Ciprofloxacin 500 mg po × 1 (only if contraindication to third-generation cephalosporins *and* susceptibility is demonstrated on culture *or* <5% local resistance rate *and* test for cure available)
- Always treat for chlamydia as well as often coinfected

Key Points
- MSM—ceftriaxone is the preferred treatment
- Pharyngeal infections—ceftriaxone is the preferred treatment
- Test for cure in kids <14 years, in case of pregnancy, and if nongenital source

HPV

Etiology
- Human papilloma virus (>50 subtypes)
  - 16 and 18—oncogenic
  - 6 and 11—warts

Symptoms
- Asymptomatic
- Warts (condyloma acuminate) visible or palpable on external genitalia
- Postcoital bleeding

Diagnosis
- Clinical
  - Visible, flesh-coloured papules
  - Aceto-white reaction

Prevention
- Vaccination with Gardasil (quadrivalent—6, 11, 16, 18)
  - Girls age 9 to 26 years
  - Boys age 9 to 26 years—not covered by any provincial vaccination program currently

- Vaccination with Cervarix (bivalent—16, 18)
  - Girls age 9 to 26 years
  - Condom use not shown to limit transmission

Complications

- Cervical cancer, vulvar and vaginal cancer, genital warts, anal cancer, pharyngeal cancer

Treatment

Only helps speed resolution of the warts, does not eradicate the infection with HPV

- Imiquimod 5% cream: three times per week for up to 16 weeks
  - Apply at night then wash off 6 to 10 hours later with soap and water
- Cryotherapy—generally safest in pregnancy
- Laser
- Surgery
- Trichloracetic acid (80%–90%)
  - Apply until white
  - Applied by physician once every 1 to 2 weeks until lesions are gone
- Podophyllin (10%–25%)—contraindicated in pregnancy
  - Apply petroleum jelly to surrounding tissue for protection
  - Leave podophyllin for 4 to 6 hours then wash off
- Podofilox (0.5%)
  - Home treatment, applied with cotton swab bid for three consecutive days, repeat every week

Key Points

- Ensure regular cervical cancer screening
- MSM at higher risk of anal warts and anal cancer

HSV

Etiology

- Herpes simplex virus (I and II)
  - Type I: oral
  - Type II: genital
  - Viral shedding can occur at any time, but is increased during the prodrome and while lesions are present

Symptoms

- Prodrome—genital pruritus, tingling, burning, or pain
- Vesicles on an erythematous base leading to ulcerations

Diagnosis

- Usually clinical diagnosis, onset 2 to 21 days after exposure
- Viral swabs of vesicular fluid for culture, antigen testing, or PCR

Prevention

- Condoms can reduce transmission rate by approximately 50%
- Suppressive therapy for HSV II positive partner in a serodiscordant pair

Treatment

- First episode
  - Acyclovir 400 mg po tid × 5 to 7 days
  - Valacyclovir 1000 mg po bid × 5 to 7 days

- Subsequent episodes
  - Acyclovir 400 mg po tid × 5 days
  - Valacyclovir 1000 mg po bid × 3 days
- Suppressive therapy given if >6 episodes/year
  - Acyclovir 400 mg po bid
  - Valacyclovir 1 g po daily

Key Points

- Primary outbreak can be severe, possibly with systemic flu-like symptoms
- Possible to have HSVI infection of genitalia or HSVII infection of oral mucosa, but tend to be less severe
- Can treat with antivirals within 72 hrs of prodromal symptoms or lesion presentation
- Offer suppressive therapy to pregnant women at 36 weeks and deliver via C-section if experiencing prodromal symptoms or active lesions at time of labour onset

SYPHILIS

Etiology

- *Treponema pallidum*

Symptoms

- Primary syphilis: painless papule or ulcer
- Secondary syphilis: rash and flu-like symptoms
- Latent syphilis: asymptomatic
- Tertiary syphilis: neurologic, cardiovascular (aortic root dilatation), and tissue complications

Diagnosis

- VDRL reactive and treponemal test reaction (eg, TP-EIA) *or*
- Dark field microscopy positive *or*
- Direct fluorescent antibody positive

Prevention

- Consistent condom use

Treatment

- Primary: Benzathine Penicillin G 2.4 million units IM × 1
- Secondary: Benzathine Penicillin G 2.4 million units IM × 1
- Latent:
  - Early (<1 year from likely infection): Benzathine Penicillin G 2.4 million units IM × 1
  - Late (>1 year from likely infection): Benzathine Penicillin G 2.4 million units every week × 3 weeks
- Tertiary: Benzathine Penicillin G 2.4 million units IM × every week × 3 weeks
  - Special case—neurosyphilis: penicillin G 3 to 4 million units IV q4H × 10 to 14 days

Key Points

- Latent syphilis is diagnosed in asymptomatic patients with reactive VDRL and TP-EIA; however, testing may also be reactive if they have had previously treated syphilis
- After treatment, recheck VDRL and ensure at least four-fold decrease in titers; otherwise, consider reinfection

Keep PID on your differential diagnosis of female presenting with lower abdominal pain.

VULVOVAGINITIS (SEE PRIORITY TOPIC 97)

PELVIC INFLAMMATORY DISEASE

Etiology

- Most common are Chlamydia or Gonorrhea
- May be GI organisms

Symptoms

- Fever
- Discharge
- Abdominal/pelvic pain
- Cervical motion tenderness
- Asymptomatic (60%)

Treatment

- Cefixime 800 mg po × 1 **and** doxycycline 100 mg po bid × 14 days
- Addition: Flagyl 500 mg po bid × 14 days if mass or abscess present
- Reassess in 48 hours

Key Points

- Do not remove IUD until after treatment
- Treat partners

Bibliography

DynaMed. *Chlamydia Genital Infection.* Ipswich, MA: EBSCO Publishing; 2012, February 12. http://search.ebscohost.com/login.aspx?direct=true&site=DynaMed&id=113862; http://web.ebscohost.com.cyber.usask.ca/dynamed/detail?vid=9&hid=21&sid=f693f962-f812-4ab7-bdf3-40973d062e32%40sessionmgr14&bdata=JnNpdGU9ZHluYW1lZC1saXZlJnNjb3BlPXNpdGU%3d#db=dme&AN=114223.

DynaMed. *Herpes Genitalis.* Ipswich, MA: EBSCO Publishing. 2012, March 22. http://search.ebscohost.com/login.aspx?direct=true&site=DynaMed&id=113862; http://web.ebscohost.com.cyber.usask.ca/dynamed/detail?vid=3&hid=21&sid=2e1251fa-304f-48b9-ab96-202194d757cf%40sessionmgr14&bdata=JnNpdGU9ZHluYW1lZC1saXZlJnNjb3BlPXNpdGU%3d#db=dme&AN=114875&anchor=suppressive.

Health Canada. Public Health Agency—Canadian guidelines on sexually transmitted infections. Public Health Agency of Canada Issued Important Notice on gonococcal infection; 2011. http://www.phac-aspc.gc.ca/std-mts/sti-its/alert/2011/alert-gono-eng.php.

Health Canada, Healthy Living. Human papilloma virus (HPV). 2010. http://www.hc-sc.gc.ca/hl-vs/iyh-vsv/diseases-maladies/hpv-vph-eng.php.

Hick C. Diagnostic testing for syphilis. In: Rose B, ed. *UpToDate.* 2012. http://www.uptodate.com/contents/diagnostic-testing-for-syphilis?source=search_result&search=syphilis+treatment&selectedTitle=4~150.

Sparling F, Hicks C. Pathogenesis, clinical manifestations, and treatment of late syphilis. In: Rose B, ed. *UpToDate.* 2012. http://www.uptodate.com/contents/pathogenesis-clinical-manifestations-and-treatment-of-late-syphilis?source=search_result&search=syphilis+treatment&selectedTitle=2~150#H22.

Wald A. Prevention of genital herpes virus infections. In: Rose B, ed. *UpToDate.* 2012. http://www.uptodate.com/contents/prevention-of-genital-herpes-virus-infections?source=search_result&search=prevention+of+hsv&selectedTitle=5~150.

Yingming A, Tran C, eds. *Toronto Notes.* 27th ed. Toronto, ON: Toronto Notes for Medical Students Inc; 2011.

Breast Lump

Priority Topic 11

Definition

- Any lump or mass noted on clinical examination or noted by patient

Physical Examination

- Findings suggestive of benign breast disease
  - Smooth
  - Rubbery
  - Discrete
  - Nontender
  - Mobile
  - Well circumscribed
  - Hormone dependent (cyclic)
  - No skin or nipple changes
  - Young age
- Findings concerning for breast cancer
  - Firm
  - Indistinct/not well circumscribed
  - Skin or nipple changes (retraction)
  - Peau d'orange
  - Fixed
  - Increasing size

Risk Factors for Breast Cancer

- Female
- Age >40
- Prior history of breast cancer
- Prior breast biopsy (regardless of pathology results)
- First-degree relative with breast cancer
- Menarche before age 12
- Menopause after 55
- Nulliparity
- First pregnancy after age 30
- Radiation
- HRT for >5 years duration
- OCP use*
- Alcohol*
- Sedentary lifestyle*
- Obesity*

Many of the risk factors are a result of prolonged estrogen exposure.

*Investigations

- Imaging
  - Women <30 years: ultrasound is investigation of choice due to denser breasts
  - Women >30 years: diagnostic mammography (may require U/S for more information)
  - Possible MRI—case-by-case basis, especially if dense breasts

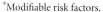

*Modifiable risk factors.

■ Tissue sample
  • Fine needle aspiration (FNA)
  • Core biopsy
  • Surgical excision

Screening

■ Breast cancer screening for average risk women
  • Women 50 to 74: routine screening mammography Q2 to 3 years
  • No routine screening for women <50 years old or >74 years old
  • No routine clinical breast examination alone or in conjunction with mammography
  • Do not advise women to perform routine breast self-examinations as there is no benefit and possible harm due to increased benign biopsies and no increased survival rates
    ○ Women who should have diagnostic mammographies rather than screening mammographies
      ▫ Post surgical biopsy
      ▫ Post benign core biopsy
      ▫ Breast implants
      ▫ Pregnant or breastfeeding
      ▫ Breast cancer survivors
      ▫ Women <40 years

Breast cancer screening for higher risk women (BRCA 1 or 2 positive, etc) requires earlier and more frequent screening.

BRCA 1 and 2 are tumor suppressor genes.

If inherited, a mutation in these genes increases a women's risk of breast, ovarian, colon, cervical, and uterine cancer.

Men that inherit a harmful BRCA 1 mutation also have an increased risk of breast cancer.

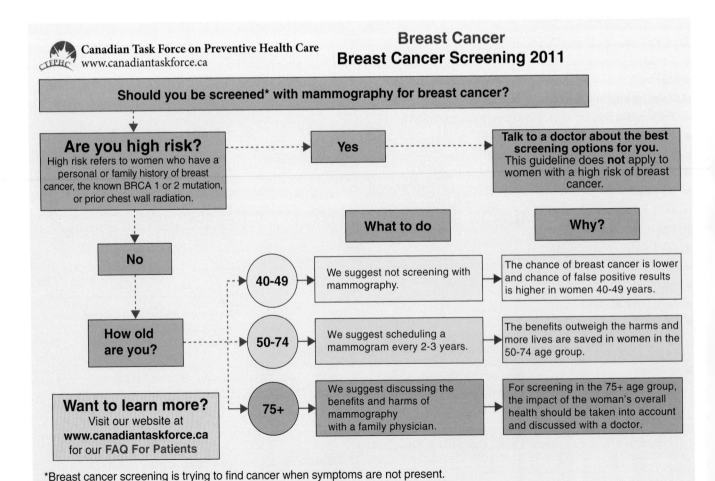

*Breast cancer screening is trying to find cancer when symptoms are not present.

Treatment of Breast Cancer

- Lumpectomy + radiation
- Mastectomy
- Sentinel node biopsy
- Node dissection
- Hormone therapy
- Chemotherapy
- Metastases
  - Nodal status is the most important prognostic factor
  - Bone > lung > pleura > liver > brain
  - Monitor for symptoms of metastases in cases of known breast cancer

Complications of Breast Cancer

- Lymphedema possibly from nodal metastases or after node dissection
- Generalized aches and pains
- Side effects from radiation and chemotherapy

Differential Diagnosis

Benign Breast Lumps

- Fibrocystic changes
  - Age 30 years to menopause
  - Focal areas of nodularity or cysts
  - A normal variant, but does increase baseline risk of breast cancer slightly
- Fibroadenoma
  - Age <30 years
  - Most common breast lump in young women
  - Solid
  - Most often in upper-outer quadrant of breast
  - Cannot differentiate from cancer on physical examination or on U/S
  - Will need biopsy to ensure not cancerous
- Fat necrosis
  - Due to trauma
  - Firm
  - Ill-defined mass
  - Skin or nipple retraction possible
- Abscess
  - Hot, firm, erythematous overlying skin
  - Common during breast-feeding due to blockage of ducts causing mastitis
  - Most common pathogen is *Staphylococcus aureus*
  - Fever and leukocytosis usually present
  - Must consider inflammatory breast cancer
- Intraductal papilloma
  - Solitary
  - Intraductal
  - Benign polyp
  - Unilateral bloody nipple discharge
  - 10% risk of transformation to DCIS

Inflammatory Breast Cancer

- Aggressive cancer defined by dermal lymphatic invasion
- May or may not be associated with a mass
- Skin hot, red, painful, peau d'orange
- Generally have normal WBC and no fever
- If concerned, arrange for urgent mammography and obtain at least two skin punch biopsies

Bibliography

Chen YA, Tran C. *Toronto Notes—Comprehensive Medical Reference & Review for MCCQE I and USMLE II.* Toronto, Canada: Toronto Notes for Medical Students Inc; 2011.

Michel J, Gabriela L. Recommendations on screening for breast cancer in average-risk women age 40–74 years. *CMAJ.* 2011;183(18):2146-2146. DOI: 10.1503/cmaj.111–2101.

Taghian A, El-Ghamry M, Merajver S. Inflammatory breast cancer: clinical features and treatment. In: Rose B, ed. *UpToDate.* 2011. Available from http://www.uptodateonline.com. http://www.uptodate.com/contents/inflammatory-breast-cancer-clinical-features-and-treatment?source=search_result&search=inflammatory+breast+cancer&selectedTitle=1~34

10

Women's Health

Contraception
Priority Topic 16

LOW-DOSE ESTROGEN <35 μg

1. **Contraindications (CI) to OCP**
   - Active or past VTE
   - Undiagnosed vaginal bleeding
   - Smoking >35 years >15 cigarettes/day
   - Known/suspected breast cancer
   - Hypertension
   - Heart disease
   - Diabetes with retinopathy, nephropathy, or neuropathy
   - Stroke
   - Less than 4 to 6 weeks postpartum (coagulation/fibrinolysis normalizes 3 weeks postpartum)
   - Known/suspected pregnancy
   - Liver cirrhosis or tumor
   - Migraine with aura

2. **Relative contraindications to OCPs**
   - HTN if controlled
   - Migraine and age >35
   - History of or OCP-related cholestasis or active cholecystitis
   - Older age (>35) and obese (↑ DVT risk)
   - Bariatric surgery (may ↓ absorption)

3. **Risks of OCP use**
   - VTE
   - MI/stroke (arterial clot)
   - Increased cervical cancer in women with persistent HPV (decreased ovarian cancer and endometrial cancer)
   - Gallbladder disease (theoretical)

4. **Signs/symptoms of**

Estrogen deficiency:
- Early spotting (days 1-9)
- Continuous bleeding
- Vasomotor symptoms (hot flush, sweats, flushing)
- Amenorrhea

Estrogen excess
- Hypermenorrhea
- Dysmenorrhea
- Breast tenderness ($\uparrow$ size)
- VTE
- UTI
- HTN

Progesterone deficiency
- Late spotting (days 10-21)
- Late withdrawal bleeding

Excess progestin
- Fatigue
- Depression
- Breast tenderness
- Weight gain
- $\uparrow$ appetite
- $\downarrow$ libido
- Dizziness

Generally try a pill for 3 months before considering switching to a new pill.

5. **Reduced OCP efficacy with**
- Many antiepileptics which increase OCP metabolism
- Some antibiotics (Rifampin and possibly other antibiotics decrease OCP efficacy)
- Vomiting or malabsorption (bariatric surgery)
- Poor compliance (theoretical failure rate 0.3%, typical use failure 3%-8%)

6. **Other options**

Progestin injection q 12 weeks
- $\downarrow$ endometrial cancer risk
- $\downarrow$ drug interactions with anticonvulsant medications

Contraindications: pregnancy, unexplained vaginal bleeding, current breast cancer, current thrombophlebitis or venous thromboembolic disorders (DVT, PE)

Adverse effects: weight gain, $\downarrow$ bone density (affect on peak BMD unknown), delayed recovery of fertility (2-12 months)

Best option for patients with the following:
- Migraine
- Breast feeding
- CI to estrogen
- Smoker age $\geq$35
- Sickle cell anemia
- Anticonvulsant
- $\uparrow$ VTE risk

Theoretical failure 0.3%; typical use failure = 3% to 6%

Progestin-only pill (Micronor)
- Similar adverse effects and contraindications as injection
- Decreased efficacy, therefore scheduled adherence important
- Theoretical failure 0.5% typical use failure 5% to 10%

If late in taking Micronor by >3 hours, back-up contraception is required.

Patch (Evra Patch) and ring (Nuva Ring)

- Similar CI as OCP
- Patch ↓ effective in women >90 kg
- Theoretical failure: 0.3% to 0.8%, typical use failure = 8%

IUD: types include copper IUD and levonorgestrel-releasing IUD (Mirena)

Contraindications

- Active pelvic infection (STI, endometritis) (may consider leaving IUD in place for treatment of pelvic infections)
- Known or suspected pregnancy
- Unexplained vaginal bleeding
- Anatomic abnormalities (bicornuate uterus/fibroids)
- Current breast cancer (only for levonorgestrel-releasing IUD)
- Cervical or endometrial cancer
- Wilson disease or copper allergy (copper IUD) (Dean and Goldberg, 2012)
  - May be inserted immediately following abortion
    - At the time of TOP, providing long-acting reversible contraception, especially with IUD, is associated with a reduction of repeat abortion over the next 2 years
    - Failure (copper): 0.8% perfect and typical use
    - Failure (IUD-LNG): 0.2% perfect and typical use

TABLE 10-1	Efficacy of Other Contraceptive Methods
METHOD	**TYPICAL FAILURE RATE (%)**
Condom	Male 18; female 21
Diaphragm	~12.5
Spermicides	28
Sponge	~18
Coitus interruptus	22
Breast feeding	5
Female sterilization	<1
Vasectomy	<1
No method	85
Zieman, 2012	

7. **Emergency contraception**
   - General: use if unprotected sex, failure of barrier method, ↓ efficacy of usual contraceptive
     - No physical examination or pregnancy test is required to provide this medication
     - No medical contraindications to this therapy
     - Confirm that intercourse was consensual
     - Advise patients to take antiemetic prior to oral method of emergency contraception (Yuzpe method only)
   - Plan B (levonorgestrel 1.5 mg po × 1)
     - Works best if <72 hours postcoital, but may be given up to 120 hours (less effective as time increases). Less side effects than Yuzpe method and is available without prescription
     - 75% effective if taken within 72 hours

Always advise that condoms should be used in addition to OCP, to decrease STI risk.

- Yuzpe (200 mg estradiol + 1 mg levonorgestrel). Generally no longer used due to side effects of nausea and vomiting.
  - Works best <72 hours postcoital but again may be given up to 120 hours
- Copper IUD
  - Can be used up to 5 days postcoital

8. **Approach to contraceptive selection**
   - Assess absolute and relative contraindications to contraceptive use
   - Assess for STI exposure
   - Assess barriers to selected method of oral contraception (personal, financial, or cultural)
   - Discuss/manage common side effects (breakthrough bleeding, breast tenderness, nausea, weight gain, acne, headache, and chloasma)
   - Obtain BP and BMI
   - Advise about risks of ↓ efficacy (medications, bariatric surgery, late initiation) and availability of emergency contraception

9. **Approach to missed OCP**
   - Ovulation rarely occurs after 7 days of combined oral contraceptive use
   - To prevent unintended pregnancy, the hormone-free period should not extend beyond 7 days in combined oral contraceptive users
   - If the hormone-free interval >7 days, consider emergency contraception to prevent unintended pregnancy + back up × 7 days
   - Miss one pill in <24 hours in week 2 or 3 take ASAP. No back up required.
   - Miss, more than two pills, use back up or quit and start a new cycle after breakthrough bleed

Important to review missed dose guidelines for all contraceptive forms, in order to counsel patients correctly.

Bibliography

Dean G, Goldberg AB. Overview of intrauterine contraception. *Up to Date*. 2012. http://www.uptodate.com/contents/overview-of-intrauterine-contraception?source=preview&anchor=H23833369#H23833369.

Jensen B, Regier LD, eds. *Rx Files: Drug Comparison Charts*. 8th ed.2010.

Rose SB, Lawton BA. Impact of long-acting reversible contraception on return for repeat abortion. *Am J Obstet Gynecol*. 2012;206(1):37.e1-37.e6.

Zieman M. Overview of contraception. *Up to Date*. 2012. http://www.uptodate.com/contents/overview-of-contraception?source=preview&anchor=H31#H31.

Pregnancy

Priority Topic 77

General Definitions

1. Trimesters:
   a. T1: 0 to 12 weeks
   b. T2: 12 to 28 weeks
   c. T3: 28 to 40 weeks
2. Normal pregnancy: 37 to 42 weeks
3. Active labour: regular contractions that result in cervical change and descent of the presenting part of the fetus.

Investigations

1. Confirm pregnancy with urine or serum pregnancy test
2. Establish desirability of pregnancy
3. Establish accurate dates and maternal risk factors (medical and social)
4. In high-risk patients, rescreen for HIV at 28 to 36 weeks
5. Complete appropriate prenatal screening and visits. See Prenatal Care Flowsheet (Table 10-2) for all prenatal visit information.

TABLE 10-2 Prenatal Care Flowsheet: Page 1

At least 2-3 months preconception *Ref: Joint SOGC-Motherisk Guideline Dec 2007.*		• Start **folic acid 0.4–1 mg od** in women without risk factors • **Folic acid 5 mg od** for hx of previous baby with defect (NTD, facial cleft, heart/urinary tract/limb defect), family hx NTD, DM, smoking, obesity, poor diet, substance abuse, epileptics on valproic acid or carbamazepine, or if forgets to take vitamins regularly
<12 weeks	Visits q monthly until 28 weeks	**Obstetrical ultrasound** for dating, if indicated
12 weeks		Start listening for fetal heart with handheld Doppler
8-14 weeks		• **Routine prenatal blood work**: *ABO blood group, Rh and Ab, CBC, HIV, rubella, syphilis, HepB sAg, U/A, Hep C Ab, NAAT for GC/Chlamydia* • ***Consider:*** *VZV Ab (if no history of varicella), A1c/FBG for high risk of DM* • Physical examination • **Pap** smear, if not done in past 6 months and >21 years old • Fill out prenatal forms, refer if needed
11-13 weeks + 6 days	**CVS** done at 11-13 weeks 6 days in Calgary, risk of loss 1%, allows for earlier diagnosis than amniocentesis	**1st trim. integrated serum screen*** (part 1 of 2) offered to all women (preferred option) for Trisomy 18, 21
		and if indicated, NT ultrasound (see reverse for indications for NT U/S)
16 weeks		Gestation at which **therapeutic abortion** is not available in all provinces
15-17 weeks		**Amniocentesis** routinely offered to all women >40 years and >35 years with multiple gestation (results take 10-14 days) loss risk 1:400
15-20 weeks + 6 days Best at 16-18 weeks		**2nd trim. serum screen*** (part 2 of 2) (85% detection) or **quad screen** done *without 1st trim. Serum screen in late presenters* (77% detection, false positive 5.2%) (for trisomy 19, 21, and ONTDs)
18-24 weeks		**Routine ultrasound** for dates/anomalies *Note: **Earliest** ultrasound establishes dates, **not** the most recent ultrasound.*
20 weeks		Start measuring **SFH** routinely
26-28 weeks	**BG targets:** Fasting 3.8-5.2 1 hour PP 5.5-7.7 2 hours PP 5.0-6.6	Screen for **gestational diabetes**: **50 g nonfasting GCT** **<7.8** = normal **75 g OGTT results:** **7.8-10.2** requires 75 g OGTT **≥5.3/10.6/8.9** at 0,1,2 h **≥10.3** = GDM 1 of 3 = IGT; 2 of 3 = GDM
28 weeks	Visits q 2 weeks 28-36 weeks	• Repeat **CBC** or Hg by fingerpoke • **Rh neg**: repeat type and screen for alloantibodies before administering **RhIg (WinRho) 300 mcg** IM • **Rh Pos**: repeat **type and screen** for alloantibodies; however, this is *not* necessary if there are two previous results on file
30-32 weeks		**Ultrasound** to rule out **IUGR** in women with initial weight >90 kg or BMI>30.0 (obese)
28-36 weeks		Repeat **HIV, GC/Chlamydia, syphilis** testing if at risk
35-37 weeks		**GBS swab** (results valid for 5 weeks), *send results to delivering hospital*
38+ weeks	Visits q 1 week until term	• Consider **cervical examination** at prenatal visit • May offer **sweeping of membranes** to prevent postterm gestation
41-42 weeks		**Induction** to prevent postterm gestation vs **expectant management** (requires fetal monitoring with NST and AFI twice weekly) *Ref: SOGC Guideline Sept 2008*
DELIVERY		• **Rh negative mother: WinRho 300 mcg** IM within 72 h of delivery if infant Rh+ • **Rubella** immunization to nonimmune women (Public Health) • **BCG** for baby, routinely offered to high-risk populations, mother must have negative HIV result

PRENATAL CARE FLOWSHEET: PAGE 2

Indications for nuchal translucency ultrasound*	Indications for first trimester ultrasound* *Ref: SOGC Guideline Oct 2003 (reaffirmed Dec 2008)*
Multiple gestation HIV positive Maternal age ≥ 40 at EDD Personal or family history of Down syndrome, trisomy 18, or trisomy 13 Age >35 years with ≥ 3 miscarriages	Threatened abortion, incomplete abortion Prior to termination Suspected multiple gestation, ectopic pregnancy, molar pregnancy, and suspected pelvic masses Increased risk for major fetal congenital malformations Very uncertain dates

Use of diagnostic imaging is not limited to these indications.

Gestational diabetes screening in pregnancy: *Ref: SOGC guideline Nov 2002, Can Diabetes Assoc. 2008*

Test	Standard screen is **1 h 50 g** nonfasting glucose challenge test at **24 to 28 weeks**
Early Testing	Start screening in first trimester if multiple risk factors present, **and repeat in subsequent trimesters**
Risk Factors	• Aboriginal, Hispanic, South Asian, Asian, African • Previous history of GDM or glucose intolerance • Previous macrosomia (>4000 g) • Previous unexplained stillbirth • Previous neonatal hypoglycemia, hypocalcemia, or hyperbilirubinemia • Advanced maternal age (≥ 35 years) • Obesity • Repeated glucosuria in pregnancy • Polyhydramnios • Suspected macrosomia • PCOS • Acanthosis nigricans • Corticosteroid use
Postpartum	If GDM is diagnosed in pregnancy, a **75 g OGTT** should be done at **6-12 weeks postpartum** to screen for persistent DM or impaired glucose tolerance.

Group B Streptococcus Screening: *Ref: Prevention of Perinatal Group B Streptococcal Disease, CDC guidelines, August 16, 2002:*

Vaginal and rectal GBS screening cultures at **35-37 weeks** in **all** pregnant women (unless patient had GBS bacteriuria during the current pregnancy or previous infant with GBS disease).

Intrapartum prophylaxis indicated:	Intrapartum prophylaxis not indicated:
• Previous infant with invasive GBS disease • GBS bacteriuria during current pregnancy • Positive GBS screening culture in current pregnancy • Unknown GBS status and (1) delivery at <37 weeks or (2) ROM >18 hours or (3) intrapartum temp >38°C *(if amnionitis suspected, use broad-spectrum antibiotic instead)*	• Previous pregnancy with positive GBS culture (unless culture also positive in current pregnancy) • Planned cesarean delivery in absence of ROM or labour • Negative GBS culture in current pregnancy, regardless of intrapartum risk factors

Recommended antibiotics for intrapartum prophylaxis:

Recommended:	**Penicillin G, 5 million units IV** initial dose, then **2.5 million units IV q 4 h** until delivery
Alternative:	**Ampicillin, 2 g IV** initial dose, then **1 g IV q 4 h** until delivery (broader spectrum, better for amnionitis, but potential for increased antibiotic-associated adverse effects)
If penicillin allergic:	**Not at high risk for anaphylaxis**: • **Cefazolin**, 3 g IV initial dose, then 1 g IV q 8 h until delivery. **High risk for anaphylaxis**: • **Clindamycin**, 900 mg IV q 8 h until delivery, or (must do susceptibility testing anenatally) • **Erythromycin**, 500 mg IV q 6 h until delivery (must do susceptibility antenatally) **GBS resistant to clindamycin or erythromycin or susceptibility unknown:** • **Vancomycin**, 1 g IV q 12 h until delivery

BV in Pregnancy *Ref: SOGC Guideline Aug 2008*	**UTI and asymptomatic bacteriuria in pregnancy**
Do not routinely screen for and treat BV in asymptomatic women **not** at increased risk for preterm birth. If at increased risk of preterm birth, treatment may reduce risk of low birth weight. **Risks of BV in pregnancy:** preterm birth, PPROM, spontaneous abortion, chorioamnionitis, postpartum endometritis, C-section wound infection. **Treatment:** (SOGC Aug 2008) • **Metronidazole 500 mg bid** × 7 days or • **Clindamycin 300 mg bid** × **7 days** (topical agents not recommended, since **not** associated with risk reduction)	Treat both **asymptomatic bacteriuria** (midstream culture positive >10⁵ cfu/mL) and **symptomatic UTI** (symptoms + midstream culture positive >10² cfu/mL) to reduce risks. Repeat culture 1-2 weeks after treatment. **Treatment options:** • **Nitrofurantoin (Macrobid)** 100 mg bid × 7days *(avoid at labour and delivery because of hemolytic anemia)* • **TMP-SMX** 1 DS tab bid × 3 days *(avoid in first trimester and near term)* • **TMP** 100 mg bid × 7 days *(avoid in first trimester)* • **Amoxicillin** 500 mg tid × 7 days *or* **Ampicillin** 250 mg tid × 7 days • **Amoxicillin-clavulanate** 500 mg bid × 7 days • **Cephalexin** 250 mg qid × 7 days **Effective for GBS in urine:** amoxicillin, ampicillin, nitrofurantoin, TMP, TMP/SMX

Courtesy of Lisa Friesen.

COMMON MEDICAL CONDITIONS IN PREGNANCY

Hypertensive Disorders in Pregnancy

Definitions

1. Gestational hypertension (GHTN): DBP >90 occurring after 20 weeks gestation
2. HELLP syndrome: gestational hypertension may progress to HELLP syndrome. The syndrome includes hemolysis, elevated liver enzymes, and low platelets in the setting of gestational hypertension.

HELLP Syndrome
Hemolysis
Elevated Liver Enzymes
Low Platelets

Symptoms

1. RUQ pain
2. Headache
3. ↓ urine output
4. Nausea +/− vomiting
5. Visual disturbance
6. Hyperreflexia

Risk Factors

1. Primigravid
2. Medical history or family history of GHTN
3. First child with new partner
4. DM
5. Extremes of age (<18 or >35)
6. IUGR
7. Oligohydramnios
8. Twin gestation

Investigations

- Hb, platelets, coags, ALT, AST, LDH, U/A (proteinuria)

Treatment

1. If stable: treat with labetalol or methyldopa until term. Monitor growth and placental flow by Doppler U/S
2. Pregnancy less <34 weeks GA or unstable mother should be managed by obstetrician
3. Hb and platelets
4. Start IV
5. Assess status of fetus
6. Laboratory work including blood type, crossmatch
7. Control blood pressure and treat if >160/105 mm Hg
   a. Labetalol 20 mg IV, then 40 mg IV, then 80 mg IV × 2 at 10 minute intervals to achieve target BP (max dose 220 mg/day)
   b. Hydralazine 5 mg IV, repeat 5 to 10 mg IV q 20 minutes to max dose of 20 mg/day or BP controlled
   c. Nifedipine 10 mg po and repeat with 20 mg in 30 minutes
8. Urgent delivery and ICU postpartum may be needed

Gestational Diabetes

Definition

Onset of DM 2 during pregnancy

Complications

1. Maternal
   a. HTN
   b. Polyhydramnios
   c. Retinopathy
   d. Hypoglycemia
   e. Pyelonephritis/UTI

2. Fetal
   a. Macrosomia
   b. IUGR
   c. Hypoglycemia
   d. Polycythemia
   e. Fetal lung immaturity

Risk Factors

1. Obesity
2. Previous pregnancy with gestational DM 2 or IGT
3. Family history of DM

Diagnosis

1. If risk factors for diabetes II, conduct fasting glucose at initial prenatal visit
2. If low risk for DM II, screen for GDM at 24 to 28 weeks GA with 50 g OGTT
3. Screening at 24 to 28 weeks GA
   a. 1 hour 50 g OGCT
      i. <7.8 mmol/L is normal
      ii. 7.8 to 10.2 mmol/L → indication for a 2 hour 75 g OGTT
      iii. ≥ 10.3 = GDM
   b. 2 hour 75 g OGTT
      i. FPG ≥5.3 mmol/L
      ii. At 1 hour ≥10.6 mmol/L
      iii. At 2 hour ≥8.9 mmol/L
   c. Impaired glucose tolerance
      i. Fasting: 6.1 to 6.9 mmol/L
      ii. 75 g OGTT: 7.5 to 11.0 mmol/L

Treatment

1. Blood glucose targets for GDM (see Table 10-3)
2. Induce by 40 weeks gestation
3. Blood sugars hourly during labour
4. Follow up 75 g OGTT 6 weeks to 6 months postpartum as gestational DM mothers have 50% increased risk of developing DM 2
5. Dietary advice
6. Pharmacotherapy, insulin, metformin, and/or glyburide

TABLE 10-3	Glucose Targets	
	DM	GDM
A1C	≤7	≤6
FPG (mmol/L)	4 to 7	3.8 to 5.2
2 h PPG (mmol/L)	5 to 10	5.0 to 6.6

COMMON PROBLEMS ENCOUNTERED DURING LABOUR

Dystocia
Definitions
1. Labour dystocia is prolongation of labour. Consider three Ps (Power, Passage, Passenger). Clinical definitions:
   a. >4 hours of <0.5 cm/hour dilation or
   b. >1 hour of no descent with active pushing
2. Shoulder dystocia: impaction of the anterior shoulder of fetus against symphysis after fetal head has been delivered. **This is a life-threatening emergency.**

Risk Factors for Shoulder Dystocia
1. Obesity
2. DM
3. Macrosomia
4. Instrument delivery (currently or previously)
5. Most women with shoulder dystocia have no identifiable risk factors. Be prepared.

Uterine Rupture
Definition
Potentially catastrophic complication of pregnancy whereby the uterus tears during labour

Symptoms
1. Shock
2. Acute onset of abdominal pain
3. Acute change in station
4. Abnormal FHR
5. Vaginal bleeding

Risk Factors
1. Uterine scar
2. Hyperstimulation (usually from pharmacological agents for IOL)
3. Grand multiparity

Diagnosis
1. Stable patients can usually be evaluated with ultrasound to confirm diagnosis
2. Unstable patients usually warrant emergent delivery

Treatment
1. Rule out placenta abruption
2. Maternal stabilization
3. Emergent delivery

Placental Abruption
Definition
Potentially catastrophic complication of pregnancy where the placenta prematurely separates from the uterine wall

Symptoms
1. Painful vaginal bleeding
2. ↑ uterine tonicity/contractions
3. +/− fetal distress

ALARMER
Ask for help
Legs flexed (McRoberts)
Apply suprapubic pressure
Release posterior shoulder
Manual Corkscrew
Episiotomy
Rollover (hands and knees)

Use mnemonic ALARMER for shoulder dystocia.

Risk factors

1. Abdominal trauma
2. Cocaine abuse
3. Polyhydramnios
4. Hypertension (essential, pregnancy induced, preeclampsia)
5. Premature rupture of membranes (PROM)
6. Chorioamnionitis
7. Thrombophilia
8. Previous abruption
9. Maternal age
10. Smoking during pregnancy
11. Parity

Diagnosis

Clinical diagnosis as ultrasound not sensitive

Investigations/Management

1. Establish IV access
2. WBC, Hb, platelets, blood type and Rh status, C&M, coagulation studies, Kleihauer-Betke test
3. Abdominal U/S
4. Foley catheter to monitor urine output
5. Continuous EFM

Treatment

1. Delivery indicated (if GA >34 weeks) or watchful waiting if maternal and fetal stability confirmed
2. Cesarean section indicated if non-reassuring fetal heart rate (FHR) or ongoing maternal blood loss
3. If stable, vaginal delivery is a reasonable option, induce and augment

Chorioamnionitis

Definition

Infection of the chorion or amniotic fluid from ascending organism

Symptoms

1. Maternal fever
2. Maternal/fetal ↑ HR
3. Foul/purulent discharge
4. Uterine tenderness

Risk Factors

1. Prolonged rupture of membranes
2. Prolonged labour
3. Multiple vaginal examinations
4. Bacterial vaginosis, STI, GBS
5. Intrauterine or fetal monitoring devices

Diagnosis

Clinical

Treatment

1. IV ampicillin 2 g q 6 hours and gentamycin 1.5 mg/kg q 8 hours in patients with normal renal function
2. Expedient delivery
3. Higher risk of PPH

Rupture of Membranes

Definitions

1. Premature rupture of membranes (PROM): rupture of membranes before the onset of labour
2. Preterm PROM (PPROM) ≤37 weeks GA (may require steroids if <34 weeks GA)
3. Prolonged rupture of membranes: rupture of membranes >18 hours

Symptoms

1. Gush clear or yellow fluid from the vagina
2. Intermittent constant leakage of fluid from the vagina
3. Overdiagnosed based on history of per vaginum (PV) fluid

Diagnosis/PE Findings

1. Sterile speculum and fluid pooling in vaginal vault
2. Positive Nitrazine
3. Ferning on microscopic examination
4. U/S for AFI and BPP

Differential Diagnosis

1. Urinary incontinence
2. Vaginal discharge
3. Perspiration

Management/Treatment

1. If <34 weeks gestation, betamethasone 12 mg IM q 24 hours × 2
2. Consider expert consultation (OBS, NICU)
3. Admit with vitals q 4 hours daily BPP and WBC count
4. Cultures for STI and GBS
5. Consider antibiotics
6. Emergent delivery if fetal distress

Endometritis

Definition

Endometrial infection (may be intrapartum, postpartum, or following TOP).

Symptoms

1. Rising fever
2. Uterine tenderness postpartum day 2 to 3

Risk Factors

1. Prolonged labour, prolonged ROM (>18 hours), amnionitis
2. Meconium-stained amniotic fluid
3. Maternal age <17
4. Manual placental removal
5. Bacterial vaginosis during pregnancy

Diagnosis

Rule out other causes of post-operative fever

Treatment

1. Provide anaerobic coverage (clindamycin 900 mg IV q 8 hours + gentamicin 5 mg/kg q 24 hours)
2. Give cefazolin prophylactically after C/S

Postpartum Hemorrhage

Definition

Loss of >500 mL of blood after SVD or 1000 mL after C/S. Early PPH occurs within 24 hours of delivery, and late PPH occurs after 24 hours and within 6 weeks of delivery.

Etiology (four Ts)

1. **Tone**: uterine atony secondary to prolonged/augmented labour, infection, GHTN, grand multiparity, macrosomia, and polyhydramnios
2. **Tissue**: retained placenta
3. **Trauma**: vaginal, cervix, or uterus
4. **Thrombin**: coagulopathy

Risk Factors

1. May occur in women without any risk factors
2. History of postpartum hemorrhage
3. Preeclampsia
4. Placenta previa
5. Multiple gestation
6. Obesity
7. Macrosomia
8. Induced labour and other intrapartum interventions
9. Chorioamnionitis
10. Prolonged labour

Diagnosis

1. Based on blood volume lost
2. Decline in postpartum hematocrit >10%

Prevention

1. Active management in the third stage of labour (oxytocin with delivery of the anterior shoulder, controlled cord traction to deliver placenta, and uterine massage)

Treatment

1. Stepwise approach is required
2. Labs: cross match, CBC, Coags
3. Uterine massage
4. Pharmacotherapy (uterotonics)
   a. Oxytocin 10 units IM or add 40 units to 1 L NS and run IV until bleeding controlled
   b. Carboprost 0.25 mg IM q 15 to 90 minutes (maximum eight doses)
   c. Misoprostol 800 to 1000 mcg sublingual or rectally
   d. Methylergonovine 0.2 mg IM or intrauterine. May repeat at 2 to 4 hour intervals (avoid if hypertensive, Raynaud syndrome, or scleroderma)
5. If bleeding not controlled following use of uterotonics, consider the following:
   a. Foley catheter (full bladder may prevent uterine contraction)
   b. R/O genital tract lesion/trauma
   c. Examine placenta for missing parts
   d. If under shock consider hematoma, uterine rupture, partial inversion
   e. Uterine tamponade
6. Obtain expert consult for manual removal of retained placenta or exploratory laparotomy or hysterectomy

4T'S OF POSTPARTUM HEMORRHAGE

Tone
Tissue
Trauma
thrombin

Blood loss estimates for PPH are notoriously incorrect

Retained Placenta

Definition

Placenta not delivered within 30 minutes of delivery

Types

1. Trapped placenta—placenta caught behind a closed cervix
2. Placenta adherens—easily removed manually from the uterine wall
3. Placenta accreta—placenta pathologically invading into the myometrium

Symptoms

1. No lengthening of the umbilical cord
2. No gush of blood from the vagina (no separation)
3. Failure of the fundus to contract

Risk Factors

1. Prior manual removal
2. Infection
3. Placenta previa
4. Uterine scar

Diagnosis

1. Usually a clinical diagnosis
2. Ultrasound may be used to differentiate between placenta adherens and accrete but is rarely used

Treatment

1. Treat for postpartum hemorrhage as patient may bleed
2. +/− manual removal or D&C

COMMON PROBLEMS POSTPARTUM

Postpartum Blues and Postpartum Depression

Definitions

1. Postpartum blues: onset day 3 to 10 postpartum characterized by increased anxiety, irritability, weariness, ↓ concentration, and sleep disturbance. Self-limited and does not last >2 weeks. Normal hormonal changes.
2. Postpartum depression (PPD): Major depressive episode within 1 month of childbirth. Suspect if blues last >2 weeks or severe in first 2 weeks. Psychosis can occur within in the first month postpartum.

Symptoms

1. Tearfulness
2. Fatigue
3. Irritability
4. Mood liability
5. ↓ affect
6. Sensitive to criticism
7. Occasional homicidal/infanticidal ideation

Risk Factors

1. History of depression
2. Family history of depression
3. Inadequate social support
4. Psychosocial stress
5. Pregnancy loss

Treatment

1. SSRI
2. Psychotherapy
3. Supportive care
4. ECT

FETAL HEART RATE MONITORING

Definitions

1. Normal FHR baseline: 110 to 160 bpm. High baseline (maternal/fetal/placental etiologies): fever, hyperthyroid, anemia, hypoxia.
2. Variability (normal 5-25 bpm). If ↓ or absent for >40 minutes, fetal wellbeing must be assessed. There is ↓ variability with maternal dehydration or infection.
3. Accels: increase of ≥15 bpm lasting ≥15 seconds in response to fetal movement of uterine contractions.
4. Decels:
   a. Early: uniform in shape with onset early in contraction and returns to baseline by the end of the contraction. Due to vagal response to head compression.
   b. Variables: most common. Variable in shape, onset, and duration. Secondary to cord compression or forceful pushing. Non-reassuring = rule of 60s: decels <60 bpm, >60 bpm below baseline, >60 seconds in duration with slow return to baseline.
   c. Late: uniform in shape with late onset in contraction, return to baseline after end of contraction. Must see three in a row to define as late decels. Abrupt decrease in FHR secondary to fetal hypoxia, academia, maternal hypotension, uterine hypertonus, or uteroplacental insufficiency.
5. Reassuring FHR: at least two accelerations of FHR >15 bpm from baseline lasting >15 seconds in a 20-minute strip.

Early decels are benign.

Management

1. Decelerations:
   a. Call for help
   b. Roll to LLDP
   c. 100% O_2 to mother via non-rebreather mask
   d. Stop oxytocin
   e. Fetal scalp electrode
   f. Vaginal examination to r/o prolapse
   g. C/S if needed

Bibliography

Anath CV, Kinzler WL. Clinical features and diagnosis of placental abruption. *Up to Date*. http://www.uptodate.com/contents/clinical-features-and-diagnosis-of-placental-abruption?source=preview&anchor=H4#H8. Accessed March 16, 2012.

Dynamed. Metritis (postpartum). 2011. http://web.ebscohost.com/dynamed/detail?sid=1f5fe243-c64d-4d09-9738-7f312e001a51%40sessionmgr12&vid=4&hid=21&bdata=JnNpdGU9ZHluYW1lZC1saXZlJnNjb3BlPXNpdGU%3d#db=dme&AN=113859. Accessed March 17, 2012.

Dynamed. Postpartum hemorrhage. 2011. http://web.ebscohost.com/dynamed/detail?vid=6&hid=21&sid=1f5fe243-c64d-4d09-9738-7f312e001a51%40sessionmgr12&bdata=JnNpdGU9ZHluYW1lZC1saXZlJnNjb3BlPXNpdGU%3d#db=dme&AN=114247. Accessed March 17, 2012.

Weeks A. Diagnosis and management of retained placenta after vaginal birth. *Up to Date*. 2011. http://www.uptodate.com/contents/diagnosis-and-management-of-retained-placenta-after-vaginal-birth?source=search_result&search=retained+placenta&selectedTitle=1~24. Accessed March 15, 2012.

Vaginal Bleeding
Priority Topic 96

Always rule out pregnancy first

Factors to consider with vaginal bleeding:

- Pregnancy status
- Age
- Timing (cycle, acute vs chronic)
- Systemic disease
- Medications (hormones)

If pregnant and bleeding always consider: ectopic pregnancy, placental abruption, abortion, trophoblastic disease, and treat hemodynamic instability.

Definitions

1. Normal menses: average menses lasts 7 days, approximately 35 mL of blood loss, wide range of normal
2. Menorrhagia—excessive bleeding during menses
3. Metrorrhagia—uterine bleeding at irregular intervals
4. Oligomenorrhea—menses occurring at intervals >35 days

Never conduct a pelvic examination on a woman with PV bleeding in the second or third trimester without r/o vasa or placenta previa.

NONPREGNANT VAGINAL BLEEDING

TABLE 10-4	Causes and Treatment of Vaginal Bleeding		
	ETIOLOGIES	SYMPTOMS	TREATMENT/MGMT
Ovulatory	Anatomic: • Cervix (polyp, inflammation, PID, IUD) • Uterus (fibroid, cancer)	Menorrhagia	Treat specific etiology
	Concurrent disease: coagulopathy, thyroid, renal, hepatic	Menorrhagia and/or metrorrhagia	Treat specific etiology
	Foreign body	Foul odour	Removal of foreign body
	Medications: anticoagulation, antipsychotic, corticosteroids, SSRI, tamoxifen, ginseng, ginkgo, soy	Metrorrhagia	Correct coagulopathy, change contraceptive delivery, discontinue offending medication/ product.
Anovulatory	OCP: inadequate estrogen or poor adherence (compliance)	Metrorrhagia	Trial of OCP with higher estrogen
	Hypothalamic: PCOS, ↓ thyroid, excess androgen, ↑ cortisol or prolactin, stress, WT loss, puberty, perimenopause	Menorrhagia, oligomenorrhea, or amenorrhea Spotting	Treat specific etiology
Postmenopause (age >40)	Vaginal: atrophic Cervix: polyps, erosion, cancer Uterus : polyp, fibroid, endometrial cancer	Spotting or menorrhagia (postmenopausal)	Considered to be endometrial cancer until proven otherwise. Evaluate endometrium before treatment.

Management

1. Stabilize ABC
2. r/o pregnancy
3. Laboratory investigations: β-hCG, CBC (Hg, WBC, platelets), INR, PTT, TSH, prolactin, glucose, PAP smear, G+C urine PCR, (signs of androgen excess? → DHEA, free testosterone)
4. Endometrial assessment—biopsy or D+C
   a. All women >35 with changing menstrual bleeding pattern or postmenopausal bleed
   b. Women <35 with 2 to 3 year of untreated anovulatory bleed especially if obese
5. Imaging:
   a. Transvaginal ultrasound (detect pregnancy with quantitative β-hCG of 1500 mIU/mL and in experienced hands detect placenta previa)
   b. Hysteroscopy—if unresponsive to treatment
   c. CT pelvis

Treatment

1. Treat hemodynamic instability
2. Acute heavy bleeding with hypovolemia or Hg <70 units
   a. High dose of oral estrogen (OCP tid × 7 days) or IV estrogen
   b. Tranexamic acid 1300 mg po tid for 5 days during menstruation
   c. Ferrous gluconate 325 mg tid duration (re-evaluate in 6 weeks)
   d. If bleeding continues—IV DDAVP +/− D&C, hysteroscopy
   e. Consider transfusion if severe hemorrhage or medical comorbidities
3. Chronic frequent or heavy bleeding
   a. Treat underlying cause
   b. NSAIDs—promote platelet aggregation
   c. Severe/refractory—consider ablation/hysterectomy
   d. Postmenopausal
      i. Hyperplasia and not cancer/atypia—IM medroxyprogesterone and repeat endometrial evaluation q 3 to 6 months for hyperplasia
      ii. Atypical hyperplasia—D&C or hysterectomy
      iii. Atrophic—consider OCP or HRT

ENDOMETRIAL CANCER

Etiology
Estrogen (↑ unopposed estrogen → hyperplasia → cancer)

Types
Adenocarcinoma ≥ 80% of endometrial cancers

Risk Factors

1. Obesity
2. DM
3. HTN
4. HRT with unopposed estrogen
5. Tamoxifen >5 years
6. Nulliparous
7. Early menarche/late menopause

8. Pelvic radiation
9. Family history of breast or ovarian cancer
10. Family history of HNPCC

Symptoms

1. Abnormal uterine bleeding
2. Vaginal discharge
3. Rarely, bladder symptoms due to pressure, back pain radiating anteriorly, increased abdominal girth, dyspareunia

Diagnosis

1. Invasive approaches:
   • D&C
   • Endometrial biopsy
   • Hysteroscopy and directed biopsy
2. Noninvasive approach includes ultrasonography (Brand et al., 2000)

Treatment

Based on biopsy results:

1. Unsatisfactory or unable to obtain biopsy—high risk for cancer → D&C if low risk → transvaginal ultrasound
2. Negative biopsy but ongoing symptoms → repeat biopsy or transvaginal US
3. Hyperplasia with no atypia
   a. IM medroxyprogesterone
   b. Repeat biopsy in 3 months (if follow-up biopsy unchanged, hysterectomy or IM medroxyprogesterone q 6-12 months)
3. Atypical hyperplasia—hysterectomy (D&C or ablation are also options but they are not recommended if unwell or comorbidities)
4. Atrophic—consider OCP or HRT
5. Cancer—hysterectomy + node sampling + peritoneal sampling
   a. Radiation if stage 1B (chemotherapy for palliative cases only as endometrial cancer not very responsive)

Guideline Summary (SOGC - Brand et al., 2000)

1. In woman with abnormal vaginal bleeding where endometrial cancer is expected, the diagnostic method of choice is office endometrial biopsy.
2. Patients who are not candidates for endometrial biopsy should be evaluated based on risk. Low-risk patients should proceed to transvaginal ultrasound. Those at high risk (obese, history of tamoxifen, DM 2, postmenopausal, nulliparous) should proceed directly to D&C.
3. There is no cut off for endometrial thickness in the diagnosis of endometrial cancer in postmenopausal women; however 4 mm to 8 mm has been found in the literature. Clinicians should bear in mind that the lower the thickness used the higher the sensitivity but lower the specificity.
4. Ongoing bleeding despite previous negative investigations warrants additional investigation.
5. Patients who continue to have vaginal bleeding after 6 months of combined HRT should undergo endometrial biopsy.

VAGINAL BLEEDING IN PREGNANCY

Always consider ectopic pregnancy, abruption, and abortion (see Table 10-5).

TABLE 10-5	Vaginal Bleeding in Pregnancy		
	ETIOLOGIES	**SYMPTOMS**	***MGMT/TREATMENT**
First trimester	Ectopic pregnancy	Abdominal/pelvic pain Vaginal bleeding Missed period	See separate topic below
	Spontaneous abortion	Vaginal bleeding Complete passage of products of conception Open cervix	No D&C Expectant management
	Threatened abortion	Vaginal bleeding +/– cramping Cervix closed	US viable fetus <5% abort Watch and wait
	Inevitable abortion	Vaginal bleeding Cramping +/– ROM Cervix closed until products expelled	Watch and wait Misoprostol 400-800 mg PO/PV D&C
	Molar pregnancy	Vaginal bleeding Enlarged uterus Hyperthyroidism	Abnormally elevated β-hCG U/S suggestive of molar pregnancy Expert consult: • evacuation of molar pregnancy • serial β-hCG until 3 weekly normal values
Second or third trimester	Placenta abruption	See topic under pregnancy	
	Vasa previa	Vaginal bleeding Sonographic or clinical evidence of vasa previa	Emergent C/S
	Placental previa	Painless vaginal bleeding	ABCs r/o abruption Determine placental location with transvaginal US Expert consult <34 weeks GA: consider hospitalization, steroids, and decide on delivery method at 36 weeks GA Low lying (>2 cm from cervical os) may be candidates for vaginal delivery
	Bloody show	Term or near-term gestation Vaginal bleeding +/– contractions +/– cervical changes	Prepare for delivery
	Cervical: neoplasia, infection, polyps	See specific topics	

*If Rh negative, give Rh (D) immune globulin 300 mcg IV/IM.

ECTOPIC PREGNANCY

Fertilized ovum implanted outside the endometrium

Symptoms
1. Pelvic pain
2. PV bleeding
3. Amenorrhea

Risk Factors
1. Previous ectopic pregnancy
2. IUD
3. Damaged fallopian tubes (STI history, PID, tubal surgery)
4. DES exposure in utero

PE Findings
1. One-third women have no physical signs (Dynamed, 2012)
2. Pelvic examination may reveal adnexal mass

Diagnosis

Positive β-hCG with abnormal doubling time

Imaging

Visualization of ectopic pregnancy on ultrasound or surgery (intrauterine pregnancy visible on abdominal U/S when β-hCG >2000)

Treatment

1. If hemodynamically unstable, stabilize and prepare for surgery
2. Methotrexate therapy is an option for stable patients if fetal pole <3 cm on U/S. Follow with serial β-hCG
   - Methotrexate 50 mg/m^2 IM ×1; measure serum β-hCG levels on days 4 and 7; if needed repeat dose on day 7 (Barnhart, 2009)
3. Surgery
4. Rh D immunoglobulin if indicated

Guideline Summary (Ectopic Pregnancy)

1. There is no difference between methotrexate therapy and tube sparing laparoscopic surgery in overall tube preservation, recurrence of ectopic pregnancy, or future pregnancy
2. An increase in serum β-hCG of <53% in 48 hours confirms abnormal pregnancy
3. In patients with β-hCG >5000 mIU/mL, multiple or higher doses of methotrexate may be appropriate
4. Methotrexate can be used in women with confirmed or highly suspected to have ectopic pregnancy, who are stable with an unruptured mass
5. If β-hCG does not fall by at ≥15% from day 4 to day 7 of methotrexate therapy, this is considered a treatment failure and repeat methotrexate therapy or surgery is warranted
6. Posttreatment β-hCG levels should be monitored until a nonpregnancy level is reached
7. In Initial β-hCG levels <200 mIU/mL, 88% resolve spontaneously (ACOG, 2008)

Bibliography

American College of Obstetricians and Gynecologists (ACOG). *Medical Management of Ectopic Pregnancy*. Washington (DC): American College of Obstetricians and Gynecologists (ACOG); 2008 Jun. 7:ACOG practice bulletin; no. 94

Barnhart KT. Clinical practice. Ectopic pregnancy. *NEJM*. 2009 Jul 23;361(4):379-387. Review. PubMed PMID: 19625718.

Brand A, Dubuc-Lissoir J, Ehlen Y, Plante M. *Diagnosis of Endometrial Cancer in Women with Abnormal Vaginal Bleeding*. SOGC Clinical Practice Guidelines. 2000. http://www.sogc.org/guidelines/public/86E-PS-February2000.pdf.

Dynamed. Ectopic pregnancy. 2012. http://web.ebscohost.com/dynamed/detail?vid=3&hid=127&sid=b865201a-68c5-480e-a862-f82f04138595%40sessionmgr111&bdata=JnNpdGU9ZHluYW1lZC1saXZlJnNjb3BlPXNpdGU%3d#db=dme&AN=115772&anchor=other-medications.

Vaginitis

Priority Topic 97

Definition

Nonspecific symptom complex of inflammation of the vagina often associated with pruritus, discharge, and or pain

Symptoms

Include the following irrespective of etiology:

- Burning
- Pruritus

- Erythema
- Increase in quantity, colour, odour of vaginal discharge
- Dyspareunia
- Irritation
- Foul odour
- Dysuria (when urine comes in contact with inflamed areas)

Types

Usual causes are inflammation or infection; however, symptoms are similar despite etiology.

1. Vulvar lesions
2. Vaginal atrophy
3. Infectious (increased vaginal discharge)
4. Inflammation (bubble baths, chemical irritants, allergies)

Develop an age-based approach to vaginitis

VAGINAL DISCHARGE

Testing for the causes of vaginitis (see Table 10-6) is important as they account for over 90% of all causes of vaginitis in premenopausal women

TABLE 10-6   Vaginal Discharge

	CANDIDIASIS	BACTERIAL VAGINOSIS	TRICHOMONIASIS	PHYSIOLOGIC
Organism	*Candida albicans* (90%)	*Gardnerella vaginalis*	*Trichomonas vaginalis*	Lactobacillus
Vaginal discharge	Whitish, "Cottage Cheese," minimal	Thin, grey, "dish water"	Yellow-green, malodorous	White or transparent, thick or thin, mostly odourless
Signs/ symptoms	1/5 asymptomatic Pruritus Inflamed/swollen vulva Vulvar burning, dysuria, dyspareunia	Up to ¾ asymptomatic Fishy odour Absence of vulva/vaginal irritation	¼ asymptomatic Petechia on vagina/cervix Occasional irritated/tender vulva Dysuria, frequency	None or mild/transient Normal quantity of discharge 1 = 4 mL/24 h
Vaginal pH	4.0-4.5	>4.5	5.0-6.0	4.0-4.5 (premenopause) ≥ 4.7 (premenarche and post-menopausal)
Saline wet mount	Hyphae Budding yeast (non albicans)	> 20% clue cells + Whiff test	Motile, flagellated, trichomonads	PMN rare, squamous cells
Treatment	• Clotrimazole, butoconazole, miconazole, terconazole, nystatin of various durations • Fluconazole 150 mg orally × 1 • Usually topical treatment in pregnancy • Consider topical boric acid suppression for recurrent infections • Treat only if symptomatic. No adverse outcome for untreated woman in pregnancy (Cotch et al., 1998)	• Evidence conflicting but treat if high risk for pregnancy loss • **Oral** : Metronidazole 500 mg po bid × 7 days • **Vaginally**: Metronidazole gel 0.75% 5 g PV daily × 5 days Clindamycin 2% 5 g PV qhs × 7 days	• Always treat • Metronidazole 2 g po single dose or 500 mg po bid × 7 days • Pregnant: metronidazole 2 g po single dose • Co-treat partners	• Rule out pathologic causes • If investigations normal, advise patient that discharge is normal to reduce anxiety and discourage multiple consults • Advise patient that changes in sexual activity, diet, hormone levels, and medications can affect quantity of discharge

Baxter and McSheffrey, 2010, p25; Sobel, 2012.

VAGINAL ATROPHY

Vestibule thin, dry, pale, or mildly erythematous on physical examination

- Occurs with menopause, anorexia, or prolonged breast feeding
- For dyspareunia and vaginal dryness, a trial of nonhormonal vaginal lubricants and moisturizers is recommended (Replens or KY jelly)
- If nonhormonal treatment fails in those treated for vaginal atrophy (with menopause), low-dose vaginal estrogen therapy is recommend:
  - Premarin 0.625 mg conjugated estrogen/g of cream, 0.5 g of cream intravaginally twice weekly
  - Vagifem 10 mcg estradiol/tablet, one tablet intravaginally daily for 2 weeks followed by twice weekly
  - Estring 7.5 mcg of estradiol released daily over 90 days
  - Estrace 100 mcg estradiol/g of cream, 2 to 4 g daily for 1 to 2 weeks, then gradually half dose over similar timeframe. Maintenance dose of 1 g intravaginally 1 to 3 times/week.
  - In women with intact uteruses, using vaginal estrogen replacement therapy, the decision as to whether to provide progesterone protection of the endometrium should be based on vaginal estrogen doses (and therefore systemic absorption of estrogen). Protection is not required in ladies who have had a hysterectomy.
  - Use caution in patients with breast cancer
- Progressive mechanical vaginal dilatation (vaginal dilators) can also be used for treatment

VULVOVAGINITIS

Rule out vaginal lesions

- Lichen sclerosis—bluish-white papula → white plaque. Thin parchment-like skin (subepithelial fat is diminished → thin atrophic labia). Usually occurs in postmenopausal women. Diagnosis is confirmed by biopsy and treatment is with potent topical steroids (0.05% clobetasol ointment daily at night for 6-12 weeks then 1-3 times/week for maintenance).
- Vulvar cancer—average age is >65 years. Three types: squamous cell (associated with HPV), Paget disease (red lesion, postmenopausal white women, associated with cancer of the GI, GU, and breast), and melanoma. Diagnosis is confirmed by biopsy and treatment is vulvectomy with node excision.

KEY POINTS–VAGINAL DISCHARGE

1. In patients with no alarm features on history, physical examination, and negative test, make the diagnosis of physiologic discharge and communicate this to the patient to avoid recurrent presentation and unnecessary treatment and investigation in the future.

2. In children with vaginal discharge, rule out sexually transmitted diseases and foreign bodies. If candida infection is diagnosed, look for underlying illness such as diabetes or other immunocompromised state.

3. In nonpregnant, asymptomatic patients, electing not to treat BV/candida is appropriate.

Bibliography

Bachmann G, Santen RJ. Treatment of vaginal atrophy. *Up to Date.* 2011. http://www.uptodate.com /contents/treatment-of-vaginal-atrophy?source=search_result&search=vaginal+atrophy&selected Title=1~62#H16.

Chen YA, Tran C *Toronto Notes—Comprehensive medical Reference & Review for MCCQE I and USMLE II.* Toronto, Canada: Toronto Notes for Medical Students Inc; 2008.

Cotch MF, Hillier SL, Gibbs RS, Eschenbach DA. Epidemiology and outcomes associated with moderate to heavy Candida colonization during pregnancy. Vaginal Infections and Prematurity Study Group. *Am J Obstet Gynecol.* 1998 Feb;178(2):374-380. PubMed PMID: 9500502.

Martin KA, Barbieria RL. Preparations of postmenopausal therapy. *Up to Date.* 2011. http://www .uptodate.com/contents/preparations-for-postmenopausal-hormone-therapy?source=preview& anchor=H5#H18.

Priestley CJ, Jones BM , Dhar J, Goodwin L. What is normal vaginal flora? *Genitourinary Medicine.* 1997. http://www.ncbi.nlm.nih.gov/pmc/articles/PMC1195755/pdf/genitmed00001-0030.pdf.

Sobel JD. Evaluation of Women with Symptoms of Vaginitis. *Up to Date.* 2012. http://www.uptodate.com /contents/evaluation-of-women-with-symptoms-of-vaginitis?source=search_result&search=vaginitis &selectedTitle=1~150.

Menopause

Priority Topic 64

Definition

One year after the last menstrual period

Types

1. Physiologic: average age 52 (Canada)
2. Premature ovarian failure: occurs before 40 years of age
3. Iatrogenic (surgical/radiation/chemotherapy)

Symptoms

1. Vasomotor instability: hot flashes, night sweats, nausea, sleep disturbance
2. Urogenital atrophy: vaginal, urethral, bladder; leading to dyspareunia, itch, vaginal dryness, bleeding, urinary frequency, urgency, incontinence
3. Skeletal: osteoporosis, joint and muscle pain
4. Skin and soft tissue: ↓ breast size, skin thinning
5. Psychological: mood disturbance, ↓ libido, fatigue, irritability, memory loss

Diagnosis

- This is a clinical diagnosis that does not require laboratory testing
- Alternative diagnosis should be considered if atypical symptoms occur

Treatment

1. Vasomotor symptoms: hormone therapy (HRT), SSRI, venlafaxine (Effexor), gabapentin, propranolol
2. Vaginal atrophy: oral or vaginal estrogens or vaginal moisturizers
3. Assess, prevent, and treat osteoporosis: calcium and vitamin D, smoking cessation, exercise, SERM, bisphosphonate
4. ↓ Libido: vaginal lubrication, counseling, testosterone (cream or oral/systemic)
5. Specifically inquire regarding use of alternative therapies: black cohosh (hot flushes), soy (hot flushes), St. John's Wort (mood), gingko biloba (memory loss), valerian (sleep), evening primrose oil, ginseng, dong quai

No evidence for alternative therapies in treatment of menopausal symptoms and some drug interactions exist, especially with St. John's Wort

6. HRT contraindications (remember ABCD):
   a. **A**ctive liver disease
   b. **B**leeding (undiagnosed vaginal bleed)
   c. **C**ancer (hormone sensitive)
   d. **D**VT

HRT Contraindications (Remember ABCD)

A – Active liver disease

B – Bleeding (undiagnosed vaginal bleed)

C – Cancer (hormone sensitive)

D – DVT

7. HRT considerations:
   a. Establish the risks and benefits of HRT
   b. No risk of breast cancer if used <5 years, after 5 years ↑ by 2% year. Within 5 years of stopping risk returns to baseline
   c. Benefits of HRT: ↓ colon cancer, ↓ osteoporosis
   d. Risks of HRT: ↑ coronary disease, stroke, DVT, breast cancer
   e. Only indications for HRT are vasomotor or vaginal symptoms
   f. Women with uteruses must treat all systemic HRT with progestagens (estrogen creams may also require progesterone therapy)
   g. Vaginal moisturizers are good alternatives (use three times/week) for HRT-contraindicated women

Guideline Summary

1. The primary indication for HRT should be for the management of moderate to severe menopausal symptoms
2. HRT should not be prescribed for the prevention of dementia or primary or secondary prevention of cardiovascular disease
3. For vulvovaginal symptoms alone, topical HRT alone is recommended
4. Nonhormonal prescriptions such as gabapentin and antidepressants can be prescribed as alternatives to HRT for vasomotor symptoms
5. Any vaginal bleeding that occurs after 12 months of amenorrhea is considered postmenopausal bleeding and should be investigated
6. If prescribing HRT to older postmenopausal women, ultra-low or low dosing regimens should be used
7. Routine progesterone co-therapy is not required for endometrial protection in woman receiving vaginal estrogen in **appropriate doses**
8. HRT should be offered to premature ovarian failure patients and those with early menopause and is recommended until the normal age of menopause
9. Health care providers may prescribe HRT to patients with DM to relieve menopausal symptoms
10. All unscheduled bleeding should be investigated as no HRT therapy is entirely protective against endometrial carcinoma
11. Healthcare providers may prescribe HRT therapy to women at increased cancer risk for menopausal symptoms provided they have received adequate counseling and surveillance

Bibliography

Chen YA, Tran C. Comprehensive medical reference & review for MCCQE I and USMLE II. *Toronto Notes.* Toronto, Canada: Toronto Notes for Medical Students Inc; 2008.

Henneber E. Canadian Consensus Conference on Menopause, 2006. SOGC Clinical Practice Guidelines. http://www.sogc.org/guidelines/public/171E-CONS-February2006.pdf.

11
Musculoskeletal Medicine

Fractures
Priority Topic 40

Life-Threatening Fractures
- Major pelvic fracture
- Traumatic amputations
- Massive long bone fracture
- Vascular injury proximal to knee/elbow

Limb-Threatening Fractures
- Fracture/dislocation ankle
- Crush injuries
- Open fracture
- Dislocation knee/hip
- Compartment syndrome
- Fracture above knee/elbow

COMMON INJURIES/CONDITIONS

Open Fracture
- Communication between fracture site and external surface of skin
- Risk of osteomyelitis
- To OR in 6 to 8 hours

Shoulder Dislocation
- Anterior dislocation is most common
  - Patient holds in internal rotation
- Risks injury to axillary and musculocutaneous nerve
- Posterior dislocation often associated with seizures and risks damaging radial artery

Anterior talofibular ligament is the most common ligament injured in inversion ankle sprain.

Colles Fracture
- Distal radius fracture with dorsal displacement
- Often caused by fall on outstretched hands (FOOSH)
- "Dinner fork" deformity

Scaphoid Fracture
- Anatomical snuff box tenderness
- X-ray may be normal initially. If clinical suspicion is high, place in thumb spica cast and repeat x-ray in 1 to 2 weeks.

6P's of Compartment Syndrome
Pallor
Pain out of proportion
Paralysis
Parasthesia
Pulse discrepancy
Polar

Compartment Syndrome

- Increased interstitial pressure in anatomical compartment (forearm, calf) resulting in decreased perfusion and potential muscle/nerve necrosis
- Excessive pain: resistant to analgesia, worse with stretching
- Six P's: **p**allor, **p**ain (out of proportion), **p**aralysis, **p**aresthesia, **p**ulse discrepancy, **p**olar
- Treatment: early recognition/suspicion, remove constrictive casts, consult ortho—fasciotomy may be required emergently

INVESTIGATIONS

Follow Ottawa x-ray rules when deciding need to x-ray a patient

- Ottawa Knee Rules: x-ray if one or more of following:
  - Age ≥ 55
  - Tenderness at head of fibula
  - Isolated tenderness of patella
  - Inability to flex to 90 degrees
  - Inability to bear weight both immediately and in ER
- Ottawa Ankle Rules (see Figure 11-1)
- Ottawa Foot Rules (see Figure 11-1)
- If x-ray is normal and have suspicion of fracture (scaphoid fracture, stress fracture, fracture in elderly, growth plate fracture) consider casting and repeating x-ray in 1-2 weeks, or CT/bone scan to confirm diagnosis.

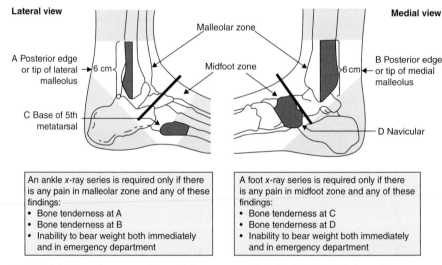

FIGURE 11-1: Ottawa ankle and foot x-ray rules. Stiell, IG, et al. A study to develop clinical decision rules for the use of radiography in acute ankle injuries. *Ann Emerg Med* 21(4);384-390. Reprinted with permission from Elsevier.

MANAGEMENT

- Dependent on fracture type, location, displacement of fragment
- Immobilize in splint or cast and refer to orthopedics if unsure

Bibliography

Brukner P, Khan K. *Clinical Sports Medicine*. 3rd ed. New York, NY: McGraw-Hill; 2009.

Stiell IG, Greenberg GH, Wells GA, et al. Derivation of a decision rule for the use of radiography in acute knee injuries. *Ann Emerg Med*. 1995;26:405-413.

Stiell I, Wells G, Laupacis A, et al. A multicentre trial to introduce clinical decision rules for the use of radiography in acute ankle injuries. *BMJ*. 1995;311:594-597.

Yingming A. Chen. *Toronto Notes 2011: Comprehensive Medical Reference Review for MCCQE I USMLE II*. 27th ed. Toronto, ON: Toronto Review; 2008.

Joint Disorders
Priority Topic 55

OSTEOARTHRITIS

Definition
- "Wear and tear" arthritis

Risk Factors
- Family history
- Advanced age (80% of 85 year olds)
- Female >male
- Trauma in past
- Obesity

Signs/Symptoms
- Asymmetric joint pain relieved with rest
- Joint pseudoinstability secondary to pain
- Short duration of stiffness (<10 minutes) after immobility
- Loss of function
- Crepitus with passive ROM
- Insidious onset of pain that is gradually progressive

Most Common Sites
- Knees
- Hips
- Hands (DIP = Heberden nodes, PIP = Bouchard nodes, first MCP)
- Spine (L4-5, L5-S1)

Investigations
- Blood work not needed unless considering diagnosis of other arthropathies (eg, RA)
- X-ray: joint space narrowing, subchondral sclerosis, subchondral cyst formation, osteophytes

Treatment
- Conservative:
  - Weight loss (minimum 5-10 lbs), rest, physiotherapy, low-impact exercise programs
  - Unloader braces for knees
  - Walking aids—cane
- Medications:
  - Acetaminophen
  - NSAIDs
  - Glucosamine—some evidence for effectiveness, low cost, no known risks
  - Topical NSAIDs/capsaicin
  - Corticosteroid joint injections
  - Hyaluronate injections (Neovisc, Synvisc, Durolane)
- Surgical: joint replacement

SEPTIC JOINT

Definition
- Invasion of a joint by an infectious agent
- Most common organisms: Staphylococcus and Streptococcus
  - Consider Gonorrhea in the sexually active people

- Cause: spontaneous or hematogenous spread; rarely direct contamination
  - Higher risk in immunocompromised, diabetics, etc
- **Always consider sepsis in a patient with a joint replacement**
  - Can have a very low grade, innocuous presentation

Symptoms
- Severe pain
- Erythema
- Warmth
- Swelling
- Inability to bear weight
- Joint will be held in position that provides largest volume of joint capsule, patient **very** unwilling to move from that position
  - Knee—flexed ~30 degrees
  - Hip—flexed ~30 degrees, externally rotated ~30 degrees, abducted ~30 degrees
- Fever, but not always

Investigations
- X-ray
- ESR, CRP, WBC, blood cultures
  - CRP + ESR are extremely sensitive markers, but poorly specific
- Joint aspirate absolutely essential—**must aspirate joint before giving antibiotics**
  - Knees, elbows, wrists, ankles can be done in ER by primary care physicians
  - Hips require fluoroscopic guidance by radiologist
  - Observe the fluid
    - Colour
      - Bright yellow—gout
      - Murky white with stringy material—pus
    - Homogeneity
      - Very homogenous—gout
      - Inhomogeneous—pus
  - Send for:
    - Cell count—general rule <50,000 white cells, not bacterial sepsis
    - Gram stain
    - Crystal analysis—to differentiate from gout/CPPD
    - Culture and sensitivity
- A decision must be made based on story, examination, observing fluid, ESR, CRP, cell count, Gram stain, and crystal analysis
- Septic arthritis is a **surgical emergency** and requires appropriate *incision and drainage* as soon as possible. One **must not** wait for the culture and sensitivity to come back.

Treatment
- Orthopedic consultation is **mandatory**
- Surgical debridement is often required for large joints
- IV antibiotics

RHEUMATOID ARTHRITIS

Definition
- Symmetric, erosive, polyarthritis of small peripheral joints
- Autoimmune disorder of unknown origin

All acute monoarticular arthritides require an aspiration!!!
"Aspirate or litigate"

Monoarticular septic arthritis + migrating polyarthralgia + rash + tendon pain = disseminated *Neisseria gonnorrhea*

Signs/Symptoms

- Morning stiffness >1 hour
- Pain aggravated by rest and improved with use
- Joint instability, crepitus
- Typical deformities: swan neck, boutonniere, radial deviation of wrist, ulnar deviation of MCP, hammer toe, mallet toe, claw toe, flexor contractures
- Constitutional symptoms often present: fatigue, myalgias

Risk Factors

- Females > males (3:1)
- Genetic predisposition (HLA-DR4/DR1)

Felty syndrome: Arthritis, splenomegaly, neutropenia

Investigations

- +RF (approximately 80% sensitive)
- Elevated ESR/CRP
- X-ray: loss of joint space, synovial inflammation

Treatment

- Rheumatologist consultation
- Conservative:
  - Education, PT, OT, vocational counseling
- Medications:
  - NSAIDs, acetaminophen, opioids, local/systemic corticosteroids for symptom relief (do not alter disease progression "non-DMARDS")
  - Disease modifying anti-rheumatic drugs (DMARDs)—standard of care
    - Start DMARDS within 3 months of diagnosis
    - Nonbiologics (eg, methotrexate [gold standard], hydroxychloroquine, sulfasalazine)
    - Biologics (infliximab, etanercept)
- Surgical: synovectomy, joint replacement/reconstruction/fusion

SYSTEMIC LUPUS ERYTHEMATOSUS

Definition

- Chronic inflammatory multisystem disease
- Characterized by production of autoantibodies

Symptoms

- Diagnosis is with +ANA Plus 3 symptoms from "MD SOAP BRAIN" mnemonic

Risk Factors

- Genetics/family history
- Female > male (10:1)
- Age
- Race (African American, Hispanic, Asian)

SLE Symptoms (MD SOAP BRAIN)

Malar rash (sparing of nasolabial folds)

Discoid rash (may cause scarring)

Serositis (pleuritis/pericarditis)

Oral ulcers (aphthous—usually painless)

ANA (+)

Photosensitivity

Blood (hemolytic anemia, thrombocytopenia)

Renal (nephrotic glomerulonephritis)

Arthritis (two joints, nonerosive)

Immune (Antiphospholipid, Anti-Ro, Anti-DS DNA, Anti-Smith)

Neurologic (seizures, psychosis)

Investigations

- +ANA (98% sensitive)
- Anti-dsDNA (95%-99% specific)
- C_3/C_4 (to monitor treatment response)

Treatment

- Rheumatologist consultation
- Patient education (avoid UV light, use sunscreen)
- Treat early and avoid long-term steroid use
- Treatment is highly varied and tailored to organ system involvement

Reiter Syndrome Triad
Arthritis
Conjunctivitis
Urethritis

Pediatric Hip Disorders by Age of Presentation
Dysplasia—birth
Septic hip—toddler
Transient Tenosynovitis—3-6 years
Legg-Calve-Perthes—4-10 years (boys>girls)
SCFE—obese 12-14 years (boys>girls)

Pediatric Bone Tumours
Osteogenic Sarcoma
• Location: around knee
• X-ray: sunburst pattern
• Age: 10-25 years (male > female)
Ewing
• Location: diaphysis of long bones
• X-ray: onion skinning
• Age: 5-15 years

SCFE can lead to irreversible changes to the morphology of the hip joint, and in turn early degenerative changes, if not treated promptly and accurately.

REACTIVE ARTHRITIS (REITER SYNDROME)

Definition

- Sterile arthritis following an infection (typically 1-4 weeks post-infection)—usually GI (*Shigella, Salmonella, Campylobacter, Yersinia*) or GU (*Chlamydia, Mycoplasma*)

Symptoms

- Triad of arthritis, conjunctivitis, urethritis (Chlamydia) = 99% specific
- May also have skin and/or mucosal membrane involvement (GI)

Treatment

- Antibiotics for nonarticular infections
- NSAIDs
- Physiotherapy, exercise

SLIPPED CAPITAL FEMORAL EPIPHYSIS

Definition

- Slipped capital femoral epiphysis (SCFE) is most common childhood/adolescent hip disorder
- Failure/slip of the growth plate in the femoral head during the time of physeal closure, resulting in slippage of epiphysis on metaphysis

Risk Factors

- Almost exclusively males
- Often obese
- Usually **not** traumatic in nature

Symptoms

- Sudden, severe pain with limp
- Restricted ROM (inability to internally rotate femur)

Investigations

- AP/lateral/frog-leg x-ray. Will show abnormalities in cortical alignment from metaphysis to epiphysis.
  - **Lateral view is most telling**—look for apex anterior "buckling" of the physis

Treatment

- Restrict weightbearing **immediately**
- Surgical consultation and management required

LEGG-CALVE-PERTHES

Definition

- Self-limited avascular necrosis of the femoral head
- Usually occurs in kids 4 to 10 years of age

Risk Factors

- Family history
- Low birth weight
- History of hip trauma

Symptoms

- Spontaneous hip pain and/or limp
- Flexion contracture/decreased internal rotation of hip

Diagnosis
- X-ray: collapse of femoral head is diagnostic
- Often normal early in disease progression, so will need to repeat if clinical suspicion high

Treatment
- Conservative = physiotherapy, ROM exercise, bracing
- Surgical = femoral or pelvic osteotomy

A new onset limp in a child always warrants pediatric and/or orthopaedic consultation.

SCOLIOSIS

Definition
- Lateral curvature of the spine
- 90% idiopathic

Symptoms
- Back pain may or may not be present
- Asymmetric shoulder height when bent over for Adam's forward bend test
- Positive Adam's test = rib hump when bent forward
- Apparent leg length discrepancy

Investigations
- Standing, full length, spine x-ray

Treatment
- Pediatric orthopedic consultation
- Depends on degree of curvature
- Observe if <20 degrees
- Bracing if >20 degrees
- Consider surgery if >40 degrees or respiratory compromise

POLYMYALGIA RHEUMATICA

Definition
- PMR results in pain and stiffness in girdle area

Diagnosis PMR Criteria
1. Age >50
2. Bilateral aching/morning stiffness >1 month
3. Elevated ESR (>40)
4. Prompt response to low-dose corticosteroids (within 48 hours of treatment)

15% of patients with PMR develop temporal arteritis.

Symptoms/Investigations
- Morning stiffness of proximal muscles that is symmetrical
- Can have constitutional symptoms (fever, malaise)
- Elevated ESR and CRP

Treatment
- Rheumatology consultation
- Low-dose steroids (15-20 mg po daily)
- Often need to treat for 2 years or longer (50% relapse rate once off treatment)

PMR vs. Polymyositis
PMR
- Pain, stiff in girdle area
- ESR >40
Polymyositis
- Symmetric, prox muscle weakness
- Increased CK and ESR

Bibliography

Brukner P, Khan K. *Clinical Sports Medicine*. 3rd ed. New York, NY: McGraw-Hill; 2009.

Chen AY, Tran C. *Toronto Notes*. Toronto, ON: Type & Graphics Inc; 2011.

Simon C, Everitt H, van Dorp F. *Oxford Handbook of General Practice*. Oxford, UK: Oxford University Press; 2010.

Low Back Pain
Priority Topic 61

GENERAL

- Acute back pain: <12 weeks
- Chronic back pain: >12 weeks

RED FLAGS

1. Cancer: night pain, weight loss, history of cancer, age >50
2. Compression fracture: acute boney tenderness, osteoporosis
3. Osteomyelitis: fever, chills, sweats, IV drug use
4. Spinal cord: neurological symptoms (motor/sensory)
5. Cauda equina (**Emergency**): loss of sphincter tone, fecal incontinence, perineal numbness, leg weakness, change in sexual function, acute urinary retention, or overflow incontinence
6. Other: worsening symptoms

DIFFERENTIAL DIAGNOSIS OF BACK PAIN

- Pyelonephritis
- Ruptured AAA
- Cancer
- Cauda equina
- Compression fracture
- Osteomyelitis
- Mechanical/MSK back pain
- Spondylosis/spondylolisthesis
- Disc herniation
- Spinal stenosis

COMMON CAUSES OF BACK PAIN

- Herniated disc:
  - Protrusion of nucleus pulposus
  - Most common secondary to flexion/lifting injury
  - Pain can be back dominant (central herniation) or leg dominant (lateral herniation)
  - Abrupt onset of pain
  - Worse with sitting, walking, standing, coughing, flexion
  - Numbness/weakness may be present in nerve root distribution
- Lumbar spinal stenosis: neurogenic claudication
  - Narrowing of spinal canal → nerve compression
  - Age >60 is risk factor
  - Pain is:
    - Radicular +/− back pain
    - Progresses proximal to distal
    - Gradual onset

Lower Limb Movements and Myotomes
- L2 = Hip flexion
- L3 = Knee extension
- L4 = Ankle dorsiflexion
- L5 = Great toe extension
- S1 = Ankle plantar flexion
- S2 = Knee flexion

Sciatica refers to pain, numbness, and leg weakness caused by pressure on the sciatic nerve. (L4-S3). Multiple diagnoses should be considered when a patient presents with sciatica.

- ○ Aggravated by extension
- ○ Poor walking/standing tolerance
- ○ Leg pain often subsides with lying/sitting
- ■ Mechanical back pain:
  - Most common causes of mechanical back pain are degenerative disc or facet processes, and muscle- or ligament-related injuries
  - No red flags present on history or physical examination
  - Generally investigations are not needed
  - Most improve in 1 month with conservative treatment

TREATMENT OF MECHANICAL BACK PAIN

Acute
- Educate (most resolve in 2-3 weeks)
- Self-care strategies
- Early return to work/activity
- Analgesia

- Physio/chiro/massage

Chronic
- Team approach (physio, etc)
- +/− physiatrist referral
- Analgesia
- Referral to neurosurgeon if appropriate

Analgesia

Acute
| Acetaminophen
| NSAIDs
| Muscle relaxant (short course)
▼ Short-acting opioids*

Chronic
| Acetaminophen
| NSAIDs
| Low-dose TCA
| Cyclobenzaprine
| Tylenol #3
▼ *Opioids

*If using opioids—find the lowest dose and switch to sustained release. Short acting opioids—use only as prn/breakthrough.

INVESTIGATIONS

Indications for lumbar spine x-ray:
1. No improvement in 1 month
2. Fever
3. Weight loss
4. History of cancer
5. Prolonged steroid use
6. Significant trauma
7. Progressive deficits
8. Other red flags

Consider CT/MRI if neurological deficits or differential diagnosis includes infection or cancer

TABLE 11-1	Low Back Pain Memory Cues/Key Findings
DIAGNOSIS	SIGNS
Compression #	• Local pain (spinal) • No pain radiation
Herniated disc	• Positive straight leg raise • Worse with flexion
Spinal stenosis	• Worse with extension
Vascular claudication	• Worse with walking set distance • Better when stop walking (<2 minutes) • Muscular cramping pain
Neurogenic claudication	• Worse with walking or standing (distance variable) • Better when change position (>10 minutes)
Mechanical back pain	• Resolves in 2-3 weeks • No red flags • Often paraspinal pain

Bibliography

Brukner P, Khan K. *Clinical Sports Medicine*. 3rd ed. New York, NY: McGraw-Hill; 2009.

Yingming A. Chen. *Toronto Notes 2011: Comprehensive Medical Reference Review for MCCQE I USMLE II.* 27th ed. Toronto, ON: Toronto Review Notes; 2008.

Neck Pain

Priority Topic 66

APPROACH TO PATIENT WITH NECK PAIN

1. History
2. Inspect
3. Palpate
4. ROM
5. Strength
6. Reflexes
7. Special tests

Neck Pain - Strength and Motor Innervation

Motor testing	Nerve Root
Neck flexion	C1, C2
Side flexion	C3
Shoulder elevation	C4
Shoulder abduction	C5
Elbow/wrist flexion	C5
Elbow/wrist extension	C7
Thumb Extension	C8
Hand Intrinsics	T1

DIFFERENTIAL DIAGNOSIS OF NECK PAIN

- Carotid dissection (most common cause of stroke in young adults)
- Referred pain from ACS
- Retropharangeal abscess, epiglottitis (infection)
- Spinal stenosis/spinal cord compression
- Disc herniation
- Nerve impingement
- Whiplash
- Lymphoma
- Pseudotumor cerebri (referred pain from idiopathic intracranial HTN)
- Muscular neck pain (posture, stress, etc)

Spinal Cord Compression

Increased pain with recumbency, movement, and Valsalva

Patient will have neurological symptoms (sensory +/− motor)

Risk factors = cancer, osteoporosis

Diagnosis with MRI

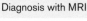

INVESTIGATIONS

- Follow C-spine rules (see Figure 11-2) to determine if x-ray is needed
- Complete AP, lateral, and odontoid views

- Xray: ensure visualization of C1-T1 vertebrae before clearing C-spine. Repeat x-ray with swimmer's view or CT scan if C7/T1 is poorly visualized.
- Consider MRI if neurological symptoms are present

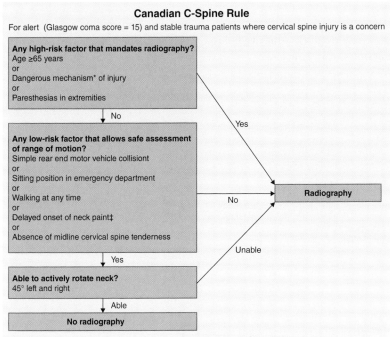

Canadian C-Spine Rule

For alert (Glasgow coma score = 15) and stable trauma patients where cervical spine injury is a concern

Any high-risk factor that mandates radiography?
Age ≥65 years
or
Dangerous mechanism* of injury
or
Paresthesias in extremities

→ No →

Any low-risk factor that allows safe assessment of range of motion?
Simple rear end motor vehicle collisiont
or
Sitting position in emergency department
or
Walking at any time
or
Delayed onset of neck paint‡
or
Absence of midline cervical spine tenderness

→ Yes →

Able to actively rotate neck?
45° left and right

→ Able →

No radiography

Yes → **Radiography**
No → **Radiography**
Unable → **Radiography**

Rule not applicable if: non trauma cases, Glasgow coma score <15, unstable vital signs, age <16 years, acute paralysis, known vertebral disease, or previous surgery of cervical spine.

*Fall from elevation ≥0.9 m (3 feet)/five stairs, axial load to head—for example, diving, motor vehicle collision high speed (>100 km/h), rollover, ejection, motorised recreational vehicles, bicycle struck or collison.

†Excludes: Pushed into oncoming traffic, hit by bus or large truck, rollover, hit by high-speed vehicle.

‡Not immediate onset of neck pain.

FIGURE 11-2: Canadian C-spine rule. Reprinted from Stiell, IG, et. al. BMJ, 2009; 339:b4146.

MANAGEMENT

- Dependent upon diagnosis
- Use multidisciplinary, conservative approach for chronic neck pain secondary to muscular issues or degenerative disc disease

Bibliography

Brukner P, Khan K. *Clinical Sports Medicine*. 3rd ed. New York, NY: McGraw-Hill; 2009.

Filate W, Ng D, Leung R, Sinyor M. *Essentials of Clinical Examination Handbook*. 5th ed. University of Toronto: The Medical Society Faculty of Medicine; 2005.

Stiell IG, Clement CM, Grimshaw J, et al. Implementation of the Canadian C-Spine Rule: a prospective 12-centre cluster randomized trial. *BMJ*. 2009 Oct 29;339:b41-b46.

Yingming A. Chen. *Toronto Notes 2011: Comprehensive Medical Reference Review for MCCQE I USMLE II*. 27th ed. Toronto, ON: Toronto Review Notes; 2011.

Lifestyle

Priority Topic 58

- Always ask about lifestyle behaviours that affect health at every visit (ie, diet, exercise, EtOH/substance use, safe sex, injury prevention).
- Ensure that you know if your patient is ready to make appropriate lifestyle modifications.

- Explore your patient's context (ie, financial, cultural, family, etc) to guide lifestyle recommendations, so as to avoid making recommendations that your patient cannot comply with (unaffordable, etc).
- Review lifestyle modifications at each encounter, understanding that behaviours may change over time.
- Reinforce positive behaviour modifications, and demonstrate how they have improved health (ie, improved blood pressure, glucose management, lipids, renal function, stroke risk, etc).
- Recommend 30 minutes of activity daily.

Bibliography

Working Group on the Certification Process. Priority topics and key features with corresponding skill dimensions and phases of the encounter. The College of Family Physicians of Canada; 2010. http://www.cfpc.ca/uploadedFiles/Education/Certification_in_Family_Medicine_Examination/Definition%20of%20Competence%20Complete%20Document%20with%20skills%20and%20phases.pdf.

Obesity

- **BMI = weight (kg)/height (m)^2**
  - Normal BMI (adults) = 18.8 to 25
  - Overweight = 25 to 29
  - Obese = 30 to 39
  - Morbidly obese= 40 to 49
  - Children (>2 years): BMI >95th percentile for age and gender = obese
- Obesity is associated with:
  - Increased risks of CV death and overall mortality
  - Increased morbidity for hypertension, CAD, stroke, diabetes mellitus, hyperlipidemia, sleep apnea, gallbladder disease, GERD, knee osteoarthritis, low back pain, neoplastic diseases (colon, renal, gallbladder)

Treatment

1. Counseling and behaviour interventions can change eating patterns and increase exercise
   - Five A's:
     - **Ask**   Determine patient's understanding, awareness of obesity
     - **Assess**   Determine patient's readiness to make necessary changes to lose weight
     - **Advise**   Appropriate dietary, exercise, support measures
     - **Assist**   Facilitate patient resources as needed
     - **Arrange**   Discuss progress and readjust plan according to patient needs
2. Medications (orlistat, SSRIs, sympathomimetics) only if diet and exercise have failed and patient has significant comorbidities. Used for short-term management only
3. Surgery (gastric bypass/banding): consider if BMI >40 or >35 + significant comorbidities

Lifestyle modification, prevention of DM 2 and CVD

If Caloric intake is reduced by 500-1000 kcal/day, it will result in 1 to 2 lb weight loss/week (assuming the same total daily energy expenditure).

Bibliography

Working Group on the Certification Process. Priority topics and key features with corresponding skill dimensions and phases of the encounter. The College of Family Physicians of Canada; 2010. http://www.cfpc.ca/uploadedFiles/Education/Certification_in_Family_Medicine_Examination/Definition%20of%20Competence%20Complete%20Document%20with%20skills%20and%20phases.pdf.

Gout

Definition
Monosodium urate crystals infiltrating joints, soft tissue, or renal tissues

Signs/Symptoms
Abrupt onset, excruciating pain, localized erythema/warmth/swelling, recurrent, +/− loss of joint mobility, Tophi (urate deposits from previous attacks), renal calculi/nephropathy

Typical joints: first MIP, ankle, knee

Four stages of gouty arthritis:

1. Asymptomatic hyperuricemia
2. Acute gouty arthritis
3. Intercritical gout
4. Chronic tophaceous gout (tophi—erosions—nephropathy/calculi)

Risk Factors
Males>females, high purine diet, obesity, family history of hyperuricemia, CKD, HTN, hyperlipidemia

Precipitants
Medications = **FACT: F**urosemide, **A**SA/EtOH, **C**ytotoxic drugs, **T**hiazide (and loop) diuretics/Theophylline

Foods = **SALTS: S**hellfish, **A**nchovies, **L**iver, **T**urkey, **S**ardines

Investigations
Definitive: joint aspartate yielding, needle-shaped, negatively birefringent monosodium urate crystals

Presumptive: acute monoarthropathy + hyperuricemia + dramatic response to NSAID/colchicine

Treatment
Acute attack

1. NSAIDs (first line)
2. Colchicine
3. Intra-articular steroid injection

Maintenance/Prophylaxis

1. First attack—lifestyle changes and remove precipitating drugs
2. Treat if one of the following:
   a. Serum uric acid >800 umol/L
   b. Three or more attacks per year
   c. Chemotherapy
   d. Advanced disease
3. Medication Choices:
   a. Allopurinol (first line)—do not start or adjust during an acute attack
   b. Colchicine (low dose, <0.6mg) + probenecid

PSEUDOGOUT (CHONDROCALCINOSIS)

Definition
- Acute inflammatory arthritis due to phagocytosis if IgG-coated calcium pyrophosphate dihydrate (CPPD) crystals—inflammatory mediated release

Risk Factors

- Females = males, advanced age, advanced osteoarthritis, neuropathic joints, diabetes mellitus, hypothyroidism, hemochromatosis, elevated PTH, decreased magnesium, decreased phosphate

Triggers

- Dehydration, illness, surgery, trauma

Signs/Symptoms

- Polyarticular > monoarticular, slower onset (than gout), self-limited (up to 3 weeks)

Typical Joints

- Knee, wrist, MCP, first MTP

Investigations

- Aspirate to rule out septic arthritis or acute gout—positively birefringent, rhomboid-shaped crystals
- X-ray: chondrocalcinosis

Treatment

- NSAIDs
- Colchicine—controversial for prophylaxis
- Intra-articular steroids

Bibliography

Chen AY, Tran C. *Toronto Notes*. Toronto, ON: Type & Graphics Inc; 2011.

Longmore M, Wilkinson I, Davidson E, Foulkes A, Mafi A. *Oxford Handbook of Clinical Medicine*. 8th ed. Oxford, UK: Oxford University Press; 2010.

12

Care of the Elderly

Elderly

Priority Topic 35

- Avoid medication side effects in the elderly by
  - Avoiding polypharmacy when possible
  - Reviewing medication list periodically; every time you add a new medication, consider interactions
  - Avoiding medications and OTC/herbals known to have increased risk, this includes prescription and nonprescription medications
  - Ensuring reliable pill taking (eg, bubble pack from pharmacy)
  - Inquiring about nonprescription medication use (eg, herbal medicines, cough drops, over-the-counter drugs, vitamins)
- Promote safety and prolong independence by screening for modifiable risk factors (eg, visual disturbance, impaired hearing, falls)
- Assess functional status: allow for timely discussion of changes in living arrangements and social supports available
- Fall prevention
- Consider atypical presentations of disease in the elderly patient
  - Infection—frequently do not present with fever
  - Pain—can present as restlessness, confusion, etc
  - Depression—often presents as somatic complaints (changes in weight, sleep, energy) or anxiety symptoms, poor performance on cognitive tests because give up trying to answer
  - Myocardial infarction—less classic chest pain presentation, may have dyspnea or fatigue as main symptom
  - Acute abdomen—often have less symptoms, less pain for given pathology, less rebound tenderness, less fever

Bibliography

MacKay MJ. Financial and personal competence in the elderly: the position of the Canadian Psychiatric Association. *Can J Psy.* 1989;34:829.

The American Geriatrics Society 2012 Beers Criteria Update Expert Panel. American geriatrics society updated Beers criteria for potentially inappropriate medication use in older adults. *J Am Geriat Soc.* 2012. Epub ahead of print. doi:10.1111/j.1532-5415.2012.03923.

Working Group on the Certification Process. Priority topics and key features with corresponding skill dimensions and phases of the encounter. The College of Family Physicians of Canada; 2010.

Multiple Medical Problems

Priority Topic 65

- Clarify the primary reason(s) for the visit and prioritize problems through negotiation with the patient
- Consider depression, anxiety, or abuse (including physical, medication, or drug abuse) in the differential along with organic pathology
- Set limits for the frequency and duration of visits in patients with multiple visits with unchanging symptoms
- Screen periodically for depression due to higher risk if multiple chronic medical conditions are present
- Review periodically the management of patients with multiple medical conditions with goal to:
    - Simplify management (pharmacologic and nonpharmacologic)
    - Limit polypharmacy, eliminating medications that are no longer necessary/recommended
    - Minimize possible drug interactions through review of medication list including OTCs and herbals
    - Update management based on new scientific evidence
- Reassess the patient's condition and situation for possible change which will affect management
- Assist the patient with multiple medical problems (and potentially seeing many specialists) with coordination of care and management

Bibliography

Working Group on the Certification Process. Priority topics and key features with corresponding skill dimensions and phases of the encounter. The College of Family Physicians of Canada; 2010.

Dementia

Priority Topic 23

Aphasia = language disturbance

Apraxia = cannot carry out learned, purposeful movements

Agnosia = loss of ability to recognize persons, sounds, shapes, or smells

DEFINITION

Multiple cognitive deficits manifested by memory impairment and substantial decline from previous cognitive functioning plus one of the following:

- Aphasia
- Apraxia
- Agnosia
- Disturbance in executive function (eg, planning, organizing, abstracting)

PREVALENCE

- 8% people over age 65
- Most common is Alzheimer or mixed Alzheimer disease patients
- Other types of dementia include vascular, fronto-temporal, Parkinson, Lewy body

DIAGNOSIS

- Dementia is a clinical diagnosis.
- Brief cognitive tests (MoCA, MMSE) can help discriminate between dementia and normal state

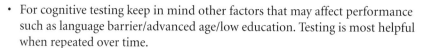
- For cognitive testing keep in mind other factors that may affect performance such as language barrier/advanced age/low education. Testing is most helpful when repeated over time.
- Montréal Cognitive Assessment (MoCA, www.mocatest.org) is for mild impairment
- Mini Mental Status Exam (MMSE): a score of 25 means mild, 19 to 10 means moderate, 9-0 means severe dementia
- Lab testing is recommended to rule out causes of chronic metabolic encephalopathy
  - CBC, TSH, electrolytes, calcium, fasting glucose, vitamin B_{12} (consider folate in patients with celiac or inadequate diet)
  - CT scan: can be used to rule in concomitant cerebrovascular disease that can affect management or rule out other conditions (eg, normal pressure hydrocephalus, bleeding, malignancy)
  - Genetic testing: consider in appropriately selected patients (eg, family with young onset disease)

DIFFERENTIAL DIAGNOSIS

- Delirium and depression (see Table 12-1)
- Brain pathology: vascular insult, infectious, metabolic insult, paraneoplastic syndrome, tumor, epileptic, hydrocephalus
- Mild cognitive impairment

Delirium differential diagnosis—**I WATCH DEATH SOB**

Infection
Withdrawal from drugs
Acute metabolic disorder
Trauma
CNS pathology
Hypoxia
Deficiencies in vitamins
Endocrinopathies
Acute vascular
Toxins
Heavy metals
Sleep
Ouch (pain)
Bowel (constipation)

RISK FACTORS AND PRECIPITATING FACTORS

- Risk factors: age over 65, male, impaired cognition, impaired functional status, sensory impairment, poor nutritional status, medications (psychoactive, anticholinergic), alcohol abuse, medical comorbidities, systolic hypertension, elevated cholesterol, head injury with loss of consciousness, low education level
- Precipitating factors: drugs (sedative hypnotic, narcotic, anticholinergic, polypharmacy, alcohol or drug withdrawal), primary neurologic disease, current illness, surgery, ICU, physical restraints, bladder catheter, pain, emotional stress, prolonged sleep deprivation

TYPES OF DEMENTIA

- **Alzheimer dementia:** progressive worsening of cognitive function
- **Frontotemporal dementia:** younger age of onset, prominent behavioural changes (eg, disinhibition) or prominent language impairment

- **Parkinson dementia:** have idiopathic Parkinson disease for 1+ year prior to onset of dementia, may have visual hallucinations and fluctuation in disease course
- **Lewy body dementia:** begins with cognitive and behavioural disorder that can have concurrent parkinsonian features, may have visual hallucinations and fluctuation in disease course
- **Vascular dementia:** typically stepwise decline, focal neurologic features often found early in course, dysexecutive syndrome

MILD COGNITIVE IMPAIRMENT (MCI)

- Definition: impairment in memory but no significant decrease in function and do not meet criteria for dementia
- Diagnosis: clinical—decline from previous level of functioning, gradual in onset and duration of >6 months, not due to depression/delirium/other psychiatric disorder
- Screening with MoCA helps demonstrate objective cognitive loss, monitor closely since high risk for going on to dementia
- Treatment includes: manage vascular risk factors, increased cognitive and physical activity, assess and treat sleep disorders

MANAGEMENT OF DEMENTIA

Note: cognition-enhancing medications are not part of CCFP objectives and will not be discussed here

1. Primary prevention
- Control systolic hypertension (>160 mm Hg)
- Treatment of specific medical conditions solely for dementia primary prevention is not indicated (statins, ASA, correction of carotid artery stenosis, antithrombotic therapy)
- Lifestyle factors: reduce risk of head injury, increased physical and mental activity
- Medications: none indicated for primary prevention, estrogen not indicated for prevention of dementia

2. Mild-Moderate
Disclosure of diagnosis: respect patient's autonomy/confidentiality/safety
Medical:
- Treat comorbid medical conditions
- Avoid anticholinergic medications (eg, see Anticholinergic Risk Scale)
- With sudden changes in cognition/function/behaviour search for causes of delirium
  - Dementia is a risk factor for delirium
- Assess for behavioural challenges: for example, anxiety, insomnia, depressive symptoms
  - Management is best with non-pharmacological techniques when possible
- Driving: assess both cognition and visual-spatial skills, when doubt exists send for driving examination
  - Safety to drive is based on functional "assessment", **not** on the diagnosis of any particular medical condition
  - Physicians do not take away license, but there is a duty to report to provincial motor vehicle licensing authority if we believe someone is unfit for driving and the authorities will assess
  - *CMA Driver's Guide* is a good resource
Lifestyle:
- Individualized exercise program is beneficial
- Refer to community resources (eg, adult day care, Alzheimer's Society, social worker)

- Assess risk for falls
- Inquire about advance care directives
- Caregivers are often called the hidden patient—assess needs and supports of caregiver!

3. Severe

- Goals of management: (1) improve quality of life (patient and caregivers), (2) maintain optimal function, (3) provide maximum comfort
- Assess needs for help with activities of daily living (ADLs) and living situation
- Assess every 3 to 4 months: cognition, function, behaviour, medical and nutritional status, caregiver's safety, and health
- Assess for behavioural challenges: for example, anxiety, insomnia, depressive symptoms
  - Management is best with non-pharmacological techniques when possible
  - When there is a change in behaviour, search for causes, do not assume it is a progression of dementia
- Pharmacotherapy:
  - "Start low and go slow"
  - Risperidone 1 mg/day and olanzapine 5 to 10 mg/day improve symptoms, associated with increased risk of death in this patient population
  - Lorazepam may be used short-term for behavioural emergencies
  - Depression can be treated with SSRI

ADLs (Activities of Daily Living)
- **D**ressing
- **E**ating
- **A**mbulating
- **T**oileting
- **H**ygiene

IADLs (Instrumental Activities of Daily Living)
- **S**hopping
- **H**ousekeeping
- **A**ccounting
- **F**ood preparation
- **T**ransportation

TABLE 12-1	Comparison of Dementia, Delirium, and Depression		
	DEMENTIA	**DELIRIUM**	**DEPRESSION**
Onset	Insidious	Acute	Gradual with life changes
Duration	Months to years	Hours	At least 2 weeks
Course	Stepwise	Fluctuates, more at night	Diurnal, worse in morning
Alertness	Normal	Fluctuates	Normal
Orientation	Normal or mild impairment	Always impaired	Normal
Perception	Normal	Distorted and hallucinations	Normal
Tests	MMSE	CAM (Confusions Assessment Method)	GDS (Geriatric Depression Screen)

Bibliography

Canadian Medical Association. *CMA Driver's Guide: Determining Medical Fitness to Operate Motor Vehicles.* 2006. http://www.cma.ca/determining-fitness-to-drive.

Carnahan RM, Lund BC, Perry PJ, Pollock BG, Culp KR. The anticholinergic drug scale as a measure of drug-related anticholinergic burden: associations with serum anticholinergic activity. *J Clin Pharmacol.* 2006;46(12):1481.

Chen AY, Tran C. *Toronto Notes.* Toronto, ON: Type & Graphics Inc; 2011.

Chertkow H, Massoud F, Nasreddine Z, et al. Diagnosis and treatment of dementia: 3. Mild cognitive impairment and cognitive impairment without dementia. *Can Med Assn J.* 2008;178(10):1273.

Feldman HH, Jacova C, Robillard A, et al. Diagnosis and treatment of dementia: 2. Diagnosis. *Can Med Asson J.* 2008;178(7);825.

Herrmann N, Gauthier S. Diagnosis and treatment of dementia: 6. Management of severe Alzheimer disease. *Can Med Assn J.* 2008;179(12):1279.

Hogan DB, Bailey P, Black S, et al. Diagnosis and treatment of dementia: 4. Approach to management of mild to moderate dementia. *Can Med Assn J.* 2008;179(8):787.

Hogan DB, Bailey P, Black S, et al. Diagnosis and treatment of dementia: 5. Nonpharmacologic and pharmacologic therapy for mild to moderate dementia. *Can Med Assn J.* 2008;179(10):1019.

Patterson C, Feighter JW, Garcia A, Hsiung GY, MacKnight C, Sadovnick AD. Diagnosis and treatment of dementia: 1. Risk assessment and primary prevention of Alzheimer disease. *Can Med Assn J*, 2008;178(5):548.

Working Group on the Certification Process. Priority topics and key features with corresponding skill dimensions and phases of the encounter. The College of Family Physicians of Canada; 2010. http://www.cfpc.ca/uploadedFiles/Education/Certification_in_Family_Medicine_Examination/Definition%20of%20Competence%20Complete%20Document%20with%20skills%20and%20phases.pdf

Mental Competency
Priority Topic 64

KEY POINTS

- Clues of possible cognitive decline include concerns from family/friends, difficulty managing medications, showing up on the wrong date for appointments, change in behaviour. For example, decline in personal hygiene.
- Consider competence when diagnoses are made which are associated with a higher likelihood of cognitive decline, for example, CVA, dementia, mental illness. However, a particular medical diagnosis does *not* indicate incompetency.
- Competence may change over time
- Competence is situation specific. For example, competence to care for self, to sign out AMA, to stand trial, to sign a POA, to change a will, to make financial decisions. Moreover, financial competence for CEO of company differs from financial competence to run a household.
- To be incompetent in one area does not necessarily imply incompetence in another. For example, a patient may be competent to make health care decisions but not financial decisions.

ASSESSMENT

- Standardized screening tests for cognitive decline are available (see Dementia— Priority Topic 23)
- Assessing competence
  - Type of questions depends on type of competence being assessed
  - Collect relevant collateral information as required
  - Patients can be referred for further assessment (eg, safety in kitchen cooking assessment)
  - For financial competency, questions could include: if you go to the store to buy milk and eggs how much do you expect that would cost? And who helps you pay bills?

LEGAL

- If a patient is not competent to make a decision, there is a hierarchical list of the legal substitute decision maker
  - This varies by province—be aware of the legislation in your jurisdiction
  - There may be provisions for emergency situations
- Think about the need to assess competence when the patient is making decisions, for example, filling out documents such as advance directives
  - Encourage patients to fill out documents prior to onset of impairment or early in progressive conditions

Bibliography

MacKay MJ. Financial and personal competence in the elderly: The position of the Canadian Psychiatric Association. *Can J Psych.*1989;34;829.

Working Group on the Certification Process. Priority topics and key features with corresponding skill dimensions and phases of the encounter. The College of Family Physicians of Canada; 2010. http://www.cfpc.ca/uploadedFiles/Education/Certification_in_Family_Medicine_Examination/Definition%20of%20Competence%20Complete%20Document%20with%20skills%20and%20phases.pdf

Disability

Priority Topic 28

- Monitor, diagnose, and treat patients with disability
- Assess all spheres of function including emotional, physical, and social (finances, employment, family)
- Assess patients with chronic medical conditions for disability
- Use multifaceted management to minimize impact of the disability and prevent functional deterioration, for example, orthotics, lifestyle modification, time off work, community support, social workers, OT/PT, pharmacist
  - Consider short- and long-term disability leave in your plan
- Offer primary prevention strategies for patients at risk for disability (eg, exercises, braces, counseling, work modification, hand rails, lighting)
- Risk factors for disability: elderly, mental illness, manual labour, chronic conditions

FALLS

- More than one-third of people over age 65 have a fall per year, significant morbidity and mortality are associated with falls
- Differential diagnosis for falls:
  - Visual impairment, peripheral neuropathy, CVA, TIA, joint instability, deconditioning, medication effects, environmental or home hazards, orthostatic hypotension
- Risk factors: previous falls, balance impairment, decreased muscle strength, visual impairment, more than four medications or psychoactive drugs, gait impairment and walking difficulty, depression, dizziness or orthostasis, functional limitations, age >80 years, female, incontinence, cognitive impairment, arthritis, diabetes, pain
- Assessment:
  - Quick screen: ask about falls in past year and problems with gait or balance, if yes do further assessment
  - Physical examination: gait, sensory (hearing and vision), orthostatic vital signs, neurologic and musculoskeletal assessment, depression and cognitive impairment screen, review appropriateness of footwear and gait aids
- Prevention:
  - Vitamin D 800 IU/day (NNT 14 to prevent one fall)
  - Individualized exercise program and gait aids
  - Home assessment and modification for high-risk individuals, for example, anti-slip shoe devices, hip protectors
  - Gradual withdrawal of psychotropic medications (where appropriate)

FALL RISK FACTS

Increases from 8% (no risk factors) to 78% (with four risk factors) in 1 year

Increased risk in first 2 weeks after hospital discharge

Increased falls with: antihypertensives, sedatives, antipsychotics, antidepressants, benzodiazepines, NSAIDs

Bibliography

Al-Aama T. Falls in the elderly: spectrum and prevention. *Can Fam Phy.*2011;57,771.

BMJ Best Practice. Assessment of falls in the elderly. 2011. http://bestpractice.bmj.com/best-practice/monograph/880/diagnosis/differential-diagnosis.html.

Public Health Agency of Canada. Evidence-based best practices for the prevention of falls. 2009. http://www.phac-aspc.gc.ca/seniors-aines/publications/pro/injury-blessure/falls-chutes/chap4-eng.php.

Working Group on the Certification Process. Priority topics and key features with corresponding skill dimensions and phases of the encounter. The College of Family Physicians of Canada; 2010.

Palliative Care
Priority Topic 70

DEFINITION

"Palliative care is an approach that improves the quality of life of patients and their families facing the problem associated with life-threatening illness, through the prevention and relief of suffering by means of early identification and impeccable assessment and treatment of pain and other problems, physical, psychosocial and spiritual"

—World Health Organization

PRINCIPLES OF PALLIATIVE CARE

- Indicated for all patients with terminal conditions (not just cancer)
- Goal—to enhance quality of life
- Early discussions and planning with multidisciplinary support and involvement of family/friends
- Address/clarify patient wishes for end of life issues: intubation, resuscitation, use of antibiotics, home vs hospital vs hospice. Review patient wishes often
- Identify and address possible causes of requests for hastened death: poor symptom management, depression, isolation, fear of dying, anxiety, spiritual distress
- Consider the whole patient (grief, sadness, loss, fear) and provide support to the patient and family

It is important to offer a support system to help the family cope during the patient's illness and in their own bereavement.

MEDICATIONS

- Review medications according to changes in goals of therapy
  - Stop medications no longer compatible with goals
- Monitor for side effects of medication, anticipate and manage side-effects
- **Pain:** use oral route if possible, prescribe long-acting medications with short-acting for breakthrough pain, add adjuvant pain medications (NSAIDs, steroids, bisphosphates, cannabinoids)
- **Nausea:** anticholinergics (eg, scopolamine), 5HT3 antagonists (eg, ondansetron), prokinetic (eg, metoclopramide), antihistamines (eg, dimenhydramine—less effective)
- **Dyspnea:** position and increase air circulation, opiates are drug of choice, oxygen based on symptom improvement, manage cough/secretions/anxiety
- **Constipation:** hydration, osmotic agents (PEG—tasteless and well tolerated), motility agents (senna), lubricating agents (docusate, glycerin suppository)

Bibliography
Human Resources and Skills Development Canada. Information for health care professionals: EI compassionate care. 2011. http://www.hrsdc.gc.ca/eng/publications_resources/health_care/ei_ccb.shtml. Accessed February 27, 2012.

The College of Family Physicians of Canada. Position statement: palliative care. 2011.

Working Group on the Certification Process. Priority topics and key features with corresponding skill dimensions and phases of the encounter. The College of Family Physicians of Canada; 2010. http://www.cfpc.ca/uploadedFiles/Education/Certification_in_Family_Medicine_Examination/Definition%20of%20Competence%20Complete%20Document%20with%20skills%20and%20phases.pdf.

World Health Organization. WHO definition of palliative care. www.who.int/cancer/palliative/definition/en/. Accessed February 27, 2012.

13

Travel Medicine

Travel Medicine

Priority Topic 93

- Travel medicine is the promotion of health and the prevention of disease or other adverse health outcomes when travelling internationally.
- A consult to a family physician or travel medicine clinic **6 weeks prior to travel is the minimum** period recommended in order to ensure that the minimum required vaccinations can be given on time.
- If a patient is presenting for travel vaccination advice ensure all other vaccinations are up to date (Hepatitis B, MMR, tetanus/diphtheria, varicella, pertussis, polio).

GENERAL TRAVEL/SAFETY ADVICE

Refer to www.voyage.gc.ca for more specific travel information.

- Accidents (wearing seatbelts) and vehicular trauma risks
- Safe sex practices
- Safe travel for women
- Drink water from only clean sources (no ice cubes, brush with bottled water)
- Food: only eat peeled or cooked fruit/vegetables; avoid street food, unpasteurized dairy, raw meat/seafood
- Proper hand washing and use of antiseptic gels/washes
- Sunscreen/sun protection
- Avoid intoxication and illicit drugs
- Use insect repellent
- Travel insurance and medical insurance

MEDICATIONS

- Ensure the patient has enough medication for their trip.
- Medication should always travel with the patient. If required for narcotics or needles, a letter documenting the need and number of medications and supplies should always be with the patient.
- A list of medications and indications should be kept in the patient's wallet.
- Ensure that the patient has an adequate understanding of how to manage medications and their chronic illnesses.

Risk Assessment "5Ws"

- Who—healthy? allergies? medications? age? pregnancy? breastfeeding?
- Where—the exact location(s) being traveled to (urban/rural, low-medium-high risk) and where you will be staying?
- What—what exact activities will you be doing there?
- When—when are you leaving and when are you coming back?
- Why—group travel? visiting family/friends? military? religious?

COMMON CONDITIONS ASSOCIATED WITH TRAVEL

Altitude Sickness

- Patients may exhibit symptoms above 10,000 feet including headache, SOB, change in mentation, nausea, vomiting, and decreased urinary output. (Major concern is developing cerebral edema.)
- Slow and gradual ascent is recommended, if symptomatic, stop and descend
- Prophylactic treatment: acetazolamide 24 to 48 hours prior to ascent until 48 hours after peak altitude or symptoms disappear

Traveler's Diarrhea

- Most common problem for travellers to developing countries
  - Usually a self-limiting problem → no treatment necessary. See also Table 13-1.
  - Common pathogens: enterotoxigenic *Escherichia coli* (ETEC), campylobacter, salmonella

TABLE 13-1	Traveler's Diarrhea: Severity and Management	
SEVERITY OF ILLNESS	SYMPTOMS	TREATMENT
Mild-moderate	Less than three bowel movements (BM)/day and no blood	Peptobismol, loperamide, oral rehydration (OR)
Moderate-severe	Three to five BM/day and no blood	OR and antibiotics (ciprofloxacin or azithromycin)
Severe	More than five BM/day or blood in stool ± fever	OR and antibiotics (ciprofloxacin, or azithromycin)

- ETEC/cholera oral vaccine (Dukoral) has been shown to provide moderate, short-term protection against diarrhea caused by ETEC and cholera caused by *Vibrio cholerae*. It is not recommended as a complete prevention strategy as not everyone will be fully protected by the vaccine.

Malaria

- Mosquito-borne parasitic disease caused by Plasmodium species: *falciparum* (most common + lethal) or *Plasmodium vivax, P. ovale, P. malariae, P. knowlesi*. Results in infection/lysis of liver cells and RBCs.
- Clinical features
  - Starts 8 days to months post anopheles mosquito bite
  - Paroxysmal/cyclical fever and chills (timing of fevers can help in diagnosing species)
  - Abdominal pain, diarrhea, headache, hepatosplenomegaly, thrombocytopenia, cerebral involvement—seizures/coma
- Investigations: thick/thin blood smear (Giemsa stain)
- Prevention: use treated bed-nets, avoid mosquitos, avoid dusk-dawn activities, use insect repellant with DEET and chemoprophylaxis
- Treatment/chemoprophylaxis:
  - Chloroquine (*Plasmodium falciparum* is resistant)
  - Mefloquine

- Doxycycline and quinine
- Atovaquone/proguanil (Malarone)

UPON RETURN

- In patients returning from travel with illness or a fever of unknown origin ensure to take into account the risk of an infection acquired abroad that may have lain dormant or have an atypical presentation.

- For up to date information on geographic and seasonal patterns of disease and travel advisories, check the website for the United States Centers for Disease Control and Prevention (wwwnc.cdc.gov/travel) or Foreign Affairs Canada (voyage.gc.ca). Also available is Well on Your Way, A Canadian's Guide to Healthy Travel Abroad (http://www.phac-aspc.gc.ca/tmp-pmv/pdf/bon_depart-on_your_way-eng.pdf).

Bibliography

Centres for Disease Control and Prevention. Yellow Book 2012. http://wwwnc.cdc.gov/travel/page/yellowbook-2012-home.htm. Accessed March 19, 2012.

Chen YA, Tran C, ed. *The Toronto Notes*. 27th ed. Toronto, ON: Toronto Notes for Medical Students;2011.

Committee to Advise on Tropical Medicine and Travel, Health Canada. Statement on New Oral Cholera and Travellers' Diarrhea Vaccination. http://www.phac-aspc.gc.ca/publicat/ccdr-rmtc/05vol31/asc-dcc-7/index-eng.php. Accessed March 19, 2012.

Public Health Agency of Canada. Travel Medicine. http://www.phac-aspc.gc.ca/tmp-pmv/index-eng.php. Accessed March 19, 2012.

Immigrant Health
Priority Topic 48

- Foreign born individuals account for almost 20% of the Canadian population.
- Immigrants are eligible for health care coverage under the Canada Health Act. However, there are sometimes specified wait times of up to 90 days and this is an active area of federal legislation and controversy.

IMMIGRANT HEALTH EXAMINATION

- All immigrants undergo an Immigration Medical Examination (IME) preceding arrival in Canada. The purpose of the IME is to assess the potential burden of illness and a limited number of public health risks. It is not designed to provide clinical preventive screening. The first visit examination should therefore include deficits from the IME examination.

- The IME includes:
  a. Complete physical examination including vision and hearing screen
  b. CXR (age 11 and older) to screen for TB
  c. Syphilis serology
  d. Urinalysis (age 5 and older), dipstick for protein, glucose, blood, and if positive, microscopy
  e. HIV testing (age 15 and older, as well as for children who have received blood or have a known HIV+ mother)

THE FIRST VISIT—ONCE IN CANADA

- The patient–doctor communication and relationship can be more challenging than with a traditional "Canadian" patient. Modify your approach when possible to accommodate cultural differences.

- Language—if possible have an interpreter present during visits. Be aware of the limitations of nonmedical and family interpreters.

- Document all findings but take note of cultural/ritualistic scarring versus scars from possible torture.
- When patient presents with illness, inquire about the use of alternative therapies/herbal remedies.
- Other items to include in new immigrant first visit examination:
  - Tuberculosis:
    - Test if from a country with high prevalence
    - Investigations: CXR; PPD/Mantoux test (not a marker of disease activity); sputum for acid fast bacteria
    - Symptoms/signs: night sweats, weight loss, fatigue, chronic cough, hemoptysis
    - Treatment (empiric): RIPE (rifampin, INH, pyrazinamide, ethambutol) + vitamin B_6
  - Other infectious diseases:
    - Malaria—do not routinely screen/test only if symptoms.
    - Screen for the following:
      - HEP B/C—screen using serology
      - HIV—if from a country with high rates and immigrated to Canada before age 15
      - Intestinal parasites
    - Chronic diseases—screen for the following:
      - DM
      - Iron deficiency anemia
      - Sickle cell disease
  - Mental health:
    - Depression
      - Immigrants are at a higher risk than the general public
      - Monitor for and link new immigrants with resources that can aid in transition to Canada
    - Torture/abuse—inquire about past history as appropriate
  - Women's health—discuss contraceptive options, cervical cancer screening, and immunization for HPV
  - Screening—bring patient up to date with Canadian screening guidelines (mammography, FIT testing for colon cancer, etc)
  - Vaccination:
    - Assess vaccination status and plan a schedule to bring patient up to date
    - The following vaccinations should be considered:
      - Hepatitis A/B
      - If patient tests positive for sickle cell or beta-thalassemia:
        - Pneumococcal (polysaccharide and conjugated)
        - HIB
        - Meningococcal
        - Influenza
      - Varicella—high rate of adult VZV in temperate climates
    - If vaccination status unknown:
      - Start on primary immunization schedule according to age
      - No concerns about adverse events for revaccination for MMR, polio, *Hemophilus influenza* B, pneumococcal, meningococcal, Hepatitis A/B, varicella, influenza

Bibliography

Citizenship and Immigration Canada. http://www.cic.gc.ca/english/department/what.asp. Accessed November 18, 2012.

Health Canada, Healthy Living, Just for You—Immigrants. http://www.hc-sc.gc.ca/hl-vs/jfy-spv/immigrants-eng.php. Accessed November 18, 2012.

Pottie K, Greenaway C, Feightner J, et al. Evidence-based clinical guidelines for immigrants and refugees. *Can Med Assoc J.* 2011;183:E824-E925;doi:10.1503/cmaj.090313. http://www.cmaj.ca/cgi/collection/canadian_guidelines_for_immigrant_health. Accessed November 18, 2012.

The Foundation for Medical Practice Education. New Immigrants and refugees: screening and health care. *Educational Module.* 2011 Nov;19(12). www.fmpe.org. Accessed November 18, 2012.

Hepatitis

Priority Topic 45

Definition

Inflammation of the liver, characterized by the presence of inflammatory cells in the tissue of the organ. The condition can be self-limiting or progress to fibrosis and cirrhosis. Chronic hepatitis is defined as hepatitis persisting for >6 months.

Etiology

Hepatitis viruses (most cases of hepatitis worldwide), toxins (alcohol, medications, some industrial organic solvents, and plants), other infections, obstruction, and autoimmune diseases

Cause:	Transmission:
Hepatitis A/E	Fecal-oral
Hepatitis B/C	Blood/sexual
Alcohol	Excess intake
Autoimmune	Idiopathic
Drug-induced	Acetaminophen, INH, tetracyclines, anti-epileptics, phenytoin

Symptoms

Flu-like illness, RUQ pain, jaundice, pruritus, change in bowel habit, arthralgia, fatigue, fever

Risk Factors

IVDU, travel to hepatitis-endemic areas, contaminated foods (hepatitis A), blood/bodily fluid contacts, alcohol intake, pharmacological history, toxic ingestions, high-risk sexual activity, transfusion prior to 1990, newborn from infected mother, tattoos, HIV status *(key for Hepatitis B or C)*

Vaccination

Vaccinate individuals at high risk for Hepatitis A/B and offer post-exposure prophylaxis for Hepatitis A/B along with harm reduction measures

No vaccine is available for Hepatitis C. Diagnose and treat early for improved cure rates

Investigations

Blood Work

- Liver function tests (see Table 13-2)
  - Raised AST/ALT from liver damage; if >1000 increased likelihood of viral/drug-induced ischemia
  - ALP + GGT raised is likely cholestasis
- PT/INR (sensitive for hepatic protein synthesis)
- Bilirubin

Ultrasound should be performed if obstructive cause is being considered

- To AST with alcohol – Alcohol related hepatitis: AST:ALT > 2:1
- virAL – viral related hepatitis: ALT>5x normal

TABLE 13-2	Hepatitis: Liver Function Testing		
TEST	NORMAL	HEPATOCELLULAR	OBSTRUCTIVE
Direct bilirubin	0-5 mmol/L	▲	▲
Total bilirubin	2-20 umol/L	▲	▲
ALT	10-40 u/L	▲	Transient ▲
AST	15-40 u/L	▲	–
Alk phos	30-155 u/L	▲	▲▲▲

Chronic Hepatitis

Serum transaminases increased for 6 months from any cause

Specific Causes

Obstructive Causes

- Diagnosis and treatment requires **prompt** imaging (US)
- ERCP can also be used to visualize and treat definitively
- Percutaneous drainage (for obstruction far from sphincter)

Hepatitis A

- Etiology: fecal-oral transmission with 4 to 6 week incubation period
- Prognosis
  - Possible relapse but never chronic
  - Can acutely cause hepatic failure and death

Hepatitis B (See Table 13-3)

- Etiology: maternal → fetal, sexual contact, blood-borne transmission, IVDU
- Prognosis
  - Age at infection is inversely related to risk of chronic infection
  - Cirrhosis develops in 15% to 20% of cases with chronic Hepatitis B
  - Hepatocellular carcinoma (HCC) develops in 10% to 15% of cases with chronic Hepatitis B

TABLE 13-3	Hepatitis B Seromarkers			
	HBSAG	ANTI-HBS	HBEAG	ANTI-HBE
Acute Hepatitis B	+	–	+	–
Chronic (high infectivity)	+	–	+	–
Chronic (low infectivity)	+	–	–	+
Resolved	–	+/–	–	+/–
Immunization	–	+	–	–
HBsAg, Hepatitis B surface antigen; Anti-HBs, antibody against Hepatitis B surface antigens; HBeAg, a Hepatitis B core antigen.				

- Infectivity/transmissibility is assessed using HBeAg or HBV DNA (PCR)
- Protective function is assessed using anti-HBs
- Carrier state/active infection is assessed by continued presence of HBsAg
- Past infection or immunization is assessed by anti-HBs

Hepatitis C

- Etiology: blood-borne transmission (IVDU), blood transfusion prior to 1992
- Clinical manifestations occur about 2 months after infection
- Diagnosis: positive serum HCV-RNA (positive 2 weeks post-infection). Note: serum HCV-RNA levels inversely correlate with response to treatment.
- Prognosis:
  - Chronic Hepatitis C develops in 80% of those exposed
  - Of those who develop chronic Hepatitis C, 20% go on to develop cirrhosis
  - Of those who develop cirrhosis, 1% to 4% go on to develop HCC (hepatocellular carcinoma)
- Chronic Hepatitis C
  - Refer for specialist care
  - Consider treatment with alpha-interferon and ribavirin—especially if liver fibrosis/cirrhosis, consistently raised liver enzymes, age <50, Hepatitis C genotype 2 or 3
  - HCV-RNA should be measured at 1 and 3 months after treatment is commenced
  - If patient is not a candidate for treatment, monitor for HCC: ultrasound and serum alfa-fetoprotein levels

Hepatitis D

- Coinfection with Hepatitis B only (ie, cannot have Hepatitis D without having Hepatitis B)
- Treat with interferon
- Transplant for end stage disease

Hepatitis E

- Rarely seen in North America, usually a self-limiting disease
- Etiology: fecal-oral transmission
- Consider in patients returning from endemic areas with hepatitis symptoms
- High mortality rate in pregnant patents

Following Patients

Always continue to monitor for complications of chronic hepatitis (B/C) such as HCC and cirrhosis

Continue to monitor liver enzymes until stable

Ascites—80% of cases due to chronic liver disease (cirrhosis or alcoholic hepatitis)

Bibliography

Yingming A. Chen. *Toronto Notes 2011: Comprehensive Medical Reference Review for MCCQE I USMLE II.* 27th ed. Toronto, ON: Toronto Review; 2008.

Jaundice

Supplementary Topic

Definition

A yellowish pigmentation of the skin, the conjunctiva, and other mucous membranes caused by hyperbilirubinemia

Signs and Symptoms

Dark urine and pale stools, RUQ pain, pruritus (if painless—pancreatic Ca)

Investigations

CBC, bilirubin, liver enzymes and function tests, amylase

TABLE 13-4	Differential Diagnosis for Causes of Jaundice	
UNCONJUGATED HYPERBILIRUBINEMIA	CONJUGATED HYPERBILIRUBINEMIA
Hemolysis Drugs Neonatal Gilbert/Crigler-Najjar syndromes	Hepatocellular disease Primary sclerosing cholangitis Primary biliary cirrhosis Sepsis Gallstones Biliary stricture Malignancy Metastases

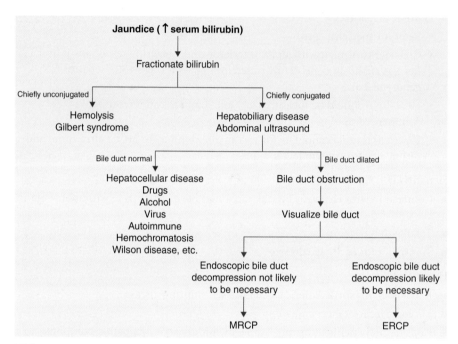

FIGURE 13-1:   Approach to jaundice. *Source:* Chen YA and Tran C. *The Toronto Notes,* 27th ed., 2011.

NEONATAL JAUNDICE

Visible clinically at bilirubin of 85 to 120 μmol/L in the mucous membranes, sclera, and tip of the nose

Newborns are at high risk for developing jaundice for multiple reasons:

- Physiological jaundice occurs on day 2 to 3 and resolves over the first week of life; worse in premature infants. Causes include immature hepatocytes, and increased bilirubin load due to high fetal RBC volume and decreased fetal RBC survival.
- Breast feeding jaundice is due to a lack of breast milk and consequent dehydration, which worsens a physiological jaundice. Onset is around 7 days with a peak at 2 to 3 weeks of life.
- Breast milk jaundice is rare and caused by an inhibitor of glucuronyl transferase in breast milk with onset at 1 week and peaks at 2nd to 3rd week.
- Pathologic jaundice: jaundice in the first 24 hours is **always** pathological
  - Unconjugated jaundice—see Figure 13-1
  - Conjugated jaundice—see Figure 13-1

Treatment

- Purpose—to prevent kernicterus
- Treatment is guided by Bhutani nomogram that illustrates the treatment in relation to the bilirubin levels

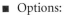

- Options:
  - Phototherapy
  - Exchange transfusion if severe hyperbilirubinemia
  - If jaundice is secondary to dehydration—increase feeds either with expressed breast milk or formula supplements
  - For Breast milk jaundice—switch feeds to formula feeding temporarily

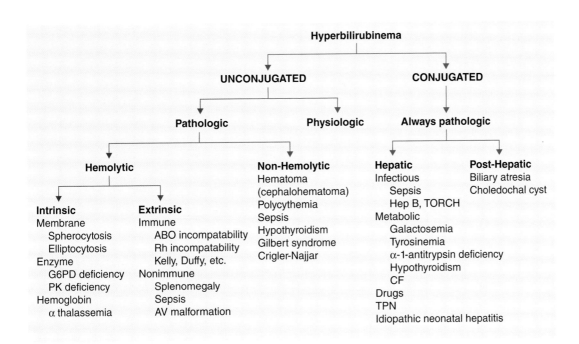

Bibliography

Chen YA, Tran C, ed. *The Toronto Notes*. 27th ed. Toronto, ON: Toronto Notes for Medical Students; 2011.

14
Social Medicine/Psychology

Domestic Violence
Priority Topic 30

- Domestic violence includes sexual, physical, and/or psychological abuse
- Screen **all** patients, regardless of gender/sexual orientation—asking is the strongest predictor of disclosure
- Twenty five percent of females have intimate partner violence in lifetime

Risk Factors
- Low SES
- Pregnancy
- Disability
- Age 18 to 24
- History of abuse
- Substance use

Cycle of Abuse
1. Increasing tension—breakdown of communication, victim becomes fearful but still wants to appease abuser, abuser becomes angrier, tension builds
2. Incident—verbal/emotional/physical abuse, anger, humiliation, blame, threats
3. Reconciliation—abuser may apologize for/minimize/deny abuse, promise it will not occur again, or blame the victim
4. Honeymoon phase—no abuse occurring, incident forgotten, victim hopeful no further abuse will occur

Cycle can lead to helplessness, guilt, low self-esteem, feeling worthless, depression, suicidal ideation, shame, substance abuse, with impact directly on patient and children.

Management
- Determine immediate and long-term risk to patient and children → ask about weapons in home
- Make safe exit plan for all involved → safe place to go, essentials together if needing a quick exit
- Involve shelter, social worker, counseling, domestic violence advocate
- Marital counseling **not** appropriate while abuse occurring

- Reassure patient is **not to blame**!
- Report suspected or confirmed child abuse
- Document all information clearly for medico-legal purposes
- Provide emergency numbers to patient
- Advise about escalating nature of domestic violence, especially during pregnancy!

Marital violence is a criminal act, but is not reportable without the victim's permission.

Bibliography

The College of Family Physicians of Canada. http://www.cfpc.ca/uploadedFiles/Education/Priority%20 Topics%20and%20Key%20Features.pdf.

Walker Lenore E. *The Battered Woman*. New York, NY: Harper and Row; 1979.

Rape/Sexual Assault
Priority Topic 78

Consider sexual assault for patients presenting with mental health disorders (anxiety, depression) or somatization.

History

- Ensure patient is not left alone
- Ensure adequate time (usually 1-2 hours)
- Ask for consent to contact police and collect evidence
- Ask about gynecological history and post-assault activities (shower, etc)
- Document observations/medically pertinent information only

Physical Examination

- Use sexual assault kit if <72 hours since assault
- Examine head to toe for signs of injury/trauma, particularly oral/vaginal/anal areas
- Collect samples ideally before urination or defecation (seminal stain swabs, pubic hair cuttings, and combings)
- Only use water for lubrication on pelvic examination

Investigations

- Serum β-hCG
- Full STI screen
  - Urine PCR for Gonorrhea, Chlamydia
  - Serum VDRL
  - HIV
  - HBsAg + anti-HAV, anti-HCV/HCV-RNA (anti-HCV positive at 4-6 weeks; HCV-RNA: if acute, positive at 2 weeks)
- Blood group, Rh type

Management

- Primary, secondary, tertiary assessment. Manage serious injuries first.
- Only report if patient consents or <16 years old
- Involve local assault team and provide counseling to **all** involved. Offer counseling periodically after incident and provide close follow-up.
- Tetanus update
- Assume positive for Chlamydia and Gonorrhea and treat (azithromycin 1 g PO × 1 + cefixime 400 mg PO × 1)

- May start prophylaxis for hepatitis B and HIV
- Offer pregnancy prophylaxis. Ideally these methods are used <72 hours post-coital, but may work up to 120 hours after.
  - Plan B (Levonorgestrel 0.75 mg)
  - Yuzpe (estradiol/norgestrel)
  - Copper T IUD
- Provide pre- and post-HIV test counseling
- Psychological: have patient change and shower after examination, follow-up with MD in rape crisis centre in 24 hours. Patient should **not** leave emergency room alone.
- Keep high index of suspicion for domestic violence. Assess danger to return home, ask about kids in home, document findings, plan safety (*see priority topic domestic violence*).
- Make follow-up appointment!

Bibliography

Chen YA, Tran C. *Toronto Notes—Comprehensive Medical Reference & Review for MCCQE I and USMLE II.* Toronto, Canada: Toronto Notes for Medical Students Inc; 2008.

The College of Family Physicians of Canada. http://www.cfpc.ca/uploadedFiles/Education/Priority%20 Topics%20and%20Key%20Features.pdf. Accessed March 19, 2012.

Violent/Aggressive Patient
Priority Topic 98

- Possible when dealing with psychiatric/intoxicated/demented or confused patients, or those with a history of violence.
- **Safety first!** For yourself and staff: be able to access exit quickly, ask security or other staff to accompany you if necessary.
  - Anticipate possibility of violence (familiarize yourself with environment and eliminate potential dangers/anything that can be used as a weapon).
  - Recognize warning signs (body language, tone of voice, verbal threats).
- Rule out an underlying medical or psychiatric cause (eg, hypoglycemia, hypoxia, schizophrenia, delirium, infection).
- Consider physical or chemical restraints if necessary (eg, injectable or sublingual benzodiazepines/antipsychotics).
- In the outpatient setting, have a plan ready for patients who are verbally or physically aggressive and make sure this is well communicated to staff and that it can be carried out.

Bibliography

The College of Family Physicians of Canada. http://www.cfpc.ca/uploadedFiles/Education/Priority%20 Topics%20and%20Key%20Features.pdf. Accessed March 19, 2012.

Stress
Priority Topic 87

- For vague symptoms with multiple etiologies (eg, headache, fatigue, pain), inquire about stress as a cause/exacerbating factor.
- If present, identify the impact of stress on functionality, and contributing factors to stress (eg, finances, employment, relationships).

- Discuss existing resources and potential solutions to issues.
- Assess coping skills, and factors which may contribute to poor coping skills (substance abuse, gambling, violence, eating)
- **Always** consider mental illnesses such as depression and anxiety.

Bibliography

The College of Family Physicians of Canada. http://www.cfpc.ca/uploadedFiles/Education/Priority%20Topics%20and%20Key%20Features.pdf. Accessed March 19, 2012.

Crisis
Priority Topic 19

- Ensure enough time to address patient's issues, remain calm, and ask for help if needed.
- Inquire about suicidal ideation/thoughts of harm to others, or whether the crisis may negatively affect others.
- Inquire about habits that may indicate poor coping strategies (substance abuse, gambling, violence, eating).
- Come up with a management plan, making sure that the patient is involved and in agreement.
- Offer medical therapy (if indicated) and nonmedical therapy (eg, counseling, social work, etc) with office/community resources, while ensuring appropriate patient-doctor boundaries are observed.

Bibliography

The College of Family Physicians of Canada. http://www.cfpc.ca/uploadedFiles/Education/Priority%20Topics%20and%20Key%20Features.pdf. Accessed March 19, 2012.

Family Issues
Priority Topic 37

- Use open-ended questions and inquire periodically about family issues, particularly at major events and when progressing to different stages

FAMILY LIFE CYCLE

- Living independently from family
- Committing to a relationship
- Living together
- Raising children
- Raising adolescents
- Children leaving home, empty nest
- Retirement
- Aging
  - Analyze potential conflicts between patient and family members, or even family members and physician, general family functionality, and the impact of the sick role on the family structure and function.

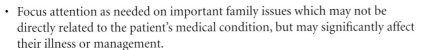

- Focus attention as needed on important family issues which may not be directly related to the patient's medical condition, but may significantly affect their illness or management.
- Provide emotional and educational support to the patient and their family; empower them to take charge of the patient's management.
- It can be helpful to have both the patient and family be willing participants in the patient's management plan for example, pregnancy as motivation to stop smoking; death of a family member and grieving leading to noncompliance with medications.
- SOO: this is important for the social and developmental context and illness experience.
- Refer if necessary for further counseling/psychotherapy/family issue management.

Bibliography

Crouch Michael A, Leonard R. *The Family in Medical Practice.* New York: Springer-Verlag; 1987.

Poon VHK, Bader E. The individual and family life cycle: predicting important transition points. In: Watson WJ, McCaffery M, eds. *Working With Families: Case-Based Modules on Common Problems in Family Medicine.* Toronto, ON: Working with Families Institute, Department of Family and Community Medicine, University of Toronto; 2003:17-25.

The College of Family Physicians of Canada. http://www.cfpc.ca/uploadedFiles/Education/Priority%20Topics%20and%20Key%20Features.pdf.

Bad News

Priority Topic 9

SKDIFF mnemonic is helpful to remember when breaking bad news—**s**etting, **k**nowledge, **d**etail, **i**nformation, **f**eelings, **f**ollow-up

1. **S**etting—appropriate, quiet and private, ensure confidentiality, ask if anyone else should be present
2. **K**nowledge—assess how much patient knows, note level of understanding, language used, potential worries
3. **D**etail—how much or little the patient wants to know; reassure patient this can change and adapt accordingly
4. **I**nformation—use language that is easy to understand, give manageable amounts of information, and check regularly for understanding; Do not rush!
5. **F**eelings—listen to patient, identify, acknowledge, and respond to feelings empathically
6. **F**ollow-up—summarize, ask about other questions/concerns, and plan a follow-up either with yourself or next appropriate caregiver

Bibliography

Buckman R, Kason Y. *How to Break Bad News—A Practical Protocol for Healthcare Professionals.* Toronto: University of Toronto Press; 1992.

Working Group on the Certification Process. *Priority Topics and Key Features With Corresponding Skill Dimensions and Phases of the Encounter.* The College of Family Physicians of Canada; 2010.

Difficult Patient

Priority Topic 27

- A high level of trust and communication are required to maintain a successful patient–doctor relationship.
- Be aware of new symptoms/signs, try to establish patient's needs, and address them as best as possible.
- Enquire about/identify any changes in patient's life/functionality that may be contributing to the difficult interaction.
- Consider an underlying personality disorder.
- Must be expected with patients suffering from chronic conditions; Be considerate, identify any personal feelings you have that may affect the situation, and try to prevent them from interfering with your patient–doctor relationship and management.
- Terminate the patient–doctor relationship if it is irreparable, in the best interest of the patient, and you are unable to provide the level of care that the patient requires.
- Seek further legal advice or guidance from the College Physician Advisory Board if unsure whether terminating the relationship is appropriate.

Bibliography

College of Physicians and Surgeons of Ontario. http://www.cpso.on.ca/uploadedFiles/policies/policies/policyitems/ending_rel.pdf. Accessed March 19, 2012.

The College of Family Physicians of Canada. http://www.cfpc.ca/uploadedFiles/Education/Priority%20Topics%20and%20Key%20Features.pdf. Accessed March 19, 2012.

15

Preparation for the SOO

The SOO—Overview, Nine Helpful Questions and How to Attack It

The SOO is a 15-minute simulated office oral examination. There are four SOOs that each examinee must complete as part of the CFPC examination and there are two problems incorporated into each SOO. The SOO is **not** a medical aspects only oral examination. It is your job to identify and manage each problem both socially and medically. The marking grid for the SOO can be divided in 11 sections (see Table 15-1)—only 4 of them are medical!!

TABLE 15-1	Simplified SOO Marking Grid
PROBLEM 1	**PROBLEM 2**
1. Identification–*medical*	5. Identification–*medical*
2. Illness experience	6. Illness experience
3. Management–*medical*	7. Management–*medical*
4. Finding common ground	8. Finding common ground
Overall SOO social and developmental context	
9. Identification of the issues	10. Integration of issues into interview/problems
11. Overall interview process and organization	

The "9 SOO things" listed below should help with the nonmedical sections.
"9 SOO THINGS" to include:
You do not have to ask these questions in any particular order but always try to ask all nine questions in each SOO.

1. Timeline of the symptoms (ie, How long have you been battling this problem?—Gives a sense of the impact on their life.)
2. What are you (the patient) worried this is? (Cancer, heart attack, brain tumor ....)
3. Family:
   - Married—doing well and good relationship?
   - Kids—doing well and good relationship?
   - Mom/Dad—alive, and good relationship?

9 SOO Questions

1. Timeline
2. What are you worried about (cancer?, etc)
3. Family
4. Social support (friends, religion, etc)
5. Job and finances
6. Disease - self limited or life long
7. Physical exam
8. Elderly: will, advance directives, etc.
9. Family meeting

Tip: Feel free to write a few things down during the SOO (they provide you with a blank paper and pen/pencil in the examination room)—it might help you summarize and make your management plan. It also can help you be a bit more personable if you aren't a person that can remember names—write it on your paper and use their name once or twice during your interview.

■ Siblings—doing well and good relationship?

■ In-laws—doing well and good relationship?

4. Social supports (family/friends/activities/religion)—ask about each of the four areas

5. Job and finances

6. Tell patient if the disease/problem is a lifelong illness or self-limited

7. Always state you're going to bring them back for a physical examination—mention what you want to do and be fairly specific, for example, "I want to bring you back for a physical and I'm going to do" … Have a differential of 2–3 diagnoses for each medical problem and list the testing you'd like to do/order to exclude/include each diagnosis

8. If the patient is an elderly make sure to ask about a will, power of attorney, and advanced directive

9. Always offer to have a family meeting or to talk to their family about whatever problem the patient is having or social situation etc

HOW TO ATTACK THE SOO–A SUGGESTED APPROACH

The SOO is not a re-enactment of a typical first encounter between a patient and their family physician. It is meant to demonstrate the various aspects that contribute to the patient's overall problem(s) and well being, and some of the factors that contribute to the development of a therapeutic bond between a patient and family physician. It may seem out of place to ask many of the questions when you are meeting a patient for the first time. If you want to do well on the SOO, you must incorporate some of these questions into your approach (see Table 15-2).

TABLE 15-2   SOO–Steps to Organizing Your Attack

STEPS TO ORGANIZE YOUR ATTACK	9 SOO THINGS
1. Introduce yourself, and state the patient's name.	
2. **HINT/CLUE 1:** The patient gives away problem 1 in their opening statement of why they came to the doctor.	
3. Attack the SOO by starting with the first problem and asking all the pertinent medical questions including Q1 and Q2 from the 9 SOO things. If you have a tentative diagnosis be sure and mention it.	1 and 2
4. Move onto social questions: how's the family (married, parents, in-laws, etc)? finances? etc ….	3, 4, and 5
5. **HINT/CLUE 2:** At approximately 5 minutes (10 minutes remaining) the patient will give a hint/clue to the second problem.	
6. Start on problem 2—often this is a social or psychiatric problem. If you haven't already, start questioning the patient about supports, and finances/job (questions 4 and 5). Make sure to still include any medical questions related to this problem. Also, if you have a tentative diagnosis, be sure and mention it.	1, 2, 3, 4, and 5
7. At 3-4 minutes left (the patient will give you a signal) summarize! An example: "It looks like we have two issues going on here, let's make a plan for each of these together."	
8. Make a management plan for each problem including a physical examination, lab testing, arranging a family meeting, prognosis for the disease/reassurance ….	6, 7, 8, and 9

Be aware, you may stumble on the second problem before the second clue is given (when you start asking the social questions after problem 1). This can result in being unsure of the exact second problem, as they won't give you the hint/clue if you've already found the problem—but remember, if it's social and there is a lot going on in the patient's life, you do not need a specific name for the problem. Example "you have two issues: one is your poor diabetes control and the second is your social situation." Additionally, the plan for most social problems is often the similar—family meeting, social work/counseling, offer follow-up, make them aware of community resources or support groups, etc.

Index